Contemporary Endocrinology

Series Editor
Leonid Poretsky, Division of Endocrinology
Lenox Hill Hospital
New York, NY, USA

Contemporary Endocrinology offers an array of titles covering clinical as well as bench research topics of interest to practicing endocrinologists and researchers. Topics include obesity management, androgen excess disorders, stem cells in endocrinology, evidence-based endocrinology, diabetes, genomics and endocrinology, as well as others. Series Editor Leonid Poretsky, MD, is Chief of the Division of Endocrinology and Associate Chairman for Research at Lenox Hill Hospital, and Professor of Medicine at Hofstra North Shore-LIJ School of Medicine.

Dimiter Avtanski • Leonid Poretsky
Editors

Obesity, Diabetes and Inflammation

Molecular Mechanisms and Clinical Management

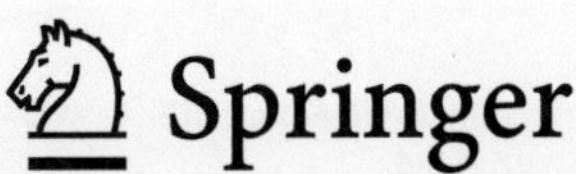 Springer

Editors
Dimiter Avtanski
Friedman Diabetes Institute
Lenox Hill Hospital
New York, NY, USA

Leonid Poretsky
Donald and Barbara Zucker School
of Medicine at Hofstra/Northwell
Hempstead, NY, USA

ISSN 2523-3785　　　　　　　　ISSN 2523-3793　(electronic)
Contemporary Endocrinology

ISBN 978-3-031-39723-3　　　　ISBN 978-3-031-39721-9　(eBook)
https://doi.org/10.1007/978-3-031-39721-9

© The Editor(s) (if applicable) and The Author(s), under exclusive license to Springer Nature Switzerland AG 2023, corrected publication 2023
This work is subject to copyright. All rights are solely and exclusively licensed by the Publisher, whether the whole or part of the material is concerned, specifically the rights of translation, reprinting, reuse of illustrations, recitation, broadcasting, reproduction on microfilms or in any other physical way, and transmission or information storage and retrieval, electronic adaptation, computer software, or by similar or dissimilar methodology now known or hereafter developed.
The use of general descriptive names, registered names, trademarks, service marks, etc. in this publication does not imply, even in the absence of a specific statement, that such names are exempt from the relevant protective laws and regulations and therefore free for general use.
The publisher, the authors, and the editors are safe to assume that the advice and information in this book are believed to be true and accurate at the date of publication. Neither the publisher nor the authors or the editors give a warranty, expressed or implied, with respect to the material contained herein or for any errors or omissions that may have been made. The publisher remains neutral with regard to jurisdictional claims in published maps and institutional affiliations.

This Springer imprint is published by the registered company Springer Nature Switzerland AG
The registered company address is: Gewerbestrasse 11, 6330 Cham, Switzerland

Preface

Although signs of inflammation were described in antiquity, its role in the pathogenesis of metabolic disease is only beginning to be understood. Obesity and diabetes are arguably the most pressing public health challenges facing the world today, affecting more than 600 million people worldwide and associated with multiple morbidities and increased mortality. A characteristic feature of these conditions is chronic low-grade inflammation of adipose tissue arising from an activated immune system and accompanied by the release of proinflammatory cytokines. Although the role that inflammation plays in the pathogenesis of obesity and diabetes is still obscure, inflammation does affect insulin sensitivity in peripheral tissues and thus may lead to the development of insulin resistance and diabetes mellitus.

In this volume, we aimed to provide a comprehensive overview of the relationships between inflammation, obesity, and diabetes. We focused on the pathogenesis and biological mechanisms of obesity, the interaction between adipose tissue and the immune system, the role of genetics and environmental factors, the progression of cardiovascular complications, and the association of obesity and inflammation with gestational diabetes as well as type 1 and type 2 diabetes. At the same time, we also included practical recommendations for preventing and managing these conditions, using both lifestyle modifications and pharmacological interventions.
This book is intended for a broad audience, including researchers, clinicians, and students of medicine at all levels. The editors would like to thank the contributing authors for their outstanding work as well as the staff of Springer Nature for their assistance in the production of this book.

New York, NY, USA
New York, NY, USA
Dimiter Avtanski
Leonid Poretsky

Contents

Chapter 1
Inflammation: Pathogenesis and Biological Markers

Nilson Tapia, Joshua Hanau, Jenny Shliozberg, and Leonid Poretsky

Abbreviations

APR	Acute phase reactants
C1-INH	C1-esterase inhibitor
CRR	C-reactive protein
ESR	Erythrocyte sedimentation rate
IFNγ	Interferon-gamma
LPS	Lipopolysaccharides
NK	Natural killer (cells)
NSAIDs	Nonsteroidal anti-inflammatory drugs

N. Tapia
Division of Allergy, Immunology and Rheumatology, University of Rochester Medical
Center, Rochester, NY, USA
e-mail: nilson_tapia@urmc.rochester.edu

J. Hanau
Division of Allergy and Immunology, Montefiore Medical Center, Albert Einstein College of
Medicine, Bronx, NY, USA
e-mail: jhanau@montefiore.org

J. Shliozberg
Division of Allergy and Immunology, Montefiore Medical Center, Albert Einstein College of
Medicine, Children's Hospital at Montefiore, Bronx, NY, USA
e-mail: jshliozb@montefiore.org

L. Poretsky (✉)
Friedman Diabetes Institute, Lenox Hill Hospital, Northwell Health, New York, NY, USA

Feinstein Institutes for Medical Research, Manhasset, NY, USA

Donald and Barbara Zucker School of Medicine at Hofstra/Northwell, Hempstead, NY, USA
e-mail: lporetsky@northwell.edu

© The Author(s), under exclusive license to Springer Nature
Switzerland AG 2023
D. Avtanski, L. Poretsky (eds.), *Obesity, Diabetes and Inflammation*,
Contemporary Endocrinology, https://doi.org/10.1007/978-3-031-39721-9_1

PCP	*Pneumocystis jirovecii* pneumonia
PCT	Procalcitonin
PRR	Pattern recognition receptors
TLR	Toll-like receptors
TNF	Tumor necrosis factor

Introduction

Although the concept of inflammation dates back to antiquity, its potential role in the pathogenesis of metabolic diseases, such as obesity and diabetes, is only now being recognized.

The details of various aspects of inflammation related to metabolic diseases are addressed in the subsequent chapters in this volume. This introductory chapter reviews general mechanisms of inflammation which apply to specific inflammatory conditions, including diabetes and obesity. We review the history of inflammation, its pathogenetic mechanisms, the role of innate and adaptive immune systems, clinically useful biomarkers, and current anti-inflammatory therapeutic strategies.

Brief History and Definitions

The term 'inflammation' is derived from the Latin *inflammare*, which means "to set on fire." This term was initially used in the first century A.D. by Roman encyclopedist Celsus who described inflammation as encompassing the four cardinal signs of *calor, dolor, rubor,* and *tumor* (i.e., heat, pain, redness, and swelling). During the nineteenth century, German pathologist Rudolf Virchow added "loss of function" as a fifth cardinal sign. The loss of function was characterized as a lack of mobility due to severe swelling [1, 2].

Inflammation can be defined as either a localized or systemic response of the body to external (e.g., trauma) or internal (e.g., ischemia, infection) triggers. Physiologically, inflammation restores the affected tissue to its preinjury state. The phases of the inflammatory response can be classified as either *acute* or *chronic*. The acute phase typically occurs within the first hours of exposure to the trigger. It is characterized by increased infiltration of neutrophils to the site of injury, in addition to changes at the microvascular level. The chronic phase can occur within months to years of trigger exposure. Unlike the acute phase, the chronic phase predominantly involves macrophages and other cells from the monocytic line (e.g., lymphocytes and plasma cells). In certain forms of vascular inflammation, mast cells can predominate, causing vasodilation and vessel wall leakage when activated [3, 4].

The term "immunity" is derived from the Latin *immunitas*. Historically, this term signified an exemption from obligations to or prosecution by the Roman state. Medically, immunity signifies protection from infections or other disease processes. Immunity can be defined as an organism's response or reaction to molecules or pathogens that are recognized as foreign or aberrant [5, 6].

The growth of immunology as a scientific discipline in both basic and clinical research began during the nineteenth century when Russian zoologist Élie Metchnikoff (1845–1916) identified phagocytic cells and described their ability to engulf and destroy foreign pathogens. This laid the foundation for innate immunity [2]. German scientists, Emil Behring (1854–1917) and Paul Ehrlich (1854–1915), discovered and characterized molecules now known as antibodies, which could protect against bacterial toxins. This work laid the ground for the concept of acquired or adaptive immunity [1]. Subsequently, these major discoveries led to the distinction and categorization of cellular vs. humoral immunity, which will be discussed in more detail later in this chapter. Briefly, humoral immunity, primarily driven by B cells, is responsible for producing antigen-specific antibodies which neutralize pathogens outside the cells. Cellular immunity involves T cells, macrophages, and cytokines to trigger apoptosis inside infected cells [5]. Major historical landmarks in the field of inflammation are summarized in Table 1.1.

Table 1.1 Historical landmarks for the concept of inflammation

Timeline	Landmark
First century A.D.	Inflammation initially described by Celsus as encompassing the four cardinal signs of *calor*, *dolor*, *rubor*, and *tumor* (i.e., heat, pain, redness, and swelling)
Nineteenth century	• Rudolf Virchow added "loss of function" as a fifth cardinal sign • Immunology grows as a scientific discipline in basic and clinical research • Elie Metchnikoff identified phagocytosis, laying the foundation for the concept of innate immunity • Emil Behring and Paul Ehrlich discover antibodies, providing groundwork for the study of adaptive immunity
1828	Johann Buchner successfully isolates salicin from willow bark
1853	Charles Frederic Gerhardt synthesizes acetyl salicylic acid
1897	• Edmund Biernacki develops the concept of the erythrocyte sedimentation rate (ESR) • Felix Hoffmann and pharmaceutical company Bayer manufacture aspirin
Twentieth century 1930	William Tillet and Thomas Francis discover C-reactive protein (CRP)
1937	French scientist Vilem Laufberger discovers ferritin
1940s	Glucocorticoids discovered
1970s	Lloyd old and colleagues identify tumor necrosis factor (TNF) molecules
1975	Leonard Deftos and Bernard Roos identify and describe procalcitonin
1998	TNF inhibitor drug, infliximab, is approved by FDA
Twenty-first century 2001	Anakinra, the first IL-1 inhibitor, is approved by FDA
2007	Eculizumab receives first approval by FDA
2009	Ustekinumab, a dual IL-12/23 inhibitor approved by FDA
2010	Tocilizumab approved as an IL-6 inhibitor by FDA
2015	Secukinumab, an IL-17 inhibitor, approved by FDA
2016	Infliximab-dyyb, the first biosimilar monoclonal antibody, is approved by FDA
2017	IL-23 inhibitor, guselkumab, is approved by the FDA

Clinical Biomarkers

Various bioactive compounds released during the inflammatory response into the circulation have been used in clinical medicine as markers of inflammation [7]. Biomarkers of inflammation produced by the liver are also called acute phase reactants (APRs). They are primarily synthesized by the hepatocytes with the assistance of various cytokines (such as tumor necrosis factors or TNFs). The most widely clinically used APRs are erythrocyte sedimentation rate (ESR) and C-reactive protein (CRP) [3, 8]. Procalcitonin and ferritin are among the additional acute phase reactants used in clinical medicine.

The concept of *ESR* was first developed in 1897 by Edmund F. Biernacki, who found that red blood cells settled in plasma faster in the presence of fibrinogen. It was noted that there was a difference in sedimentation rates between pregnant and non-pregnant women, so ESR was initially used as a marker of pregnancy. ESR measures the speed with which erythrocytes settle into the plasma of an anticoagulated blood specimen. ESR begins to rise within 24–48 h of inflammation onset [8]. Multiple confounding factors may increase or decrease ESR, creating the risk of misinterpretation. For example, anemia and pregnancy can increase ESR, while sickle cell disease is associated with low ESR.

CRP was discovered in 1930 by William Tillett and Thomas Francis in patients with pneumococcal pneumonia. This APR is produced in the liver and, like ESR, lacks specificity. CRP is responsible for the recognition and elimination of pathogens and for clearing apoptotic cells. Typically, CRP becomes elevated in the patient's serum as part of a response to inflammation or tissue injury within the first 4–6 h of the onset of inflammation, although circulating levels may vary. CRP activates the complement system (briefly reviewed below). Obesity, insulin resistance, or smoking are common non-infectious causes of elevated CRP [8].

Procalcitonin (PCT) is an inflammation biomarker that can help distinguish bacterial etiology from other causes of infection since viral infections do not increase its synthesis. PCT was initially described in 1975 by Leonard Deftos and Bernard Roos [9]. In the absence of systemic inflammation, PCT is produced by thyroid neuroendocrine cells and is not released into circulation until it is converted to calcitonin. Therefore, PCT is typically undetectable in healthy patients. In the presence of systemic inflammation and bacterial infections, PCT is produced by various tissues and released into the bloodstream without being converted to calcitonin. Typically, PCT can rise within the first 4 h of triggering onset and peaks within 48 h. Due to its levels declining over 24–36 h, PCT can be trended as inflammation resolves. This finding has guided antibiotic therapy allowing for the reduction of antibiotic overuse [10].

Ferritin is both an iron-storage protein and an acute phase reactant. It is synthesized by hepatocytes, macrophages, and Kupffer cells [11]. Ferritin is a nonspecific APR and can be elevated in various inflammatory conditions, including acute infections and malignancies [12]. Ferritin levels can fluctuate throughout the day;

therefore, its overall trend over a prolonged period has higher clinical significance than day-to-day levels.

Immunology of Inflammation

Inflammation lays the foundation of a variety of human disease states. Regardless of the type of inflammation, the immune system is always involved (Fig. 1.1). As briefly mentioned in the history section, the immune system can be divided into *innate* and *adaptive* systems. Both innate and adaptive immune functions participate in the inflammatory process. A better understanding of the cellular and molecular components of the human immune system helped uncover the pathophysiology of many human diseases and the mechanisms of many modern treatment modalities.

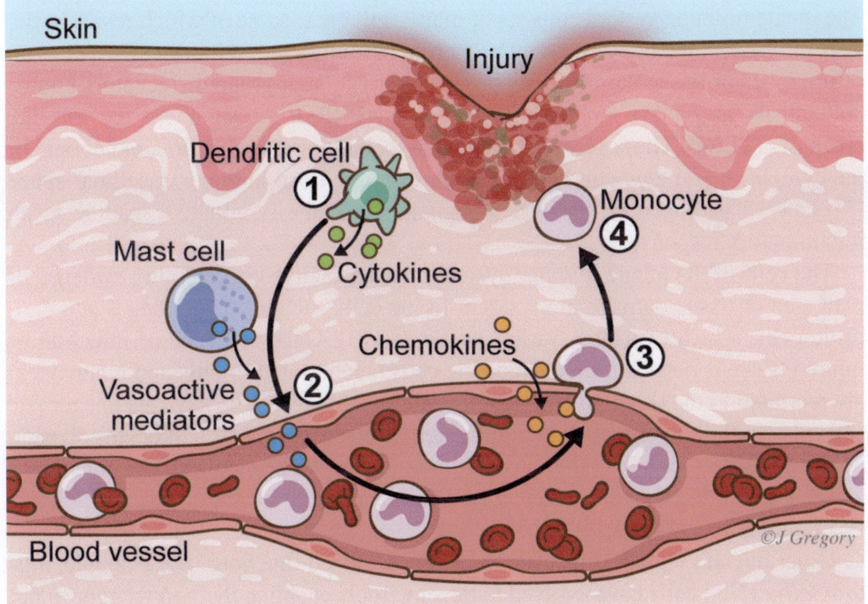

Fig. 1.1 Innate inflammatory response to tissue inflammation

When tissue injury occurs, a predictable sequence of events follows. (1) Sentinel immune cells, such as dendritic cells, are able to recognize microbes or tissue injury and release a variety of inflammatory mediators, such as the cytokines IL-1, TNFα, and IL-6. (2) The release of these cytokines and other mediators has multiple downstream effects, including enhanced production of vasoactive mediators, which lead to vessel dilation, increased vascular permeability, and, ultimately, tissue edema. (3) Effector cells of the immune system, such as neutrophils and monocytes, are recruited to the site of the injury by chemokines, which are released by local immune cells in response to the detection of cellular injury. These effector cells migrate out of circulation into the injured tissue. (4) Monocytes are activated to phagocytose and remove debris, ultimately leading to tissue remodeling

The following sections will review the cellular and molecular components of the innate and adaptive immune systems.

Innate Immune System

The innate immune system is the first line of defense against pathogens. It consists of *cellular* and *molecular* components which help detect the presence of pathogens and guide early responses against them. Unlike the adaptive immune system, the components of the innate immune system are present at birth and allow for the identification of a limited spectrum of molecular patterns associated with pathogens.

Cells of the Innate Immune System

The innate immune system consists of many cell types, some of which reside in tissues throughout the body and play a key role in immune surveillance. The presence of microbes or tissue damage is first detected by a large group of receptors known collectively as *pattern recognition receptors* (PRRs), among them the toll-like receptors (TLRs). These receptors can be associated with the plasma membrane or the cytoplasm and they can be present in a soluble form in the extracellular space [5]. Once a pathogen is detected, a signaling cascade is initiated, leading to an inflammatory response.

The cells of the innate immune system most specialized in detecting evidence of pathogen or tissue damage are resident tissue cells such as macrophages and dendritic cells, which express a variety of PRRs [13]. Once evidence of infection or injured tissue is detected, the phagocytic cells (such as neutrophils and monocytes) are recruited to the tissue to eliminate invading pathogens. The key role phagocytic cells play in fighting infection is highlighted by diseases such as leukocyte adhesion deficiency type 1 (LAD-1). In this condition, neutrophils cannot exit the circulation and migrate to tissues where they are needed, leading to increased susceptibility to severe infections [14].

Other innate immune cells also possess specialized functions. For example, *natural killer* (NK) cells have evolved to develop tools enabling them to recognize and eliminate human cells infected by viruses. *Mast cells* secrete a variety of mediators, helping to establish the inflammatory milieu needed for the effective functioning of the innate immune system. One substance released by mast cells, *histamine*, increases vascular permeability, enabling the cells and effector molecules of the innate immune system to exit the circulation and enter the tissues in which they are needed. While histamine plays a key role in enabling an effective immune response, its inappropriate release promotes a variety of allergic conditions [15].

The cells of the innate immune system participate in tissue repair once the invading pathogens have been eliminated. Macrophages, in particular, play an important role in eliminating debris. They secrete a variety of molecular mediators that promote tissue regeneration, vascular growth, and, ultimately, scar formation.

Molecular Components of the Innate Immune System

The cells of the innate immune system rely on various molecular tools to function. Among these tools is a large group of mediators, termed *cytokines*, which enable effective coordination of the immune response. Cytokines are secreted by both adaptive and innate components of the immune system. The cytokines classically associated with the innate immune response are the TNFs and the interleukins 1 and 6 (IL-1 and IL-6). These cytokines lead to physiologic changes that enable effective pathogen elimination, such as, for example, raising core body temperature [16].

Other molecular components of the immune system play a more direct role in aiding the destruction of pathogens. The *complement system* consists of a group of plasma proteins activated in a cascade that plays many roles in innate immunity, ranging from deposition on the surface of microbes and aiding phagocytosis to forming polymers that directly penetrate bacterial cell membranes and lead to cellular lysis [17]. The role played by the complement system across an array of human diseases can be illustrated by the various conditions which manifest abnormalities in the complement system. Late complement component deficiencies, such as C5-C9, are linked to increased susceptibility to *Neisseria* infections. Deficiencies in early complement components, such as C2 and C4, are linked to the development of autoimmune diseases such as systemic lupus erythematosus. C1-esterase inhibitor (C1-INH) deficiency is linked to certain types of hereditary angioedema [18].

Adaptive Immune System

The adaptive immune system is an evolutionarily advanced aspect of the immune system. It enables the development of highly specific responses against a molecular structural pattern that are learned over time and retained for future encounters with the same pattern [19]. The molecular sequences which elicit these responses are called *antigens*. The ability to develop the diversity and specificity necessary for an effectively functioning adaptive immune system depends on a specific set of molecular tools that enable the recombination of preexisting genes. These molecular tools activate a finite set of core genes to generate receptors and immunoglobulins that can identify a near-infinite number of antigens [20].

The proper functioning of the adaptive immune system involves learning to identify and target antigens associated with pathogens while avoiding generating a response targeting antigens associated with the host organism or with harmless environmental antigens. When self-antigens become targeted, autoimmune disease may develop. When harmless environmental antigens are targeted, an allergic reaction may arise [21].

Components of Adaptive Immunity

The adaptive immune system consists of two major arms – *cell-mediated immunity* and *humoral immunity*. Cell-mediated immunity involves the development of classes of lymphocytes that can identify specific antigens associated with infection and perform tasks such as the direct killing of virally infected cells or the release of cytokines which help direct an effective and coordinated immune response. Lymphocytes are the main effector cells of the adaptive immune system and can be divided into two major classes – T cells and B cells. The class of lymphocytes which plays a major role in the direct killing of virally infected cells are CD8 surface-expressing T lymphocytes, known as cytotoxic T cells. Another class of T cells, which express CD4 on their surface, are known as helper T cells (Th cells). There are many classes of helper T cells, with Th1 and Th2 cells being well-studied examples. These cells help coordinate immune responses in various ways, with Th1 cells, for example, playing a role in activating mononuclear phagocytes, which kill ingested microbes in the setting of cell-mediated immunity [22].

Humoral immunity involves the development of immunoglobulins, or antibodies, which can target-specific antigens. By doing so, certain antibodies can label larger pathogens for targeted killing by groups of phagocytes. Other antibodies bind small intracellular organisms, such as viruses, preventing them from infecting cells and thus neutralizing them [23]. The class of lymphocytes which are responsible for the production of antibodies are the B cells. CD4 T cells play a role in coordinating the humoral response with B cells and ensure that antibody production is effective.

The critical importance of the adaptive immune system is best illustrated by the natural history of untreated patients with HIV/AIDS who are at increased risk of developing various opportunistic infections. One such disease, *Pneumocystis jirovecii* pneumonia (PCP), an opportunistic infection in adults with HIV/AIDS, illustrates the critical role the T lymphocytes play. CD4+ T lymphocytes proliferate after encountering the *Pneumocystis jirovecii* organism and generate interferon-gamma (IFNγ), which recruits macrophages to the site of infection. Ultimately, these lymphocytes coordinate an effective and efficient immune response that clears pathogens and prevents significant residual tissue damage [24]. The adaptive immune dysfunction that arises in patients with AIDS contributes to many other opportunistic infections caused by viruses, fungi, and parasites [25].

Chronic Inflammation Associated with Adaptive Immunity

Various chronic inflammatory conditions are associated with the dysfunction of the adaptive immune system. Certain symptoms in autoimmune diseases directly result from the production of antibodies that target self-antigens. Graves' disease is one such example. In this condition, the production of excess thyroid hormone is stimulated by autoantibodies that target the TSH receptor on the thyroid gland [26]. Other conditions, such for example type 1 diabetes mellitus, also involve autoantibodies, although the nature of islet cell destruction includes more complex cell-mediated mechanisms as well [27].

Table 1.2 The *innate* and *adaptive* immune systems

Feature	Innate Immunity	Adaptive Immunity
Specificity	Broad in nature	Narrow in nature
Memory	Absent	Present
Speed of onset	Rapid	Delayed
Induced by	Nonspecific patterns	Specific patterns
Major cells	Polynuclear cells, monocytes, mast cells	Lymphocytes
Molecular effectors	Nonspecific effectors (e.g., complement)	Specific soluble effectors (e.g., immunoglobulins)

The inflammatory milieu that is generated in chronic inflammatory conditions is driven by cytokine signaling. Some chronic conditions, such as asthma and atopic dermatitis, are often characterized by cytokines associated with Th2-driven inflammation. These cytokines, such as IL-4, IL-5, and IL-13, have been increasingly targeted by new classes of medications which aim to control the drivers of inflammation in chronic atopic diseases [28, 29]. Diseases such as rheumatoid arthritis, on the other hand, are thought to be driven more by Th1 cytokines and therefore have increasingly been treated with agents that interfere with Th1 cytokines, such as TNFα, IL-1, and IL-6 [30].

Innate and adaptive immune systems are compared in Table 1.2.

Anti-Inflammatory Therapy

Nonsteroidal *anti-inflammatory* drugs (NSAIDs) target the cyclooxygenase enzymes. The cyclooxygenase enzyme family is the key to the production of prostaglandins and thromboxane—pro-inflammatory molecules. The history of this class of drugs can be traced back to Hippocrates (460 BC–370 BC), who used willow bark extracts and leaves to treat both fever and inflammation. In 1828, the German scientist Johann Buchner isolated salicylic alcohol glucoside (salicin) from willow bark. A decade later, Raffaele Piria, an Italian chemist, converted salicin into salicylic acid [30, 31]. In 1853, the French chemist Charles Frédéric Gerhardt synthesized acetylsalicylic acid. Finally, in 1897, Felix Hoffmann, a German scientist working with the pharmaceutical company Bayer, manufactured acetylsalicylic acid, now known as Aspirin. Aspirin continues to be widely used to treat fever, inflammation, and various cardiovascular diseases [31, 32].

Glucocorticoids are effective anti-inflammatory agents commonly used for various diseases such as asthma, systemic lupus erythematosus, or rheumatoid arthritis. Discovered in the 1940s from molecular extracts of the adrenal cortex, they were found to exert their anti-inflammatory effect by inhibiting the genes coding for various pro-inflammatory molecules, such as cytokines and chemokines [33, 34].

TNFs (discussed earlier in this chapter) are pro-inflammatory molecules commonly elevated in various disease states (e.g., inflammatory arthritis, obesity-induced type 2 diabetes mellitus, etc.). TNFs were initially identified and named in the 1970s by a group led by Lloyd Old (1933–2011), a pioneer in the field of cancer immunology. The investigators injected Bacillus-Calmette Guérin-sensitized mice with lipopolysaccharides (LPS) and found that a host factor (eventually named TNF) was responsible for the tumor-necrotizing activity in the serum. Antibodies to TNF were found to prevent *Escherichia coli*-induced sepsis and inflammation in baboons [35, 36]. This discovery led to clinical trials using *TNF inhibitors* for the treatment of chronic inflammatory disease states [35, 36]. Infliximab, a chimeric monoclonal antibody, was the first TNF inhibitor approved by the FDA in August 1998. As of this writing, infliximab is FDA-approved for the treatment of Crohn's disease, ulcerative colitis, rheumatoid arthritis, ankylosing spondylitis, psoriatic arthritis, and plaque psoriasis [37].

In addition to TNF inhibitors, other target-specific drugs have been developed. For example, IL protein inhibitors (developed against IL-1, IL-6, IL-12, IL-17, and IL-23) are efficacious in treating various inflammatory conditions such as gout, rheumatoid arthritis, and psoriatic arthritis. In addition to interleukin-specific inhibitors, Eculizumab, a C5 complement protein cleavage blocker, has been successfully used to treat paroxysmal nocturnal hemoglobinuria [38–43].

Anti-inflammatory therapy options are summarized in Table 1.3.

Table 1.3 Anti-inflammatory therapies[a]

Drug Class	Mechanism of action	Drug Name(s)
Nonsteroidal anti-inflammatory drugs (NSAIDs)	Inhibition of cyclooxygenase (COX) enzyme	Ibuprofen, naproxen, aspirin, diclofenac, indomethacin, ketorolac, meloxicam, nabumetone, oxaprozin, piroxicam
Glucocorticoids	Inhibition in expression of various pro-inflammatory cytokines and chemokines	Prednisone, triamcinolone, methylprednisolone, dexamethasone, hydrocortisone, betamethasone, halobetasol
Anti-gout agent	Disruption of tubulin protein	Colchicine
TNF inhibitors	Inhibition of TNF	Infliximab (INF), adalimumab (ADA), etanercept (ETN), golimumab, certolizumab pegol
Biosimilar TNF inhibitors	Inhibition of TNF	INF-abba, INF-dyyb, ADA-atto, ADA-abdm, ADA-adaz, ETN-szzs, ETN-ykro
IL-1 inhibitors	Inhibition of IL-1	anakinra, rilonacept, canakinumab
IL-6 inhibitors	Inhibition of IL-6	Tocilizumab, sarilumab
IL-17 inhibitors	Inhibition of IL-17	Secukinumab, ixekizumab
IL-23 inhibitors	Inhibition of IL-23	Guselkumab, risankizumab
IL-12/IL-23 dual inhibitors	Dual inhibition of IL-12 and IL-23	Ustekinumab
C5 complement protein inhibitor	Inhibits the cleavage of C5 into C5a and C5b	Eculizumab

[a]List does not represent all available drug formulations

Conclusions

Many chronic inflammatory diseases have unclear triggers but are driven by immune-mediated mechanisms. With a greater understanding of the cellular and molecular components involved in inflammation, targeted therapies that interact with cytokines or effector cells have become more common in the treatment of various chronic inflammatory conditions. As the knowledge of the immune system continues to grow, therapies that modulate the inflammatory cascade will likely play larger roles in the treatment of human disease.

This volume aims to summarize current knowledge about the role of inflammation in the development of the two most prevalent metabolic diseases of our time—obesity and diabetes.

References

1. Scott A. What is "inflammation"? Are we ready to move beyond Celsus? Br J Sports Med. 2004;38:248–9.
2. Kaufmann SH. Immunology's coming of age. Front Immunol. 2019;10:684. https://doi.org/10.3389/fimmu.2019.00684.
3. Hochberg MC, Gravallese EM, Smolen JS, der Dvan H, Weinblatt ME, Weisman ME. Inflammation and its chemical mediators. In: Rheumatology. 8th ed. Philadelphia, PA: Elsevier; 2023. p. 96–108.
4. Sompayrac L. The innate immune system. In: How the immune system works. 7th ed. Chichester: Wiley-Blackwell; 2023. p. 12–25.
5. Abbas AK, Lichtman AH, Pillai S, Baker DL. Properties and overview of immune responses. In: Cellular and molecular immunology. Philadelphia, PA: Elsevier; 2022. p. 96–108.
6. Burton G. Immunitas. Oxford Research Encyclopedia of Classics; 2015. https://doi.org/10.1093/acrefore/9780199381135.013.3267.
7. Gabay C, Kushner I. Acute-phase proteins and other systemic responses to inflammation. N Engl J Med. 1999;340:448–54.
8. Bray C, Bell L, Haykal R, Kaiksow F, Mazza J, Yale S. Erythrocyte sedimentation rate and C-reactive protein measurements and their relevance in clinical medicine. WMJ. 2016;115:317–21.
9. Deftos LJ, Roos BA, Parthemore JG. Calcium and skeletal metabolism. West J Med. 1975;6:447–58.
10. Maruna P, Nedelkikova K, Gurlick R. Physiology and genetics of procalcitonin. Physiol Res. 2000;49 Suppl 1:S57–61.
11. Wang W, Knovich MA, Coffman LG, Torti FM, Torti SV. Serum ferritin: past, present and future. Biochim Biophys Acta Gen Subj. 2010;1800:760–9.
12. Cullis JO, Fitzsimons EJ, Griffiths WJH, Tsochatzis E, Thomas DW. Investigation and management of a raised serum ferritin. Br J Haematol. 2018;181:331–40.
13. Marshall JS, Warrington R, Watson W, Kim HL. An introduction to immunology and immunopathology. Allergy Asthma Clin Immunol. 2018;14:5–14.
14. Van de Vijver E, van den Berg TK, Kuijpers TW. Leukocyte adhesion deficiencies. Hematol Oncol Clin North Am. 2013;27:101–16.
15. Thangam EB, Jemima EA, Singh H, Baig MS, Khan M, Mathias CB, Church MK, Saluja R. The role of histamine and histamine receptors in mast cell-mediated allergy and inflammation:

the hunt for new therapeutic targets. Front Immunol. 2018;9:1873. https://doi.org/10.3389/fimmu.2018.01873.

16. Fajgenbaum DC, June CH. Cytokine Storm. N Engl J Med. 2020;383:2255–73.

17. Schartz ND, Tenner AJ. The good, the bad, and the opportunities of the complement system in neurodegenerative disease. J Neuroinflammation. 2020;17:354. https://doi.org/10.1186/s12974-020-02024-8.

18. Grumach AS, Kirschfink M. Are complement deficiencies really rare? Overview on prevalence, clinical importance and modern diagnostic approach. Mol Immunol. 2014;61:110–7. https://doi.org/10.1016/j.molimm.2014.06.030.

19. Chaplin DD. Overview of the immune response. J Allergy Clin Immunol. 2010;125:S3–S23.

20. Market E, Papavasiliou FN. V(D)J recombination and the evolution of the adaptive immune system. PLoS Biol. 2003;1:e16.

21. Miller FW. The increasing prevalence of autoimmunity and autoimmune diseases: an urgent call to action for improved understanding, diagnosis, treatment, and prevention. Curr Opin Immunol. 2023;80:102266.

22. Bonilla FA, Oettgen HC. Adaptive immunity. J Allergy Clin Immunol. 2010;125:S33–40.

23. Forthal DN. Functions of antibodies. Microbiol Spectr. 2014;2:2.4.21.

24. Tasaka S. Pneumocystis pneumonia in human immunodeficiency virus-infected adults and adolescents: current concepts and future directions. Clin Med Insights Circ Respir Pulm Med. 2015;61:110–7. https://doi.org/10.4137/ccrpm.s23324.

25. Masur H, Brooks JT, Benson CA, Holmes KK, Pau AK, Kaplan JE. Prevention and treatment of opportunistic infections in HIV-infected adults and adolescents: updated guidelines from the Centers for Disease Control and Prevention, National Institutes of Health, and HIV medicine Association of the Infectious Diseases Society of America. Clin Infect Dis. 2014;58:1308–11.

26. Prabhakar BS, Bahn RS, Smith TJ. Current perspective on the pathogenesis of graves' disease and ophthalmopathy. Endocr Rev. 2003;24:802–35.

27. Burrack AL, Martinov T, Fife BT. T cell-mediated Beta cell destruction: autoimmunity and alloimmunity in the context of type 1 diabetes. Front Endocrinol. 2017;8:343. https://doi.org/10.3389/fendo.2017.00343.

28. Brusselle GG, Koppelman GH. Biologic therapies for severe asthma. N Engl J Med. 2022;386:157–71.

29. Schneider S, Li L, Zink A. The new era of biologics in atopic dermatitis: a review. Dermatol Pract Concept. 2021;11:1–6. https://doi.org/10.5826/dpc.1104a144.

30. Findeisen KE, Sewell J, Ostor AJ. Biological therapies for rheumatoid arthritis: an overview for the clinician. Biologics. 2021;15:343–52.

31. Jin JB, Cai B, Zhou J-M. Salicylic acid. In: Hormone metabolism and signaling in plants; 2017. p. 273–89.

32. Mahesh G, Anil Kumar K, Reddanna P. Overview on the discovery and development of anti-inflammatory drugs: should the focus be on synthesis or degradation of PGE2? J Inflamm Res. 2021;14:253–63.

33. Barnes PJ. Glucocorticoids. In: History of allergy; 2014. p. 311–6.

34. van der Velden VH. Glucocorticoids: mechanisms of action and anti-inflammatory potential in asthma. Mediat Inflamm. 1998;7:229–37.

35. Vilcek J. First demonstration of the role of TNF in the pathogenesis of disease. J Immunol. 2008;181:5–6.

36. Tracey KJ, Fong Y, Hesse DG, Manogue KR, Lee AT, Kuo GC, Lowry SF, Cerami A. Anti-cachectin/TNF monoclonal antibodies prevent septic shock during lethal bacteraemia. Nature. 1987;330:662–4.

37. Traynor K. FDA approves biosimilar version of infliximab. Am J Health Syst Pharm. 2016;73:604–5.

38. Cohen SB. The use of Anakinra, an interleukin-1 receptor antagonist, in the treatment of rheumatoid arthritis. Rheum Dis Clin N Am. 2004;30:365–80.

39. Gavriilaki E, de Latour RP, Risitano AM. Advancing therapeutic complement inhibition in hematologic diseases: PNH and beyond. Blood. 2022;139:3571–82.
40. Wofford J, Menter A. Ustekinumab for the treatment of psoriatic arthritis. Expert Rev Clin Immunol. 2014;10:189–202.
41. Curtis JR, Xie F, Chen R, Chen L, Kilgore ML, Lewis JD, Yun H, Zhang J, Wright NC, Delzell E. Identifying newly approved medications in Medicare claims data: a case study using tocilizumab. Pharmacoepidemiol Drug Saf. 2013;22:1214–21.
42. Blauvelt A. Safety of secukinumab in the treatment of psoriasis. Expert Opin Drug Saf. 2016;15:1413–20.
43. Bhat S, Altajar S, Shankar D, Zahorian T, Robert R, Qazi T, Shah B, Farraye FA. Process and clinical outcomes of a biosimilar adoption program with infliximab-Dyyb. J Manag Care Spec Pharm. 2020;26:410–6.

Chapter 2
Obesity and Inflammation

Sonali Sengupta and Dimiter Avtanski

Abbreviations

11β-HSD	11beta-hydroxysteroid dehydrogenase
17β-HSD	17beta-hydroxysteroid dehydrogenase
AdipoR1	Adiponectin receptor
AGT	Angiotensinogen
AMPK	AMP-activated protein kinase
AP	Adipocyte precursor (cells) (*s.* preadipocytes)
AP2	Adipocyte protein 2
APO-E	Apolipoprotein E
ASP	Acylation-stimulating protein
AT	Adipose tissue
ATDC	Adipocyte tissue dendritic cells
ATF	Activating transcription factor
ATM	Adipose tissue macrophages
AUCInsulin	Area under the curve insulin
BAT	Brown adipose tissue
BLT-1	B-leukotriene receptor 1

S. Sengupta
Department of Gastroenterology, All India Institute of Medical Sciences (AIIMS),
New Delhi, India

D. Avtanski (✉)
Friedman Diabetes Institute, Lenox Hill Hospital, Northwell Health, New York, NY, USA

Feinstein Institutes for Medical Research, Manhasset, NY, USA

Donald and Barbara Zucker School of Medicine at Hofstra/Northwell, Hempstead, NY, USA
e-mail: davtanski@northwell.edu

© The Author(s), under exclusive license to Springer Nature
Switzerland AG 2023
D. Avtanski, L. Poretsky (eds.), *Obesity, Diabetes and Inflammation,*
Contemporary Endocrinology, https://doi.org/10.1007/978-3-031-39721-9_2

BMI	Body mass index
bTG	Beta thromboglobulin
C/EBP	CCAAT enhancer binding protein
C1Q	Complement 1Q
CCL2 (*s.* MCP-1)	Chemokine (C-C motif) ligand 2
CCL3 (*s.* MIP-1α)	Chemokine (C-C motif) ligand 3
CETP	Cholesteryl ester transfer protein
CFB	Complement factor B
CFD	Complement factor D
CHOP	C/EBP homologous protein
CLS	Crown-like structures
CSF	Colony-stimulating factor
CVD	Cardiovascular disease
CXCL1 (*s.* GRO1)	Chemokine (C-X-C motif) ligand 1
db/db	Leptin receptor-deficient rodent model
DC	Dendritic cells
DIO	Diet-induced obesity
DSCG (*s.* cromolyn)	Disodium cromoglycate
eIF2α	Eucaryotic initiation factor 2 alpha subunit
ER	Endoplasmic reticulum
ERAD	Endoplasmic reticulum-associated degradation
ERK	Extracellular signal-regulated kinase
ET-1	Endothelin 1
FAI	Free androgen index
FAS	Fatty acid synthase
FFA	Free fatty acid
FGF	Fibroblast growth factor
FNDC5	Fibronectin type III domain-containing protein 5
GADD	Growth arrest and DNA damage
gp130 (*s.* CD130)	Glycoprotein 130
HDAC	Histone deacetylase
HFD	High-fat diet
HIF-1	Hypoxia-inducible factor
HMM	High molecular mass
HOMA2-IR	Homeostasis model assessment of insulin resistance
HSPA5	Heat shock protein family A (Hsp70) member 5
IAAT	Intra-abdominal adipose tissue
IFN	Interferon
Ig	Immunoglobulin
IGF-I	Insulin-like growth factor 1
IKKβ	Inhibitor of nuclear factor kappa B kinase subunit beta
IL	Interleukin
IL-6R (*s.* CD126)	IL-6 receptor

IMAT	Intermuscular adipose tissue
iNOS	Inducible nitric oxide synthase
IR	Insulin resistance
IRE-1	Inositol-requiring enzyme 1
IRS1	Insulin receptor substrate 1
JAK	Janus kinase
JNK	c-Jun N-terminal kinase
LCFA	Long-chain fatty acid
LDL-C	Low-density lipoprotein cholesterol
LMM	Low molecular mass
LPL	Lipoprotein lipase
Lp-PLA2 (*s.* PAF-AH)	Lipoprotein-associated phospholipase A2
MAPK	Mitogen-activated protein kinase
MAT	Bone marrow adipose tissue
MIF	Macrophage migration inhibitor factor
MS	Mast cells
MSC	Mesenchymal stem cells
NEFA	Non-esterified fatty acid
NF-κB	Nuclear factor kappa B
NK	Natural killer (cells)
NPY	Neuropeptide Y
ob/ob	Leptin-deficient rodent model
ObR (*ss.* LEP-R, CD295)	Leptin receptor
OLETF	Otsuka long-evans tokushima fatty rat model
PAI-1	Plasminogen activator inhibitor 1
PDGF	Platelet-derived growth factor
PERK	Protein kinase RNA-like
PF-4	Platelet factor 4
PGC-1α	Peroxisome proliferator-activated receptor gamma coactivator 1 alpha
P_{O2}	Oxygen pressure
PPAR	Peroxisome proliferator-activated receptor
PTP1B	Protein tyrosine phosphatase 1B
RBP4	Retinol-binding protein 4
RELM	Resistin-like molecule
ROS	Reactive oxygen species
SAT	Subcutaneous adipose tissue
SHP-2	Src homology 2 domain-containing protein tyrosine phosphatase 2
sIL-6R	Soluble IL-6 receptor
SOCS3	Suppressor of cytokine signaling 3
STAT	Signal transducer and activator of transcription
T2D	Type 2 diabetes
TG	Triglyceride
TGFβ	Transforming growth factor beta

Th	T helper cells
TLR	Toll-like receptor
TNFR	TNF receptor
TNFα (*ss.* cachexin, cachectin)	Tumor-necrosis factor alpha
Treg	T regulatory cells
UCP1 (*s.* thermogenin)	Uncoupling protein 1
UPR	Unfolded protein response
VAT	Visceral (*s.* intra-abdominal) adipose tissue
VEGF	Vascular endothelial growth factor
WAT	White adipose tissue
WHR	Waist-to-hip ratio
XBP-1	X-box binding protein 1
ZBTB46	Zink finger and BTB domain-containing 46

Introduction

Today, obesity is reaching epidemic proportions and is one of the most significant causes of morbidity and mortality. The disbalance between energy intake and energy expenditure leads to disproportional growth of the visceral white adipose tissue (AT), although other adipose depots are also affected. AT hypertrophy and hyperplasia result in adipocyte death and infiltration of various immune cells. Consequently, a chronic low-grade inflammatory state of the AT is reached, which is one of the characteristic features of obesity. AT and the immune system respond to obesity differently, where inflammatory factors such as cytokines play a central role in this bidirectional communication.

In this chapter, we will provide an overview of obesity-induced inflammation and briefly summarize the role of the two main types of AT—white and brown adipose. Particular attention will be paid to some of the most prominent cytokines serving as communication molecules in the interplay between the AT and the immune system, the main factors contributing to AT inflammation, and specific immune cells. Through this discussion, we aim to provide a comprehensive overview of the link between obesity and inflammation and highlight particular molecular players that can potentially be used as therapeutic targets.

Obesity

Obesity can be defined based on different criteria, but it is primarily diagnosed when body mass index (BMI $= \dfrac{\text{body weight}\,[\text{kg}]}{\text{height}\,[\text{m}]^2}$) is 30.0 kg/m^2 or above [1]. The increase in obesity incidence worldwide is dramatic, reaching epidemic levels. In the USA, from 1960 to 1994, the number of obese individuals doubled [2–5]. The main factor for the alarming increase in obesity is the excessive energy uptake and decreased energy expenditure as genetic factors (such as mutations of leptin (*LEP*), leptin receptor (*ObR*), melanocortin 4 receptor (*MC4R*), or pro-opiomelanocortin (*POMC*) genes) are rare [6–8].

Excessive body weight relates to higher morbidity and mortality rates [9–19]. Being overweight or obese increases the risk of death by 20–40% and 200–300%, respectively, in individuals 50–71 years old [20]. Epidemiological studies show that the mortality rate increases when BMI exceeds 25 mg/m^2 and is especially prominent at BMI above 30 kg/m^2 [21, 22].

Obesity causes an increase in the circulating levels of free fatty acids (FFAs), triglycerides (TGs), and low-density lipoprotein cholesterol (LDL-C). This leads to the development of metabolic syndrome, insulin resistance (IR), and type 2 diabetes (T2D) [23–26].

Adipose Tissue

Besides its energy and thermo-insulating functions, AT is an endocrine organ. It produces a variety of chemical substances: cytokines and cytokine-related proteins (leptin, tumor necrosis factor alpha (TNFα), interleukin (IL) 6 (IL-6), etc.), immune-related proteins (chemokine (C-C motif) ligand 2 (CCL2, *s*. MCP-1), etc.), fibrino-lytic proteins (plasminogen activator inhibitor 1 (PAI-1), etc.), complement and complement-related proteins (adiponectin, complement factors D and B (CFD and CFB), acylation-stimulating protein (ASP), etc.), lipids and proteins for lipid metabolism or transport (lipoprotein lipase (LPL), cholesteryl ester transfer protein (CETP), apolipoprotein E (Apo-E), non-esterified fatty acids (NEFAs), etc.), enzymes involved in steroid metabolism (cytochrome P450-dependent aromatase, 17β- and 11 β-hydroxysteroid dehydrogenases (1β-HSD and 11β-HSD), etc.), RAS proteins (angiotensinogen (AGT), etc.), and other (resistin, etc.).

There are two functionally distinct types of AT—white AT (WAT) and brown AT (BAT). Each type is distributed into separate depots and has a specific endocrine profile and function [27]. WAT is divided into two main groups: subcutaneous AT (SAT), found in the lower part of the body, and intraabdominal AT (IAAT), which comprises the visceral (*s*. intra-abdominal) fat (VAT) [28]. Within the WAT, a small number of brown-like (so-called beige) adipocytes possess distinct phenotypes and characteristics from the classical white or brown adipocytes. Adipocytes in the bone marrow are considered a separate class (bone marrow AT (MAT)) that share common characteristics with the WAT and BAT.

Obesity, characterized by WAT adipocyte hypertrophy (an increase in adipocyte size) and hyperplasia (an increase in cell number) [29], affects the entire AT. The hypertrophy and hyperplasia of WAT relate to necrotic adipocyte death induced by obesity [30, 31].

Obesity disrupts white adipocyte differentiation, hormonal production, and inflammation. BAT adipocytes respond to obesity with changes in mitochondrial function related to oxidation and energy metabolism. Obesity also affects the MAT adipocytes that balance osteogenesis by changing bone mineral density.

White Adipose Tissue and Obesity

WAT is the most abundant AT in the body. It produces a wide range of hormones, growth factors, and cytokines, including leptin, adiponectin, TNFα, IL-6, PAI-1, adipsin, resistin, visfatin, retinol-binding protein 4 (RBP4), among others. WAT endocrine function is tightly controlled by hormonal (e.g., insulin) and sympathetic (e.g., adrenergic) mechanisms [32].

Adipocytes constitute about one-third of the WAT; the rest is represented by fibroblasts, macrophages, stromal cells, monocytes, and progenitor self-renewal adipocyte precursor (AP) cells (commonly known as preadipocytes) [33]. Mature adipocytes differentiate in two steps (a process commonly known as adipogenesis): (1) generation of preadipocytes from mesenchymal stem cells (MSCs) and (2) further differentiation of the preadipocytes to adipocytes [34]. Adipogenesis requires the involvement of CCAAT enhancer binding protein (C/EBP) transcription factor and peroxisome proliferator-activated receptors (PPARs) [35, 36] as well as activation of Wnt and Hedgehog signaling pathways [37, 38]. Mature adipocytes cannot proliferate and are characterized by a single large lipid droplet (unilocular cells), unlike BAT adipocytes, which contain multiple lipid vacuoles (multilocular cells).

Preadipocytes and adipocytes have different secretory profiles. While both preadipocytes and adipocytes synthesize leptin, mature adipocytes mainly produce adiponectin. In a lean state, the balance between preadipocytes and adipocytes keeps leptin and adiponectin levels in equilibrium. However, in obese states, excessive WAT mass negatively affects the rate of adipocyte differentiation, thus disrupting WAT hormonal balance and favoring leptin production. Leptin and TNFα promote the expression of proteins involved in WAT metabolism, mimicking PPAR activation and directly suppressing adiponectin receptor (AdipoR1) expression [39].

AT metabolism is regulated by multiple microRNAs that tightly control adipogenesis and adipocytokines production [40–43]. MicroRNAs such as miR-15a, miR-101, miR-148a, miR-21, miR-320, and miR-423-5p regulate WAT production of leptin [39, 44]. Positive and negative correlations with BMI are found for many circulating microRNAs, including miR-221, miR-143, and let-7 [39]. The expression of multiple microRNAs (among them miR-17-5p, miR-132, miR-134, miR-181a, miR-27a, miR-30e, miR-140, miR-147, miR-155, miR-197, miR-210, miR-103, and miR-143) link AT dysfunction with the development of obesity-associated conditions [40, 45].

Brown Adipose Tissue and Obesity

BAT is primarily present during the neonatal period, functioning to maintain thermogenesis by triglyceride degradation [46]. In infants, it classically resides in peri-aortic, cervical, interscapular, and perirenal depots, as smaller amounts can also be dispersed within the WAT depots.

Initially, BAT was not thought to exist during adulthood because this AT is very sparsely distributed around the body, and its detection and mapping are challenging. A standard method by which BAT can be visualized is positron emission tomography (PET) and computer tomography (CT) imaging. Evidence by fluorodeoxyglucose (FDG) PET in adults indicated areas of FDG uptake corresponding to BAT localized in the supraclavicular, the neck, and in the mediastinum (para-aortic), paravertebral, and suprarenal regions [47–55]. Based on such results, Cypess et al. [56] suggested that BAT is present in a substantial percentage of adults, most distinctively as a cervical-supraclavicular depot. The thermogenic function and the energy expenditure capacity of BAT negatively correlate with aging [57, 58], as demonstrated in human and rodent models [56, 59–62]. Mancini et al. [63] found that BAT aging involves changes in the energy, nucleotide, and vitamin metabolism and detected age-related alterations in the nucleotide metabolism cluster that may be used as biomarkers for the age-dependent decline in the brown adipocyte function.

BAT is essential for the classical nonshivering and cold acclimatization-recruited noradrenaline-induced thermogenesis. Classical nonshivering thermogenesis is entirely dependent on BAT [64, 65]. The unique thermogenic functions of BAT are mediated by the mitochondrial carrier family uncoupling protein 1 (UCP1, s. thermogenin) localized in the inner mitochondrial membrane. The absence of UCP1 resulted in a complete loss of thermogenic capacity of BAT cells isolated from UCP1(−/−) mice, demonstrated by Matthias et al. [66]. Activated by long-chain fatty acids (LCFAs), UCP1 uncouples the proton gradient and increases the conductance of the inner mitochondrial membrane, thus generating heat rather than ATP (a.k.a. nonshivering s. adaptive thermogenesis) [67–69]. There is ample evidence that BAT is under temperature control, and recruitment of BAT is associated with prolonged cold exposure [54, 64, 70–79].

Similarly to WAT, BAT is a highly secretory organ producing a variety of autocrine (basement membrane proteins, adipsin, basic fibroblast growth factor, insulin-like growth factor 1 (IGF-I), prostaglandins, adenosine, etc.), paracrine (nerve growth factor, vascular endothelial growth factor (VEGF), nitric oxide, angiotensinogen, etc.), and endocrine (leptin, adiponectin, resistin, irisin, etc.) factors. Leptin and adiponectin are expressed in the brown adipocytes only under certain conditions, such as inactivity or atrophy, and are decreased after cold exposure [46, 80].

BAT is very sensitive to insulin responding with enhanced glucose uptake, hydrolysis, and ATP production, and, in this regard, it provides an essential defense against obesity [46, 81]. Exploring the differences in basal energy expenditure and its role in the development of obesity and metabolic syndrome, Almind et al. [82] compared two strands of mice: C57Bl/6 (diabesity-prone) and 129S6/SvEvTac (diabesity-resistant). Among these two strands, 129S6/SvEvTac mice showed lower weight gain on a high-fat diet (HFD) and significantly higher caloric intake on a low-fat diet. 129S6/SvEvTac mice also had lower weight gain per gram of food eaten and significantly higher oxygen consumption than C57Bl/6 mice. The authors of the study explained the observed higher basal metabolic rate in 128S6/SvEvTac mice as a result of unexpected intermuscular localizations of BAT and higher UCP1 expression.

Transgenic mice with primary deficiency of BAT develop levels of obesity comparable to those of leptin-deficient (*ob/ob*), leptin receptor-deficient (*db/db*), or hypothalamic lesion (monosodium glutamate)-induced obesity, that was reversed after regeneration of BAT [83]. Mice lacking UCP1 are cold-sensitive and lean at room temperature [84] but gain weight when placed in thermoneutral conditions [85]. Human data confirm the role of BAT in obesity. An inverse correlation of BAT prevalence and activity with BMI was observed in multiple studies [47, 55, 56, 86–90], suggesting that a high percentage of BAT may have protective effects against obesity. Using PET/CT images, Leitner et al. [91] compared the anatomic distribution and functional capacity of BAT between lean and obese healthy young men under tolerable cold exposure. The study demonstrated higher levels of cold-activated BAT volumes than previously suggested, especially in lean, compared to obese individuals. The study also suggested a previously underappreciated thermogenic potential of BAT because only less than half of it was activated by cold exposure. Activation of BAT also associates with feeding and, more specifically, with diets characterized by low protein content [46].

Taken together, the above experimental and clinical observations establish the pivotal role of BAT in regulating thermogenesis by increasing glucose uptake and energy expenditure, thus making it a potential target for treating obesity [92].

Obesity and Inflammation

Overview

A distinctive feature of obesity is the hypertrophy (an increase in adipocyte size) and hyperplasia (an increase in cell number) of WAT and the infiltration of bone marrow-derived T-cells and monocytes forming characteristic crown-like structures (CLS) [29]. Immune cell infiltration to the AT leads to the activation of various signaling cascades and low-grade inflammation [93, 94]. Subsequently, obesity-induced inflammation alters the metabolism, thus giving rise to the term *"metainflammation"* (or *"metaflammation"*) [95].

The association between augmented adiposity following excessive caloric intake and AT inflammation has been documented in both animal and human studies [96,

97]. AT from obese rodents and humans demonstrated an increased secretion of TNFα [98–100]. A characteristic feature of AT inflammation is the duration and intensity of the inflammatory response, which appears to be persistent, low-grade, and fails to resolve. AT inflammation is unique in that, despite the classical inflammation, it does not significantly increase energy expenditure [101]. AT inflammation also differs depending on the WAT-specific subtype affected, as it is more complex and intense in VAT than in SAT [101].

The initial step in WAT inflammation in obesity involves dysregulation of fatty acid homeostasis, endoplasmic reticulum (ER) stress, adipocyte death, local hypoxia, and mitochondrial dysfunction. This dysregulation culminates in the activation of the c-Jun N-terminal kinase (JNK) and nuclear factor kappa B (NF-kB) signaling pathways, which results in proinflammatory cytokine production [102, 103]. Obesity affects adipocyte differentiation and disrupts cytokine equilibrium. Preadipocytes and differentiated adipocytes are highly secretory cells but have different secretory profiles. For example, leptin is produced by both the preadipocytes and the adipocytes, but only the mature adipocytes can synthesize adiponectin. Thus, in obesity, cytokine production is shifted more toward the proinflammatory leptin. The recruitment and activation of the NF-kB signaling pathway induce the production of the suppressor of cytokine signaling 3 (SOCS3) and protein tyrosine phosphatase 1B (PTP1B), which form a negative feedback loop to block leptin receptor signaling via the Janus kinase/signal transducer and activator of transcription (JAK/STAT) pathway and promote leptin resistance. The increased proinflammatory cytokines (such as IL-6, TNFα, transforming growth factor beta (TGFβ), IL-1α, CCL2, CCL3 (s. MIP-1α), endothelial adhesion molecules, and chemotactic agents) promote further infiltration of monocytes and their maturation into proinflammatory macrophages [27, 104, 105]. Active macrophages, together with adipocytes and other cells in WAT, perpetuate a vicious cycle of monocyte/macrophage recruitment and proinflammatory cytokine production. The induction of the leptin signaling pathway leads to the activation of extracellular signal-regulated kinases 1 and 2 (ERK1/2) phosphorylation, followed by an increase in NF-κB and a subsequent release of TNFα and other inflammatory factors [106, 107]. Elevated levels of TNFα, IL-6, and inducible nitric oxide synthase (iNOS) directly suppress insulin signaling [108–110], and TNFα induces lipolysis through the activation of ERK and JNK signaling pathways [111, 112]. Another consequence of obesity is dyslipidemia, characterized by increased levels of circulating free fatty acids FFAs, triglycerides TGs, and LDL-C [113] (Fig. 2.1).

Cytokines Involved in Obesity-Induced Inflammation

Cytokines are a broad and not strictly defined group of proteins produced by the immune cells or adipocytes that are key mediators in the inflammation process. Based on their structure, cytokines are divided into four groups: (1) the four α-helix

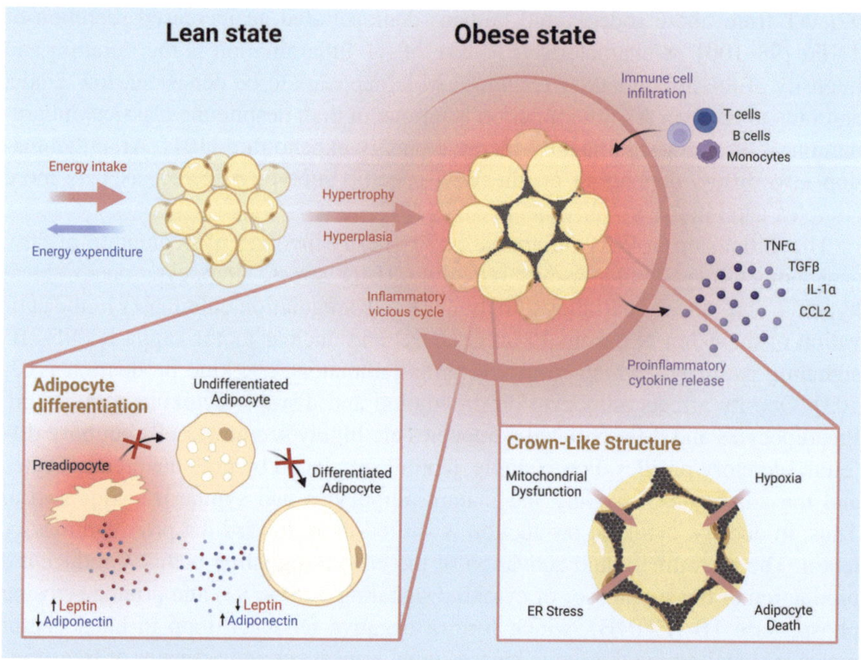

Fig. 2.1 The interplay between obesity and inflammation in adipose tissue. Obesity arises from an imbalance between energy intake and expenditure, leading to adipocyte hypertrophy (increased cell size) and hyperplasia (increased cell number), ER stress, disrupted fatty acid homeostasis, mitochondrial dysfunction, hypoxia, and adipocyte death. This results in the recruitment of various immune cells, including T and B cells, monocytes and macrophages, neutrophils, mast cells, and dendritic cells, to the adipose tissue, contributing to chronic low-grade inflammation. Immune cells infiltrating the adipose tissue form crown-like structures (CLSs) around the apoptotic adipocytes and secrete proinflammatory cytokines and growth factors, such as TNFα, TGFβ, IL-1α, and CCL2. Furthermore, the inflammatory milieu alters adipocyte differentiation and cytokine secretion, shifting the balance towards increased leptin production and decreased adiponectin release. Created with BioRender.com

bundle (*s.* α-spiral) family comprising three subfamilies (the IL-2, interferon (IFN), and IL-10 subfamilies), (2) the IL-1 family (including IL-1 and IL-18), (3) the cysteine knot cytokines (including TGFβ superfamily), and (4) the IL-17 family. However, functional classification is more useful in experimental and clinical practice, which divides the cytokines into Type 1 (those that enhance cellular immune responses) (TNFα, IFN-γ, etc.) and Type 2 (those that enhance antibody response) (TGFβ, IL-4, IL-10, IL-13, etc.). Commonly used nomenclature based on presumed function, cell of secretion, or target of action classifies cytokines into six different categories: (1) lymphokines (those produced by lymphocytes), (2) interleukins (those whose presumed targets are principally leukocytes), (3) monokines (those produced exclusively by monocytes), (4) interferons (those involved in antiviral responses), (5) colony-stimulating factors (those that support cell growth), and (6) chemokines (those that mediate chemoattraction). Cytokines synthesized in AT are commonly labeled as adipokines.

In the following sections, we will discuss only a portion of the adipokines whose balance is disrupted in obesity. WAT- and BAT-derived cytokines such as leptin, adiponectin, or irisin are critical mediators of metabolic status transmitting signals from AT to other organs. Other cytokines produced by AT, such as IL-6 and TNFα, are essential regulators of inflammatory functions modulating the immune cells to respond to traumatic events. Adipokine secretion also depends on the adipocyte size, as leptin and adiponectin are secreted more from the small adipocytes, while resistin and TNFα primarily by the enlarged adipocytes [114].

Leptin

Leptin is a pleiotropic cytokine encoded in the *ob* gene classically known to regulate satiety and energy expenditure [115, 116]. Leptin binds to a specific receptor (ObR, *s.* LEP-R or CD295), which belongs to the class I cytokine receptor family. ObR is alternatively spliced into six isoforms (ObRa-f) classified as long (ObRb), short (ObRa, c, d, and f), and secretory (soluble) (ObRe) isoforms [117–119]. All of these isoforms have a ligand binding domain (LBD) located in the N-terminus of the protein, and five of the isoforms (ObRa, b, c, d, and f) have a transmembrane domain. Of these five isoforms, ObRb long form has an intracellular domain of 303 amino acids, and the short isoforms have between 30–40 amino acids intracellular domain [119]. ObRb isoform is expressed mainly in the hypothalamus, where it participates in maintaining energy homeostasis, and in the immune cells (monocytes, polymorphonuclear, and natural killer (NK) cells), where it is involved in innate and adaptive immunity. This isoform is the dominant signaling receptor form that activates mainly JAK2/STAT but also Ras/ERK-1/2 and PI3-K/Akt/GSK3 signaling pathways [120–122]. Short ObR isoforms are believed to have mainly transporting roles (leptin internalization and degradation) [123], although they can activate the mitogen-activated protein kinase (MAPK) and JAK signaling cascades [119, 120]. Among the ObR isoforms, ObRa is most abundant and widely expressed in most cell types [123, 124].

Homozygous point mutations of the leptin gene (*ob/ob*) are associated with the early development of obesity, hyperphagia, transient hyperglycemia, glucose intolerance, and elevated plasma insulin levels. These mutations are very rare in humans [125], but *ob/ob*-mutated rodents are commonly used as a model of obesity. Point mutations of the ObR gene (*db/db*) also result in obesity as well as hyperleptinemia, an obesity phenotype, chronic hyperglycemia, pancreatic β-cell atrophy, diabetes, peripheral neuropathy, cold intolerance, myocardial disease, elevated glucosteroid hormone levels, and pubertal dysfunction, among other [119].

Leptin is mainly synthesized by the adipocytes of the WAT [126] but in smaller amounts also by the placenta, ovaries, mammary epithelium, bone marrow, and lymphoid tissues [127]. The production of leptin varies among WAT, as the adipocytes of the subcutaneous WAT express higher levels than those of the omental WAT [128]. Leptin gene expression shows sexual dimorphism (markedly higher in women) and menopausal status-dependent differences [128–131].

Plasma leptin levels are highly correlated with the percent of body fat and BMI, level of IR, and components of metabolic syndrome and T2D [132–134]. Increased leptin levels in obesity reflect peripheral leptin resistance [114]. Chronic inflammation observed in obese states seems to play a role in leptin production, and some cytokines (such as IL-1β and TNFα) have been shown to increase it [135–139]. Nevertheless, it needs to be noted that the relationship between cytokines and leptin is complex and can depend on the cellular context. For example, some studies [140] have shown that IL-1 has been shown to increase leptin production by the adipocytes, while TNFα decreases it.

In monocytes, leptin serves as a growth factor to promote proliferation and phagocytosis, the production of proinflammatory cytokines (TNFα, IL-6, and IL-12), and oxidative stress (reactive oxygen species (ROS) production), thus enabling inflammatory infiltration [141, 142]. In polymorphonuclear cells, leptin plays a role as a survival cytokine and promotes chemotaxis and oxygen radicals production [143–145]. Leptin is also necessary for the NK cells' maturation, differentiation, activation, and cytotoxicity [119]. This cytokine also plays a role in the immunomodulatory actions of mast cells (MS) [146] and the maturation and migration of the dendritic cells (DCs) [147].

Leptin production is regulated on multiple levels. Sex steroid hormones, particularly testosterone, were found to directly inhibit leptin production, as shown in a study involving male-to-female and female-to-male transgender individuals [148]. In addition, multiple microRNAs take part in the regulation of leptin synthesis, among them miR-15a, miR-101, miR-148a, miR-21, miR-320, and miR-423-5p.

Adiponectin

Adiponectin is a 244 amino acid protein hormone encoded by the ADIPOQ gene [149]. Adiponectin is secreted predominantly by the WAT adipocytes [150] but, during pregnancy, also by the placenta [151]. Interestingly, recent observations have shown that MAT is the primary source of circulating adiponectin; however, the significance of these findings is yet to be fully established [152]. Structurally, adiponectin demonstrates homologies with complement 1Q (C1Q) complex and TNFα, which is believed to be derived from a common primordial recognition molecule of the innate immune system [153].

Adiponectin circulates as low-molecular-weight (tri-, hexa-, or dodecamer) or high-molecular-weight oligomer structures, as the various oligomers may act differently [154, 155]. Adiponectin binds to either the G protein-coupled AdipoR1 and AdipoR2 or the structurally different T-cadherin (s. CDH13) belonging to the cadherin superfamily of transmembrane proteins [156, 157]. AdipoR1 is expressed predominantly in the cells of skeletal muscles, spleen, lung, heart, kidney, and liver, while the AdipoR2 receptor is mainly expressed in the liver [156, 158].

Major signaling pathways activated by AdipoR are the AMP-activated protein kinase (AMPK), PPARα, and PPARγ. However, depending on the cellular context, other signaling pathways, such as Akt and ERK, can also be activated [159–162].

Adiponectin levels negatively correlate with body weight, fat percentage, and BMI [163]. Low circulating adiponectin levels are observed in obese individuals, those with metabolic syndrome, IR, or diabetes [160, 164–168], and are associated with a higher risk of developing inflammation-related conditions, such as obesity, T2D, or cardiovascular disease (CVD). On the other hand, high adiponectin levels have been linked to a lower risk of these conditions [169].

Adiponectin is an anti-inflammatory cytokine that promotes insulin sensitivity and fat oxidation [132, 159, 170–173]. High molecular weight oligomers are thought to possess higher biological activity in glucose homeostasis [155, 174]. Adiponectin inhibits the production of TNFα and IL-6 and modulates the activity of the immune cells [175–178]. In macrophages, adiponectin functions as a regulator of polarization and the differentiation from M1 to M2 type [179]. In T cells, it suppresses their differentiation to Th1 and Th17 cells [180].

Resistin

Resistin (named for "resistance to insulin" and also known as FIZZ3, ADSF, or XCP1) is a cysteine-rich adipokine polypeptide, a member of the resistin-like molecule (RELM) hormone family, encoded by the *RETN* gene [181].

The primary source of resistin is the AT; however, it is also produced in smaller amounts by the hypothalamus, pituitary, adrenal glands, pancreas, gastrointestinal tract, myocytes, spleen, and white blood cells [182, 183]. There is sexual dimorphism and a significant difference in the resistin expression among the WAT depots (more prominent in abdominal subcutaneous and omental fat than in the thigh and breast fat tissue) [181, 184].

Resistin is secreted as a homodimer of 94-amino acid polypeptide bound with disulfide bounds and 10 conserved cysteine residues [185]. Resistin can form homo- or heterooligomer structures with another member of the RELM family, RELMα [186]. In humans, circulating resistin is found in two distinct assembly states—the disulfide-linked hexamer or high-molecular-mass (HMM) resistin (the predominant species) and a smaller complex or low-molecular-mass (LMM) resistin (the higher bioactive form) [187].

Comparative analyses show that human and mouse resistin share only 59% identity at the amino acids level and differ significantly in their mode of action [188]. While resistin is highly expressed in rodents' WAT [189], it is almost undetectable in humans [190]. In mice serum, resistin circulates as a ~ 54 kDa dimeric form that resembles the human HMM form and a smaller ~46 kDa monomer similar to the human HMW form [187]. In differentiated 3 T3-L1 mouse adipocytes, 80–90% of resistin is in the form of a dimer, and the rest is a monomer [187].

Resistin production is regulated by multiple factors. Its production is stimulated by hyperglycemia, steroid hormones (dexamethasone, androgens, estrogens), neuropeptide Y (NPY), and age [182, 191]. Factors inhibiting resistin production include insulin, fasting, thyroid hormones, growth hormone, endothelin-1 (ET-1), neurotransmitters, and PPARγ [182].

Genetic (*ob/ob*, *db/db*, tubby, agouti) and diet-induced obesity (DIO) mouse models, as well as human studies, revealed that serum resistin levels positively correlate with the level of adiposity [181, 192–196]. The expression of resistin in WAT is induced during adipocyte differentiation; on the other hand, resistin inhibits adipocyte differentiation [181, 189]. Although resistin is mainly synthesized by the adipocytes, the AT macrophages (ATMs) also secrete it [181, 190, 197].

Resistin stimulates macrophage production of proinflammatory cytokines IL-1, IL-6, IL-12, and TNFα [198, 199]. However, the effect of these cytokines on resistin production is not entirely understood. While some reports demonstrate that TNFα stimulates resistin production [200], other studies show the opposite effect [201]. Plasma resistin levels associate with markers of inflammation, including soluble TNFα receptor (TNFR) 2 (TNFR-2), IL-6, and lipoprotein-associated phospholipase A2 (Lp-PLA2, s. PAF-AH) [202–205]. Resistin activates the expression of toll-like receptor (TLR) 4 (TLR4) [206, 207], the kinases JNK and IKKβ (inhibitor of nuclear factor kappa B kinase subunit beta) [208], and the NF-κB signaling pathway [198, 199].

TNFα

TNFα (*ss.* cachexin, cachectin) is a cell signaling protein encoded by the TNFA gene that plays a role in the inflammation process by regulating the function of the immune cells [209]. This protein belongs to the TNF superfamily that currently comprises 19 members, such as TNFβ, FasL, and CDD95L [210]. Although TNFα is produced mainly by the activated monocytes and macrophages, it is also synthesized by many other cell types, including lymphocytes, NK cells, MS, neutrons, and adipocytes [211]. Initially, TNFα is synthesized in a precursor form, a 26-kDa protein called pro-TNF, a type II transmembrane protein with its N-terminus spanning the membrane with its N-terminus facing the cytoplasm, and C-terminus the intracellular space [212]. The mature soluble 17-kDa form of TNFα is derived by proteolytic cleavage in the intracellular domain by proteases belonging to the serine protease family [213]. In its active form, TNFα circulates as a homotrimer. TNFα binds to TNFRs, TNFR1, and TNFR2. The TNF receptors form a trimeric structure upon ligand binding, activating NF-κB, JNK, p38-MAPK, and other signaling pathways [214].

TNFα production correlates with the level of adiposity [98, 215, 216]. High levels of TNFα are observed in obesity, as seen in rodents [98, 217] and humans [99], while weight loss is associated with a decrease in TNFα production [218]. TNFα inhibits adipocyte differentiation and can reverse it by inhibiting the expression of PPARγ, C/EBPα, and other genes involved in maintaining the adipocyte phenotype [219–221].

IL-6

IL-6 is cyto-, adipo-, and myokine produced by activated immune (T cells, monocyte/macrophages) and stromal cells. It is coded by the *IL6* gene, which in humans is located on chromosome 7 [222]. IL-6 is a glycoprotein with a 4 α-helix bundle arrangement structurally similar to other cytokines in the interleukin family [223, 224]. IL-6 has multiple functions in the body, including regulating the immune and inflammatory responses, the promotion of angiogenesis, and the regulation of bone metabolism.

IL-6 binds to the IL-6 receptor (IL-6R, *s.* CD126), which is a type I cytokine receptor consisting of a membrane-bound α chain (IL-6Rα) receptor subunit and signal transducer glycoprotein 130 (gp130, *s.* CD130) [225, 226]. Binding to IL-6Rα provokes a homodimerization of gp130, forming a high-affinity functional receptor complex, which activates JAKs and phosphorylation of the tyrosine residues in the cytoplasmic domain of gp130. Binding to the receptor further leads to the activation of two major signaling pathways—Src homology 2 (SH2) domain-containing protein tyrosine phosphatase 2 (SHP-2)/ERK/MAPK and JAK/STAT [227].

IL-6 is produced in AT and is a well-recognized marker for visceral adiposity [228–233]. AT is estimated to contribute 15–35% of all circulating IL-6 [234]. IL-6 levels are markedly increased in obese individuals [235] showing positive correlations with BMI and waist circumference [236–238]. Interestingly, IL-6-knock-out (IL-6$^{-/-}$) mice develop a mature-onset obesity phenotype that can be partially reversed by IL-6 replacement [239]. Research demonstrated that mice with a targeted mutation of the IL-6 gene [240] did not develop age-related obesity. In the last study, IL-6$^{-/-}$ mice actually gained less weight than their wild-type counterparts and displayed no differences in WAT's LPL activity or plasma levels of leptin and TNFα. However, there was a difference in plasma adiponectin levels between the two groups, which was higher in the HFD-fed IL-6$^{-/-}$ mice.

IL-6 has a key role in inflammation and exerts pleiotropic effects. Depending on the context, it may possess both pro- and anti-inflammatory actions [241]. IL-6 is involved in the activation of the T and B cells and increases MS proliferation by suppressing the proteolytic cleavage of the soluble IL-6 receptor (sIL-6R) from IL-6R and downregulating the SOCS3 signaling pathway [242].

Irisin

Irisin is a myo- and adipokine polypeptide, a transcriptional activator of nuclear receptor peroxisome proliferator-activated receptor gamma coactivator 1 alpha (PGC-1α) that greatly increases the transcriptional activity of PPARγ [243, 244]. Irisin is a derivate of fibronectin type III domain-containing protein 5 (FNDC5), whose synthesis is induced by the muscle PGC-1α after exercise or cold exposure [243, 245–248].

Most reports show that irisin levels correlate to adiposity markers, such as body weight, BMI, waist circumference, and fat mass, and are higher in men than women [244, 249–253]. Circulating irisin levels also show a correlation with other parameters accompanying obesity, such as waist-to-hip ratio (WHR), total cholesterol, triglyceride, LDL cholesterol, the area under the curve for insulin (AUCInsulin), homeostasis model assessment of IR (HOMA2-IR), M values, and free androgen index (FAI) [254]. In obese/diabetic-prone Otsuka Long-Evans Tokushima Fatty (OLETF) rats, a significant positive correlation was detected between triceps muscle FNDC5 mRNA and leptin plasma levels [255]. In most studies, irisin levels were found to negatively correlate with daily physical activity, energy expenditure, and body weight reduction. However, other studies demonstrated no difference in irisin levels or even opposite correlations [251–253, 256–258]. Although exercise is suggested to promote irisin production, the direct link between exercise and irisin is not well understood since its effect is usually transient [244, 253, 259–266].

Mechanistically, irisin suppresses adipocyte differentiation as shown in human primary adipocyte cell culture and mouse 3 T3-L1 cells where reduction of the expression of adipocyte protein 2 (AP2), PPARγ, and fatty acid synthase (FAS) was observed [267]. These effects of irisin were partially reversed after supplementation with rosiglitazone, suggesting the role of PPARγ in mediating irisin functions in the AT [267].

Inducers of Adipose Tissue Inflammation in Obesity

ER Stress

ER stress is a chronic perturbation of the ER homeostasis caused by an imbalance between its demand for protein folding and capacity. ER stress is characterized by the accumulation of aberrant proteins caused by an increased secretory load of the ER or by a pathological process such as obesity. As a result of ER stress, cells activate a series of signaling pathways commonly labeled as unfolded protein response (UPR) that can activate triglycerides and cholesterol production. Obesity and ER stress constitute a vicious cycle since obesity both induces it and is aggravated by it [268].

Obese mice (*ob/ob*, *db/db*, or DIO) exhibit elevated markers of ER stress (increased protein kinase RNA-like endoplasmic reticulum kinase (PERK) and eucaryotic initiation factor 2 alpha subunit (eIF2α) phosphorylation, increased heat shock protein family A (Hsp70) member 5 (HSPA5) transcription) and activation of JNK signaling) [269, 270]. Human data also show a correlation between activated ER stress markers and obesity, particularly protective chaperons downstream of activating transcription factor (ATF) 6α (ATF6α) [271]. In response to ER stress, three branches of UPR are activated—those controlled by PERK, inositol-requiring enzyme 1 (IRE-1), and ATF6 [272]. Activation of the PERK branch upregulates the

NF-κB signaling pathway and a subset of translational targets (including ATF4) involved in antioxidant activities and amino acid transport. Activation of PERK also enhances the expression of the pro-apoptotic C/EBP homologous protein (CHOP) and growth arrest and DNA damage (GADD) protein 34 (GADD34), resulting in a negative feedback loop of PERK. Induction of the IRE-1 branch leads to splicing and nuclear translocation of X-box binding protein 1 (XBP-1) mRNA, which regulates the expression of ER chaperones and proteins involved in ER-associated degradation (ERAD). Additionally, IRE-1 activates JNK, ERK, and NF-κB signaling pathways. The third branch activated by ER stress, ATF6, regulates chaperone expression and is engaged in inflammatory pathways via the regulation of NF-κB activity [272].

Imbalance in Fatty Acids Homeostasis

Obesity disrupts fatty acid homeostasis, thus triggering proinflammatory cytokine generation and activation of inflammatory signaling pathways. The imbalance of fatty acids homeostasis is caused by the overconsumption of fat-rich foods (particularly those containing high levels of LCFAs). LCFAs are critical components of cell membranes and have a variety of other functions. High levels of LCFAs (such as stearic, arachidic, and behenic acids) can stimulate the generation of TNFα, IL-6, and IL-1 [273, 274]. Arachidic acid, abundant in foods such as red meat, butter, and cheese, can activate the UPR signaling pathway by activating TLR2 and TLR4 receptors [275]. Furthermore, UPR signaling can also be activated by ER stress.

Hypoxia

Hypoxia plays a crucial role in AT dysfunction in obesity. It is caused by the massive expansion of WAT, resulting in reduced blood supply (lower capillary density) and decreased oxygen concentration and pressure (P_{O2}) [276–282]. The molecular responses to hypoxia are mediated by various transcription factors, including NF-κB, cAMP response element binding protein (CREB), and C/EBP homologous protein (also identified as CHOP/GADD153) [283–285], but mainly by the hypoxia-inducible factor 1 (HIF-1), which is frequently described as *"the master regulator of oxygen homeostasis"* [286, 287]. HIF-1 is a heterodimer composed of two subunits (α and β), where β is constitutively expressed but insensitive to oxygen, and α serves as an oxygen sensor [287]. In humans, the α subunit of HIF consists of three paralogs (HIF-1α, HIF-2α/EPAS, and HIF-3α), and the β subunit–of two paralogs (ARNT and ARNT2) [288]. HIF-1α is constantly synthesized and degraded by the 26S proteasomal system in normoxic conditions. However, when activated by hypoxia, it is stabilized and translocated to the nucleus, where it binds to *cis*-acting regulatory elements of the target genes [289]. The transcriptional activity of HIF-1α is regulated by nuclear co-activators (p300 and CBP) [290, 291] and co-repressors (histone deacetylases (HDACs)) [291]. HIF-1α targets various genes regulating cellular functions, apoptosis, ECM remodeling, angiogenesis, glucose metabolism, and inflammation [282]. A main gene target of HIF-1α is VEGF which promotes angiogenesis and is required for adipocyte differentiation and AT growth [292, 293].

Obesity leads to increased expression of HIF-1α, shown in mice [294] and humans [295]. Overexpression of HIF-1α in WAT leads to weight gain [296], and weight loss downregulates AT *HIF1α* expression [297]. Surprisingly, a transgenic mouse model expressing a dominant-negative version of *HIF1α* exhibits an obese phenotype [296]. Decreased P_{O2} underpins oxidative and ER stress and induces an inflammatory response [283, 298, 299]. Obesity-induced hypoxia is associated with dysregulated adipokine production, demonstrated in various mouse models (DOI, KKAy, *ob/ob*) [294, 299, 300].

Hypoxia suppresses adipocyte expression and secretion of adiponectin and upregulates the production of leptin, PAI-1, IL-6, macrophage migration inhibitor factor (MIF), visfatin, and apelin [282, 294, 301–304]. Additionally, hypoxia inhibits adipocyte differentiation [283, 305–307], further contributing to the dysregulation of WAT cytokine production. Hypoxia-induced increase in proinflammatory cytokine secretion is attenuated by inhibiting JNK and p38 signaling [282]. Immunohistochemistry observations revealed that the areas of low P_{O2} colocalize with those with the accumulation of macrophages [300].

Hypoxia affects the expression of over a thousand genes, many related to inflammation and oxidative stress. It links to oxidative stress by increasing the generation of ROS and ER stress by increasing the production of CHOP and glucose-regulation protein 78 (GRP78) [282, 299].

Mitochondrial Dysfunction

Research on mitochondrial dysfunction is growing in popularity because of its potential to explain the underlying mechanisms of obesity. Mitochondria are responsible for energy production and play a role in regulating body weight. They are also involved in ROX production and controlling oxidative stress, which also associates with metabolic disorders, including obesity.

Multiple studies report the association of mitochondrial dysfunction with obesity and T2D [308–310]. Excessive nutrient consumption causes mitochondrial dysfunction [311, 312], while calory restriction suppresses it [313, 314]. Mitochondrial dysfunction has been hypothesized to be correlated with inflammation [315], and may cause an increase in ROS production and oxidative stress [316]. Obesity also impairs mitochondrial dynamics [317, 318]. Rodent models of obesity (*db/db* or DOI) show decreased mitochondrial biogenesis in AT [319]. In genetically obese mice, reduced mitochondrial DNA and functions have been altered with a concomitant reduction in adiponectin production [320, 321]. A decrease in mitochondrial activity has been observed in AT from obese humans [308]. Mitochondrial dysfunction has been shown to cause inflammation via JNK [321] and NF-κB signaling [322], resulting in the upregulation of inflammatory cytokines production.

Overall, the evidence suggests that mitochondrial dysfunction may be involved in the pathophysiology of obesity and metabolic disorders. Further research is needed to explore the exact mechanisms by which mitochondrial dysfunction contributes to obesity and to determine effective prevention and treatment strategies.

Adipose Tissue Inflammation and Immune System Cells

Extensive animal studies have shown that cells of both the innate (macrophages, neutrophils, dendritic cells, and MS) and adaptive (B and T cells) immune systems participate in obesity-induced AT inflammation [323].

Macrophages

As described above, obesity causes infiltration of macrophages to WAT [324–329]. The number of ATMs correlates positively with BMI and adipocyte size and decreases following weight loss [297, 330, 331]. Macrophages change their number, location, and inflammatory phenotype within WAT, and their percentage may reach up to 40–50% in obesity [330]. Within the CLSs, macrophages localize to dead adipocytes and fuse to form syncytia of multinucleate giant cells that scavenge residual adipocyte lipid droplets [325]. Obesity also changes macrophages' phenotype from anti-inflammatory M2-like to proinflammatory M1-like [332–334], a significant source of TNFα, IL-6, and CCL2, thus leading to local and systemic inflammation [195, 330]. Since M1 macrophages obtain their energy mainly by glycolysis, the M2 macrophages utilize oxidative metabolism. During local and systemic inflammatory responses, tissue-resident macrophages present antigens, which allow the recruitment of other immune cells. The currently accepted model is that tissue-resident macrophages originate from bone marrow monocytes that infiltrate tissue during physiological immunosurveillance or in response to inflammatory events. Obesity increases the circulating levels of CD11b(+) monocytes, which express the chemoattractant B-leukotriene receptor 1 (BLT-1) that sustains monocyte trafficking to WAT [335, 336]. Proinflammatory macrophages also express genes involved in myelopoiesis, affecting monocyte circulating levels [337]. Thus, obesity generates a self-feedback loop of monocyte/macrophage infiltration to sustain low-grade chronic inflammation of WAT.

Neutrophils

Neutrophils are a leukocyte subpopulation of granulocytes involved in innate immunity. They are also important modulators of inflammation. Neutrophils are the most abundant white blood cell type comprising up to 90% of all granulocytes in the blood. Although they are relatively rare in the lean AT, obesity increases their number [338]. Mice subjected to HFD feeding show recruitment of neutrophils to AT as early as 3 days after HFD initiation, remaining constant for up to 90 days [338, 339]. Watanabe et al. [340] demonstrated that neutrophils interact with the adipocytes in proinflammatory cytokine production and are required for the AT expression of chemotactic molecules responsible for macrophage attraction. Neutrophils secrete several proteases (such as elastases) that can further promote inflammation and insulin receptor substrate 1 (IRS1) dysfunction, thus causing IR [338].

Although the available evidence shows the importance of neutrophils in obesity-induced inflammation, their role must be further elucidated.

Dendritic Cells

DCs play a crucial role in the development of obesity-induced inflammation. These specialized immune cells are found throughout the body, including in WAT, where they help to regulate immune responses and maintain tissue homeostasis. Dendritic cells secrete a variety of proinflammatory mediators, including TNFα, IL-12p70, IL-23, nitric oxide, chemokines, and prostaglandins [341, 342]. In healthy individuals, dendritic cells help to maintain immune tolerance by presenting self-antigens to T cells, thereby linking innate and adaptive immunity [343]. However, in individuals with obesity, the excessive accumulation of fat in WAT and the increased production of proinflammatory cytokines activate the dendritic cells to produce more proinflammatory cytokines, which can augment the immune response.

DC comprises a substantial proportion of AT-infiltrated immune cells. AT dendritic cells (ATDCs) is a subset of DC expressing specific markers such as the Zink finger and BTB domain-containing 46 (ZBTB46) [344]. The accumulation of ATDC correlates with BMI in humans [345] and HFD exposure in mice [346, 347] and is associated with the areas of CLS [347].

The role of ATDCs in obesity-induced inflammation and IR still needs to be better understood. However, it is thought that ATDCs may regulate body weight while preserving AT function and homeostasis in obesity [344].

Mast Cells

MSs originate from multipotent hematopoietic stem cells and are part of the innate immune system [348]. They activate T lymphocytes and promote macrophage apoptosis and angiogenesis [349]. In AT, MSs affect angiogenesis and adipocyte differentiation [349].

Obesity is associated with a significant increase in the number of MSs in WAT [349], and MSs which are capable of releasing a wide range of inflammatory mediators (IL-6, INFγ, among others), promote macrophage infiltration [350], contributing further to the obesity-induced AT inflammation and IR [348]. Wang and Shi [349] demonstrated that lack of MS (using two strands of MS-deficient mice–$Kit^{W/Wv}$ and $Kit^{W-sh/W-sh}$ mice) or absence of activation of the MS (using the MS stabilizer disodium cromoglycate (DSCG *s.* cromolyn)) led to a significant reduction in body weight gain and improved glucose and insulin tolerance.

Although MSs are known to play a significant role in obesity and T2D, the complete mechanisms of their action are still vastly unclear.

B Cells

B cells are an essential component of adaptive immunity that secrete immunoglobulins (Igs) which recognize the cognate antigen. One of the IGs, IgE, is involved in the development of allergic reactions, but its production is also increased in obesity [351]. Elevated levels of IgE can provoke other immune cells (such as MS and eosinophils) to release proinflammatory molecules. In addition to synthesizing IgE, B cells can produce other types of antibodies, such as IgG and IgM. These antibodies have an additional effect on inflammation in obesity by binding to adipocytes and other cells. They also can trigger the release of inflammatory molecules and contribute to the development of chronic inflammation [352]. Furthermore, B cells can also produce cytokines (such as TNFα and IL-6) that can further promote inflammation and contribute to the development of inflammation and T2D [353, 354].

B cells are divided into two classes (B1 and B2) which display unique phenotypes, functions, and cytokine secretion profiles. B1 cells are enriched in mucosal tissues, body cavities, and fatty tissues, such as the omentum and the fat pads near the peritoneal cavity. B2 cells produce antibodies specifically to T cell-dependent antigens and are enriched in secondary lymphoid organs [354]. A sustained increase in the number of B cells has been observed in mice fed with HFD from day 90 to day 180 [355]. During the course of HFD, B cells infiltrate the AT and undergo functional changes to a proinflammatory phenotype [356]. This process peaks at around 3–4 weeks after initiation of the HFD [356].

Overall, B cells play a vital role in the development of obesity-induced inflammation through the production of antibodies and cytokines.

T Cells

T cells recognize processed antigenic peptides presented by the antigen-presenting cells. T cells are classified into two main subtypes: CD8(+) (*s.* T cytotoxic cells) and CD4(+). T regulatory cells (Tregs) (*ss.* T helper, T suppressor cells) are another group of T cells that can be considered as a subtype of the CD4(+) group. CD3(+) T cells (that can belong to both CD8(+) or CD4(+) groups) constitute the largest AT immune-cell population, following macrophages. Nishimura et al. [357] demonstrated CD8(+) T cell infiltration into the epididymal AT in mice placed on HFD. This infiltration preceded the accumulation of macrophages. The immunological and genetic depletion of CD8(+) T cells lowered macrophage infiltration and AT inflammation, while the adoptive transfer of CD8(+) T cells to CD8-deficient mice aggravated AT inflammation. Based on the obtained results, the authors of the study concluded that AT in obese mice activates CD8(+) T cells, which, in turn, promote the recruitment and activation of macrophages in this tissue [357]. CD4(+) T cells recognize major histocompatibility complex class II presented on the surface of antigen-presenting cells like dendritic cells, macrophages, and B cells, and are subclassified into pro-inflammatory T helper (Th) 1 (Th1) and Th17 cells, anti-inflammatory Th2 cells and Tregs. The number of CD3(+) CD4 (+) Th17 cells increases in obesity in an IL-6-dependent manner [358].

Conclusions

Obesity is one of the biggest health concerns in our modern society, affecting hundreds of millions of individuals. Left untreated, it results in multiple comorbidities causing suffering to millions. Although well documented, the relationship between obesity and inflammation is complex and multifaceted and not completely understood. However, our knowledge is growing rapidly. It is no doubt that a better understanding of the molecular mechanisms by which obesity induces inflammation is crucial for the development of effective strategies for the prevention and treatment of metabolic syndrome, insulin resistance, and T2D.

References

1. Obesity: preventing and managing the global epidemic. Report of a WHO consultation. World Health Organ Tech Rep Ser. 2000;894:i.
2. Flegal KM, Carroll MD, Kuczmarski RJ, Johnson CL. Overweight and obesity in the United States: prevalence and trends, 1960-1994. Int J Obes Relat Metab Disord. 1998;22(1):39–47.
3. Ogden CL, Carroll MD, McDowell MA, Flegal KM. Obesity among adults in the United States—no statistically significant chance since 2003–2004. NCHS Data Brief. 2007;1:1–8.

4. Ogden CL, Yanovski SZ, Carroll MD, Flegal KM. The epidemiology of obesity. Gastroenterology. 2007;132(6):2087–102.
5. Nguyen D, El-Serag H. The epidemiology of obesity. Gastroenterol Clin. 2010;39(1):1–7.
6. Kant AK, Graubard BI. Secular trends in patterns of self-reported food consumption of adult Americans: NHANES 1971-1975 to NHANES 1999-2002. Am J Clin Nutr. 2006;84(5):1215–23.
7. Prentice AM, Jebb SA. Obesity in Britain: gluttony or sloth? BMJ. 1995;311(7002):437–9.
8. Dietz WH, Gortmaker SL. Do we fatten our children at the television set? Obesity and television viewing in children and adolescents. Pediatrics. 1985;75(5):807–12.
9. Westlund K, Nicolaysen R. Ten-year mortality and morbidity related to serum cholesterol. A follow-up of 3.751 men aged 40-49. Scand J Clin Lab Invest Suppl. 1972;127:1–24.
10. Lew EA, Garfinkel L. Variations in mortality by weight among 750,000 men and women. J Chronic Dis. 1979;32(8):563–76.
11. Larsson B, Björntorp P, Tibblin G. The health consequences of moderate obesity. Int J Obes. 1981;5(2):97–116.
12. Kopelman PG. Obesity as a medical problem. Nature. 2000;404(6778):635–43.
13. Calle EE, Kaaks R. Overweight, obesity and cancer: epidemiological evidence and proposed mechanisms. Nat Rev Cancer. 2004;4(8):579–91.
14. Medalie JH, Papier C, Herman JB, Goldbourt U, Tamir S, Neufeld HN, et al. Diabetes mellitus among 10,000 adult men. I. Five-year incidence and associated variables. Isr J Med Sci. 1974;10(7):681–97.
15. Knowler WC, Pettitt DJ, Savage PJ, Bennett PH. Diabetes incidence in Pima indians: contributions of obesity and parental diabetes. Am J Epidemiol. 1981;113(2):144–56.
16. Colditz GA, Willett WC, Stampfer MJ, Manson JE, Hennekens CH, Arky RA, et al. Weight as a risk factor for clinical diabetes in women. Am J Epidemiol. 1990;132(3):501–13.
17. Chan JM, Rimm EB, Colditz GA, Stampfer MJ, Willett WC. Obesity, fat distribution, and weight gain as risk factors for clinical diabetes in men. Diabetes Care. 1994;17(9):961–9.
18. Colditz GA, Willett WC, Rotnitzky A, Manson JE. Weight gain as a risk factor for clinical diabetes mellitus in women. Ann Intern Med. 1995;122(7):481–6.
19. Lee ET, Howard BV, Savage PJ, Cowan LD, Fabsitz RR, Oopik AJ, et al. Diabetes and impaired glucose tolerance in three American Indian populations aged 45-74 years: the strong heart study. Diabetes Care. 1995;18(5):599–610.
20. Adams KF, Schatzkin A, Harris TB, Kipnis V, Mouw T, Ballard-Barbash R, et al. Overweight, obesity, and mortality in a large prospective cohort of persons 50 to 71 years old. N Engl J Med. 2006;355(8):763–78.
21. Physical status: the use and interpretation of anthropometry. Report of a WHO expert committee. World Health Organ Tech Rep Ser. 1995;854:1–452.
22. Manson JE, Stampfer MJ, Hennekens CH, Willett WC. Body weight and longevity. A reassessment. JAMA. 1987;257(3):353–8.
23. Poy MN, Eliasson L, Krutzfeldt J, Kuwajima S, Ma X, Macdonald PE, et al. A pancreatic islet-specific microRNA regulates insulin secretion. Nature. 2004;432(7014):226–30.
24. Gauthier BR, Wollheim CB. MicroRNAs: "Ribo-regulators" of glucose homeostasis. Nat Med. 2006;12:36–8.
25. Tay YM-S, Tam W-L, Ang Y-S, Gaughwin PM, Yang H, Wang W, et al. MicroRNA-134 modulates the differentiation of mouse embryonic stem cells, where it causes post-transcriptional attenuation of Nanog and LRH1. Stem Cells. 2008;26(1):17–29.
26. Ye JJ, Cao J. MicroRNAs in colorectal cancer as markers and targets: recent advances. World J Gastroenterol. 2014;20(15):4288–99.
27. Bjørndal B, Burri L, Staalesen V, Skorve J, Berge RK. Different adipose depots: their role in the development of metabolic syndrome and mitochondrial response to hypolipidemic agents. J Obes. 2011;2011:490650.
28. Mårin P, Andersson B, Ottosson M, Olbe L, Chowdhury B, Kvist H, et al. The morphology and metabolism of intraabdominal adipose tissue in men. Metabolism. 1992;41(11):1242–8.

29. Hirsch J, Batchelor B. Adipose tissue cellularity in human obesity. Clin Endocrinol Metab. 1976;5(2):299–311.
30. Sun K, Kusminski CM, Scherer PE. Adipose tissue remodeling and obesity. J Clin Invest. 2011;121(6):2094–101.
31. Hammarstedt A, Gogg S, Hedjazifar S, Nerstedt A, Smith U. Impaired adipogenesis and dysfunctional adipose tissue in human hypertrophic obesity. Physiol Rev. 2018;98(4):1911–41.
32. Sethi JK, Vidal-Puig AJ. Thematic review series: adipocyte biology. Adipose tissue function and plasticity orchestrate nutritional adaptation. J Lipid Res. 2007;48(6):1253–62.
33. Vázquez-Vela MEF, Torres N, Tovar AR. White adipose tissue as endocrine organ and its role in obesity. Arch Med Res. 2008;39(8):715–28.
34. Dani C, Billon N. Adipocyte precursors: developmental origins, self-renewal, and plasticity. In: Adipose tissue biology. New York, NY: Springer; 2012. p. 1–16.
35. Rosen ED, Spiegelman BM. Molecular regulation of adipogenesis. Annu Rev Cell Dev Biol. 2000;16:145–71.
36. Rosen ED, MacDougald OA. Adipocyte differentiation from the inside out. Nat Rev Mol Cell Biol. 2006;7(12):885–96.
37. Longo KA, Wright WS, Kang S, Gerin I, Chiang S-H, Lucas PC, et al. Wnt10b inhibits development of white and brown adipose tissues. J Biol Chem. 2004;279(34):35503–9.
38. Fontaine C, Cousin W, Plaisant M, Dani C, Peraldi P. Hedgehog signaling alters adipocyte maturation of human mesenchymal stem cells. Stem Cells. 2008;26(4):1037–46.
39. Meerson A, Traurig M, Ossowski V, Fleming JM, Mullins M, Baier LJ. Human adipose microRNA-221 is upregulated in obesity and affects fat metabolism downstream of leptin and TNF-α. Diabetologia. 2013;56(9):1971–9.
40. Xie H, Lim B, Lodish HF. MicroRNAs induced during adipogenesis that accelerate fat cell development are downregulated in obesity. Diabetes. 2009;58(5):1050–7.
41. Takanabe R, Ono K, Abe Y, Takaya T, Horie T, Wada H, et al. Up-regulated expression of microRNA-143 in association with obesity in adipose tissue of mice fed high-fat diet. Biochem Biophys Res Commun. 2008;376(4):728–32.
42. Esau C, Kang X, Peralta E, Hanson E, Marcusson EG, Ravichandran LV, et al. MicroRNA-143 regulates adipocyte differentiation. J Biol Chem. 2004;279(50):52361–5.
43. Kajimoto K, Naraba H, Iwai N. MicroRNA and 3T3-L1 pre-adipocyte differentiation. RNA. 2006;12(9):1626–32.
44. Cai Z, Zhang L, Chen M, Jiang X, Xu N. Castration-induced changes in microRNA expression profiles in subcutaneous adipose tissue of male pigs. J Appl Genet. 2014;55(2):259.
45. Klöting N, Berthold S, Kovacs P, Schön MR, Fasshauer M, Ruschke K, et al. MicroRNA expression in human omental and subcutaneous adipose tissue. PLoS One. 2009;4(3):e4699.
46. Cannon B, Nedergaard J. Brown adipose tissue: function and physiological significance. Physiol Rev. 2004;84(1):277–359.
47. Virtanen KA, Lidell ME, Orava J, Heglind M, Westergren R, Niemi T, et al. Functional brown adipose tissue in healthy adults. N Engl J Med. 2009;360(15):1518–25.
48. Elgazzar AH, Gelfand MJ, Washburn LC, Clark J, Nagaraj N, Cummings D, et al. I-123 MIBG scintigraphy in adults. A report of clinical experience. Clin Nucl Med. 1995;20(2):147–52.
49. Minotti AJ, Shah L, Keller K. Positron emission tomography/computed tomography fusion imaging in brown adipose tissue. Clin Nucl Med. 2004;29(1):5–11.
50. Gelfand MJ. 123I-MIBG uptake in the neck and shoulders of a neuroblastoma patient: damage to sympathetic innervation blocks uptake in brown adipose tissue. Pediatr Radiol. 2004;34(7):577–9.
51. Truong MT, Erasmus JJ, Munden RF, Marom EM, Sabloff BS, Gladish GW, et al. Focal FDG uptake in mediastinal brown fat mimicking malignancy: a potential pitfall resolved on PET/CT. AJR Am J Roentgenol. 2004;183(4):1127–32.
52. Higuchi T, Kinuya S, Taki J, Nakajima K, Ikeda M, Namura M, et al. Brown adipose tissue: evaluation with 201Tl and 99mTc-sestamibi dual-tracer SPECT. Ann Nucl Med. 2004;18(6):547–9.

53. Karabudak O, Nalbant S, Ulusoy RE, Dogan B, Harmanyeri Y. Generalized nonspecific pustular lesions in Tietze's syndrome. J Clin Rheumatol. 2007;13(5):300–1.
54. Nedergaard J, Bengtsson T, Cannon B. Unexpected evidence for active brown adipose tissue in adult humans. Am J Physiol Endocrinol Metab. 2007;293(2):E444–52.
55. Saito M, Okamatsu-Ogura Y, Matsushita M, Watanabe K, Yoneshiro T, Nio-Kobayashi J, et al. High incidence of metabolically active brown adipose tissue in healthy adult humans: effects of cold exposure and adiposity. Diabetes. 2009;58(7):1526–31.
56. Cypess AM, Lehman S, Williams G, Tal I, Rodman D, Goldfine AB, et al. Identification and importance of brown adipose tissue in adult humans. N Engl J Med. 2009;360(15):1509–17.
57. Kirkland JL, Dax EM. Adipocyte hormone responsiveness and aging in the rat: problems in the interpretation of aging research. J Am Geriatr Soc. 1984;32(3):219–28.
58. Florez-Duquet M, Horwitz BA, McDonald RB. Cellular proliferation and UCP content in brown adipose tissue of cold-exposed aging Fischer 344 rats. Am J Phys. 1998;274(1):R196–203.
59. Heaton JM. The distribution of brown adipose tissue in the human. J Anat. 1972;112(Pt 1):35–9.
60. Florez-Duquet M, McDonald RB. Cold-induced thermoregulation and biological aging. Physiol Rev. 1998;78(2):339–58.
61. McDonald RB, Horwitz BA. Brown adipose tissue thermogenesis during aging and senescence. J Bioenerg Biomembr. 1999;31(5):507–16.
62. Graja A, Schulz TJ. Mechanisms of aging-related impairment of brown adipocyte development and function. Gerontology. 2015;61(3):211–7.
63. Mancini C, Gohlke S, Garcia-Carrizo F, Zagoriy V, Stephanowitz H, Schulz TJ. Identification of biomarkers of brown adipose tissue aging highlights the role of dysfunctional energy and nucleotide metabolism pathways. Sci Rep. 2021;11(1):19928.
64. Foster DO, Frydman ML. Tissue distribution of cold-induced thermogenesis in conscious warm- or cold-acclimated rats reevaluated from changes in tissue blood flow: the dominant role of brown adipose tissue in the replacement of shivering by nonshivering thermogenesis. Can J Physiol Pharmacol. 1979;57(3):257–70.
65. Golozoubova V, Hohtola E, Matthias A, Jacobsson A, Cannon B, Nedergaard J. Only UCP1 can mediate adaptive nonshivering thermogenesis in the cold. FASEB J. 2001;15(11):2048–50.
66. Matthias A, Ohlson KB, Fredriksson JM, Jacobsson A, Nedergaard J, Cannon B. Thermogenic responses in brown fat cells are fully UCP1-dependent. UCP2 or UCP3 do not substitute for UCP1 in adrenergically or fatty scid-induced thermogenesis. J Biol Chem. 2000;275(33):25073–81.
67. Cannon B, Nedergaard J. Respiratory and thermogenic capacities of cells and mitochondria from brown and white adipose tissue. Methods Mol Biol. 2001;155:295–303.
68. Richard D, Picard F. Brown fat biology and thermogenesis. Front Biosci (Landmark Ed). 2011;16(4):1233–60.
69. Fedorenko A, Lishko PV, Kirichok Y. Mechanism of fatty-acid-dependent UCP1 uncoupling in brown fat mitochondria. Cell. 2012;151(2):400–13.
70. Hanssen MJW, van der Lans AAJJ, Brans B, Hoeks J, Jardon KMC, Schaart G, et al. Short-term cold acclimation recruits Brown adipose tissue in obese humans. Diabetes. 2016;65(5):1179–89.
71. Blondin DP, Labbé SM, Tingelstad HC, Noll C, Kunach M, Phoenix S, et al. Increased brown adipose tissue oxidative capacity in cold-acclimated humans. J Clin Endocrinol Metab. 2014;99(3):E438–46.
72. Huttunen P, Hirvonen J, Kinnula V. The occurrence of brown adipose tissue in outdoor workers. Eur J Appl Physiol Occup Physiol. 1981;46(4):339–45.
73. Milner RE, Trayhurn P. Cold-induced changes in uncoupling protein and GDP binding sites in brown fat of Ob/Ob mice. Am J Phys. 1989;257(2 Pt 2):R292–9.

74. Jacobsson A, Mühleisen M, Cannon B, Nedergaard J. The uncoupling protein thermogenin during acclimation: indications for pretranslational control. Am J Phys. 1994;267(4 Pt 2):R999–1007.
75. Cohade C, Mourtzikos KA, Wahl RL. "USA-fat": prevalence is related to ambient outdoor temperature-evaluation with 18F-FDG PET/CT. J Nucl Med. 2003;44(8):1267–70.
76. Garcia CA, Van Nostrand D, Majd M, Atkins F, Acio E, Sheikh A, et al. Benzodiazepine-resistant "brown fat" pattern in positron emission tomography: two case reports of resolution with temperature control. Mol Imaging Biol. 2004;6(6):368–72.
77. Heiba SI, Bernik S, Raphael B, Sandella N, Cholewinski W, Klein P. The distinctive role of positron emission tomography/computed tomography in breast carcinoma with brown adipose tissue 2-fluoro-2-deoxy-d-glucose uptake. Breast J. 2005;11(6):457–61.
78. Garcia CA, Van Nostrand D, Atkins F, Acio E, Butler C, Esposito G, et al. Reduction of brown fat 2-deoxy-2-[F-18]fluoro-D-glucose uptake by controlling environmental temperature prior to positron emission tomography scan. Mol Imaging Biol. 2006;8(1):24–9.
79. Christensen CR, Clark PB, Morton KA. Reversal of hypermetabolic brown adipose tissue in F-18 FDG PET imaging. Clin Nucl Med. 2006;31(4):193–6.
80. Puerta M, Abelenda M, Rocha M, Trayhurn P. Effect of acute cold exposure on the expression of the adiponectin, resistin and leptin genes in rat white and brown adipose tissues. Horm Metab Res. 2002;34(11–12):629–34.
81. Spiegelman BM, Flier JS. Obesity and the regulation of energy balance. Cell. 2001;104(4):531–43.
82. Almind K, Manieri M, Sivitz WI, Cinti S, Kahn CR. Ectopic brown adipose tissue in muscle provides a mechanism for differences in risk of metabolic syndrome in mice. Proc Natl Acad Sci U S A. 2007;104(7):2366–71.
83. Lowell BB, S-Susulic V, Hamann A, Lawitts JA, Himms-Hagen J, Boyer BB, et al. Development of obesity in transgenic mice after genetic ablation of brown adipose tissue. Nature. 1993;366(6457):740–2.
84. Enerbäck S, Jacobsson A, Simpson EM, Guerra C, Yamashita H, Harper ME, et al. Mice lacking mitochondrial uncoupling protein are cold-sensitive but not obese. Nature. 1997;387(6628):90–4.
85. Feldmann HM, Golozoubova V, Cannon B, Nedergaard J. UCP1 ablation induces obesity and abolishes diet-induced thermogenesis in mice exempt from thermal stress by living at thermoneutrality. Cell Metab. 2009;9(2):203–9.
86. van Marken Lichtenbelt WD, Vanhommerig JW, Smulders NM, Drossaerts JMAFL, Kemerink GJ, Bouvy ND, et al. Cold-activated brown adipose tissue in healthy men. N Engl J Med. 2009;360(15):1500–8.
87. Zingaretti MC, Crosta F, Vitali A, Guerrieri M, Frontini A, Cannon B, et al. The presence of UCP1 demonstrates that metabolically active adipose tissue in the neck of adult humans truly represents brown adipose tissue. FASEB J. 2009;23(9):3113–20.
88. Pfannenberg C, Werner MK, Ripkens S, Stef I, Deckert A, Schmadl M, et al. Impact of age on the relationships of brown adipose tissue with sex and adiposity in humans. Diabetes. 2010;59(7):1789–93.
89. Ouellet V, Routhier-Labadie A, Bellemare W, Lakhal-Chaieb L, Turcotte E, Carpentier AC, et al. Outdoor temperature, age, sex, body mass index, and diabetic status determine the prevalence, mass, and glucose-uptake activity of 18F-FDG-detected BAT in humans. J Clin Endocrinol Metab. 2011;96(1):192–9.
90. Bartelt A, Heeren J. Adipose tissue browning and metabolic health. Nat Rev Endocrinol. 2014;10(1):24–36.
91. Leitner BP, Huang S, Brychta RJ, Duckworth CJ, Baskin AS, McGehee S, et al. Mapping of human brown adipose tissue in lean and obese young men. Proc Natl Acad Sci U S A. 2017;114(32):8649–54.
92. Poekes L, Lanthier N, Leclercq IA. Brown adipose tissue: a potential target in the fight against obesity and the metabolic syndrome. Clin Sci (Lond). 2015;129(11):933–49.

93. Chawla A, Nguyen KD, Goh YPS. Macrophage-mediated inflammation in metabolic disease. Nat Rev Immunol. 2011;11(11):738–49.
94. Burhans MS, Hagman DK, Kuzma JN, Schmidt KA, Kratz M. Contribution of adipose tissue inflammation to the development of type 2 diabetes mellitus. Compr Physiol. 2018;9(1):1–58.
95. Hotamisligil GS. Inflammation and metabolic disorders. Nature. 2006;444(7121):860–7.
96. Lee YS, Li P, Huh JY, Hwang IJ, Lu M, Kim JI, et al. Inflammation is necessary for long-term but not short-term high-fat diet-induced insulin resistance. Diabetes. 2011;60(10):2474–83.
97. Rohm TV, Meier DT, Olefsky JM, Donath MY. Inflammation in obesity, diabetes, and related disorders. Immunity. 2022;55(1):31–55.
98. Hotamisligil GS, Shargill NS, Spiegelman BM. Adipose expression of tumor necrosis factor-alpha: direct role in obesity-linked insulin resistance. Science. 1993;259(5091):87–91.
99. Hotamisligil GS, Arner P, Caro JF, Atkinson RL, Spiegelman BM. Increased adipose tissue expression of tumor necrosis factor-alpha in human obesity and insulin resistance. J Clin Invest. 1995;95(5):2409–15.
100. Uysal KT, Wiesbrock SM, Hotamisligil GS. Functional analysis of tumor necrosis factor (TNF) receptors in TNF-alpha-mediated insulin resistance in genetic obesity. Endocrinology. 1998;139(12):4832–8.
101. Carneiro IP, Elliott SA, Siervo M, Padwal R, Bertoli S, Battezzati A, et al. Is obesity associated with altered energy expenditure? Adv Nutr. 2016;7(3):476–87.
102. Shoelson SE, Lee J, Goldfine AB. Inflammation and insulin resistance. J Clin Invest. 2006;116(7):1793–801.
103. Liu T, Zhang L, Joo D, Sun S-C. NF-κB signaling in inflammation. Signal Transduct Target Ther. 2017;2:17023.
104. Huber J, Kiefer FW, Zeyda M, Ludvik B, Silberhumer GR, Prager G, et al. CC chemokine and CC chemokine receptor profiles in visceral and subcutaneous adipose tissue are altered in human obesity. J Clin Endocrinol Metab. 2008;93(8):3215–21.
105. Pérez-Pérez A, Sánchez-Jiménez F, Vilariño-García T, Sánchez-Margalet V. Role of leptin in inflammation and vice versa. Int J Mol Sci. 2020;21(16):5887.
106. Sonnenberg GE, Krakower GR, Kissebah AH. A novel pathway to the manifestations of metabolic syndrome. Obes Res. 2004;12(2):180–6.
107. Mariano G, Stilo R, Terrazzano G, Coccia E, Vito P, Varricchio E, et al. Effects of recombinant trout leptin in superoxide production and NF-κB/MAPK phosphorylation in blood leukocytes. Peptides. 2013;48:59–69.
108. Gutierrez DA, Puglisi MJ, Hasty AH. Impact of increased adipose tissue mass on inflammation, insulin resistance, and dyslipidemia. Curr Diab Rep. 2009;9(1):26–32.
109. Hoene M, Weigert C. The role of interleukin-6 in insulin resistance, body fat distribution and energy balance. Obes Rev. 2008;9(1):20–9.
110. Perreault M, Marette A. Targeted disruption of inducible nitric oxide synthase protects against obesity-linked insulin resistance in muscle. Nat Med. 2001;7(10):1138–43.
111. Hotamisligil GS. Inflammatory pathways and insulin action. Int J Obes Relat Metab Disord. 2003;27(Suppl 3):S53–5.
112. Souza SC, Palmer HJ, Kang YH, Yamamoto MT, Muliro KV, Paulson KE, et al. TNF-alpha induction of lipolysis is mediated through activation of the extracellular signal related kinase pathway in 3T3-L1 adipocytes. J Cell Biochem. 2003;89(6):1077–86.
113. Bodkin NL, Hannah JS, Ortmeyer HK, Hansen BC. Central obesity in rhesus monkeys: association with hyperinsulinemia, insulin resistance and hypertriglyceridemia? Int J Obes Relat Metab Disord. 1993;17(1):53–61.
114. Muoio DM, Newgard CB. Obesity-related derangements in metabolic regulation. Annu Rev Biochem. 2006;75:367–401.
115. Zhang Y, Proenca R, Maffei M, Barone M, Leopold L, Friedman JM. Positional cloning of the mouse obese gene and its human homologue. Nature. 1994;372(6505):425–32.
116. Caro JF, Sinha MK, Kolaczynski JW, Zhang PL, Considine RV. Leptin: the tale of an obesity gene. Diabetes. 1996;45(11):1455–62.

117. Tartaglia LA, Dembski M, Weng X, Deng N, Culpepper J, Devos R, et al. Identification and expression cloning of a leptin receptor, OB-R. Cell. 1995;83(7):1263–71.
118. Burguera B, Couce ME, Long J, Lamsam J, Laakso K, Jensen MD, et al. The long form of the leptin receptor (OB-Rb) is widely expressed in the human brain. Neuroendocrinology. 2000;71(3):187–95.
119. Gorska E, Popko K, Stelmaszczyk-Emmel A, Ciepiela O, Kucharska A, Wasik M. Leptin receptors. Eur J Med Res. 2010;15 Suppl 2(Suppl 2):50–4.
120. Bjørbaek C, Uotani S, da Silva B, Flier JS. Divergent signaling capacities of the long and short isoforms of the leptin receptor. J Biol Chem. 1997;272(51):32686–95.
121. Sweeney G. Leptin signalling. Cell Signal. 2002;14(8):655–63.
122. Zabeau L, Lavens D, Peelman F, Eyckerman S, Vandekerckhove J, Tavernier J. The ins and outs of leptin receptor activation. FEBS Lett. 2003;546(1):45–50.
123. Uotani S, Bjørbaek C, Tornøe J, Flier JS. Functional properties of leptin receptor isoforms: internalization and degradation of leptin and ligand-induced receptor downregulation. Diabetes. 1999;48(2):279–86.
124. Morgan RC, Considine RV. Leptin. In: Encyclopedia of endocrine diseases. Amsterdam, Boston: Elsevier; 2018. p. 420–7.
125. Carlsson B, Lindell K, Gabrielsson B, Karlsson C, Bjarnason R, Westphal O, et al. Obese (Ob) gene defects are rare in human obesity. Obes Res. 1997;5(1):30–5.
126. Muoio DM, Dohm GL. Peripheral metabolic actions of leptin. Best Pract Res Clin Endocrinol Metab. 2002;16:653–66.
127. Margetic S, Gazzola C, Pegg GG, Hill RA. Leptin: a review of its peripheral actions and interactions. Int J Obes Relat Metab Disord. 2002;26(11):1407–33.
128. Montague CT, Prins JB, Sanders L, Digby JE, O'Rahilly S. Depot- and sex-specific differences in human leptin mRNA expression: implications for the control of regional fat distribution. Diabetes. 1997;46(3):342–7.
129. Maffei M, Halaas J, Ravussin E, Pratley RE, Lee GH, Zhang Y, et al. Leptin levels in human and rodent: measurement of plasma leptin and Ob RNA in obese and weight-reduced subjects. Nat Med. 1995;1(11):1155–61.
130. Rosenbaum M, Nicolson M, Hirsch J, Heymsfield SB, Gallagher D, Chu F, et al. Effects of gender, body composition, and menopause on plasma concentrations of leptin. J Clin Endocrinol Metab. 1996;81(9):3424–7.
131. Ostlund RE, Yang JW, Klein S, Gingerich R. Relation between plasma leptin concentration and body fat, gender, diet, age, and metabolic covariates. J Clin Endocrinol Metab. 1996;81(11):3909–13.
132. Vona-Davis L, Howard-McNatt M, Rose DP. Adiposity, type 2 diabetes and the metabolic syndrome in breast cancer. Obes Rev. 2007;8(5):395–408.
133. Huang L, Li C. Leptin: a multifunctional hormone. Cell Res. 2000;10(2):81–92.
134. Wajchenberg BL. Subcutaneous and visceral adipose tissue: their relation to the metabolic syndrome. Endocr Rev. 2000;21(6):697–738.
135. Saladin R, De Vos P, Guerre-Millo M, Leturque A, Girard J, Staels B, et al. Transient increase in obese gene expression after food intake or insulin administration. Nature. 1995;377(6549):527–9.
136. Leroy P, Dessolin S, Villageois P, Moon BC, Friedman JM, Ailhaud G, et al. Expression of Ob gene in adipose cells. Regulation by insulin. J Biol Chem. 1996;271(5):2365–8.
137. Kirchgessner TG, Uysal KT, Wiesbrock SM, Marino MW, Hotamisligil GS. Tumor necrosis factor-alpha contributes to obesity-related hyperleptinemia by regulating leptin release from adipocytes. J Clin Invest. 1997;100(11):2777–82.
138. Faggioni R, Fantuzzi G, Fuller J, Dinarello CA, Feingold KR, Grunfeld C. IL-1 beta mediates leptin induction during inflammation. Am J Phys. 1998;274(1):R204–8.
139. Saad MF, Khan A, Sharma A, Michael R, Riad-Gabriel MG, Boyadjian R, et al. Physiological insulinemia acutely modulates plasma leptin. Diabetes. 1998;47(4):544–9.

140. Medina EA, Stanhope KL, Mizuno TM, Mobbs CV, Gregoire F, Hubbard NE, et al. Effects of tumor necrosis factor alpha on leptin secretion and gene expression: relationship to changes of glucose metabolism in isolated rat adipocytes. Int J Obes Relat Metab Disord. 1999;23(8):896–903.

141. Napoleone E, di Santo A, Amore C, Baccante G, di Febbo C, Porreca E, et al. Leptin induces tissue factor expression in human peripheral blood mononuclear cells: a possible link between obesity and cardiovascular risk? J Thromb Haemost. 2007;5(7):1462–8.

142. Conde J, Scotece M, Gómez R, Gómez-Reino JJ, Lago F, Gualillo O. At the crossroad between immunity and metabolism: focus on leptin. Expert Rev Clin Immunol. 2010;6(5):801–8.

143. Ottonello L, Gnerre P, Bertolotto M, Mancini M, Dapino P, Russo R, et al. Leptin as a uremic toxin interferes with neutrophil chemotaxis. J Am Soc Nephrol. 2004;15(9):2366–72.

144. Yudelson J. Sustainable retail development: new success strategies. Dordrecht: Springer Netherlands; 2010. p. 1–215.

145. Sadikot RT, Zeng H, Yull FE, Li B, Cheng D, Kernodle DS, et al. p47phox deficiency impairs NF-kappa B activation and host defense in pseudomonas pneumonia. J Immunol. 2004;172(3):1801–8.

146. Caldefie-Chezet F, Poulin A, Tridon A, Sion B, Vasson MP. Leptin: a potential regulator of polymorphonuclear neutrophil bactericidal action? J Leukoc Biol. 2001;69(3):414–8.

147. Mattioli B, Straface E, Quaranta MG, Giordani L, Viora M. Leptin promotes differentiation and survival of human dendritic cells and licenses them for Th1 priming. J Immunol. 2005;174(11):6820–8.

148. Elbers JM, Asscheman H, Seidell JC, Frölich M, Meinders AE, Gooren LJ. Reversal of the sex difference in serum leptin levels upon cross-sex hormone administration in transsexuals. J Clin Endocrinol Metab. 1997;82(10):3267–70.

149. Maeda K, Okubo K, Shimomura I, Funahashi T, Matsuzawa Y, Matsubara K. cDNA cloning and expression of a novel adipose specific collagen-like factor, apM1 (AdiPose most abundant gene transcript 1). Biochem Biophys Res Commun. 1996;221(2):286–9.

150. Scherer PE, Williams S, Fogliano M, Baldini G, Lodish HF. A novel serum protein similar to C1q, produced exclusively in adipocytes. J Biol Chem. 1995;270(45):26746–9.

151. Chen J, Tan B, Karteris E, Zervou S, Digby J, Hillhouse EW, et al. Secretion of adiponectin by human placenta: differential modulation of adiponectin and its receptors by cytokines. Diabetologia. 2006;49(6):1292–302.

152. Cawthorn WP, Scheller EL, Learman BS, Parlee SD, Simon BR, Mori H, et al. Bone marrow adipose tissue is an endocrine organ that contributes to increased circulating adiponectin during caloric restriction. Cell Metab. 2014;20(2):368–75.

153. Shapiro L, Scherer PE. The crystal structure of a complement-1q family protein suggests an evolutionary link to tumor necrosis factor. Curr Biol. 1998;8(6):335–8.

154. Tsao T-S, Murrey HE, Hug C, Lee DH, Lodish HF. Oligomerization state-dependent activation of NF-kappa B signaling pathway by adipocyte complement-related protein of 30 kDa (Acrp30). J Biol Chem. 2002;277(33):29359–62.

155. Waki H, Yamauchi T, Kamon J, Ito Y, Uchida S, Kita S, et al. Impaired multimerization of human adiponectin mutants associated with diabetes. Molecular structure and multimer formation of adiponectin. J Biol Chem. 2003;278(41):40352–63.

156. Yamauchi T, Kamon J, Ito Y, TsuchLabela A, Yokomizo T, Kita S, et al. Cloning of adiponectin receptors that mediate antLabeliabetic metabolic effects. Nature. 2003;423(6941):762–9; (0028-0836 (Print) LA-eng PT-Journal Article PT-Research Support, Non-U.S. Gov't RN-0 (Adiponectin) RN-0 (Fatty AcLabels) RN-0 (Hypoglycemic Agents) RN-0 (Intercellular Signaling PeptLabeles and Proteins) RN-0 (Ligands) RN-0 (Proteins) RN):762–9.

157. Hug C, Wang J, Ahmad NS, Bogan JS, Tsao T-S, Lodish HF. T-cadherin is a receptor for hexameric and high-molecular-weight forms of Acrp30/adiponectin. Proc Natl Acad Sci U S A. 2004;101(28):10308–13.

158. Yamauchi T, Hara K, Kubota N, Terauchi Y, Tobe K, Froguel P, et al. Dual roles of adiponectin/Acrp30 in vivo as an anti-diabetic and anti-atherogenic adipokine. Curr Drug Targets Immune Endocr Metabol Disord. 2003;3(4):243–54.
159. Kadowaki T, Yamauchi T. Adiponectin and adiponectin receptors. Endocr Rev. 2005;26(3):439–51.
160. Ye R, Scherer PE. Adiponectin, driver or passenger on the road to insulin sensitivity? Mol Metab. 2013;2(3):133–41.
161. Yamauchi T, Kadowaki T. Adiponectin receptor as a key player in healthy longevity and obesity-related diseases. Cell Metab. 2013;17(2):185–96.
162. Wijesekara N, Krishnamurthy M, Bhattacharjee A, Suhail A, Sweeney G, Wheeler MB. Adiponectin-induced ERK and Akt phosphorylation protects against pancreatic beta cell apoptosis and increases insulin gene expression and secretion. J Biol Chem. 2010;285(44):33623–31.
163. Ryan AS, Berman DM, Nicklas BJ, Sinha M, Gingerich RL, Meneilly GS, et al. Plasma adiponectin and leptin levels, body composition, and glucose utilization in adult women with wide ranges of age and obesity. Diabetes Care. 2003;26(8):2383–8.
164. Arita Y, Kihara S, Ouchi N, Takahashi M, Maeda K, Miyagawa J, et al. Paradoxical decrease of an adipose-specific protein, adiponectin, in obesity. Biochem Biophys Res Commun. 1999;257(1):79–83.
165. Kern PA, Di Gregorio GB, Lu T, Rassouli N, Ranganathan G. Adiponectin expression from human adipose tissue: relation to obesity, insulin resistance, and tumor necrosis factor-alpha expression. Diabetes. 2003;52(7):1779–85.
166. Mohan V, Deepa R, Pradeepa R, Vimaleswaran KS, Mohan A, Velmurugan K, et al. Association of low adiponectin levels with the metabolic syndrome—the Chennai urban rural epidemiology study (CURES-4). Metabolism. 2005;54(4):476–81.
167. Hotta K, Funahashi T, Arita Y, Takahashi M, Matsuda M, Okamoto Y, et al. Plasma concentrations of a novel, adipose-specific protein, adiponectin, in type 2 diabetic patients. Arterioscler Thromb Vasc Biol. 2000;20(6):1595–9.
168. Phillips SA, Ciaraldi TP, APS K, Bandukwala R, Aroda V, Carter L, et al. Modulation of circulating and adipose tissue adiponectin levels by antidiabetic therapy. Diabetes. 2003;52(3):667–74.
169. Nigro E, Scudiero O, Monaco ML, Palmieri A, Mazzarella G, Costagliola C, et al. New insight into adiponectin role in obesity and obesity-related diseases. Biomed Res Int. 2014;2014:658913.
170. Hotta K, Funahashi T, Bodkin NL, Ortmeyer HK, Arita Y, Hansen BC, et al. Circulating concentrations of the adipocyte protein adiponectin are decreased in parallel with reduced insulin sensitivity during the progression to type 2 diabetes in rhesus monkeys. Diabetes. 2001;50(5):1126–33.
171. Weyer C, Funahashi T, Tanaka S, Hotta K, Matsuzawa Y, Pratley RE, et al. Hypoadiponectinemia in obesity and type 2 diabetes: close association with insulin resistance and hyperinsulinemia. J Clin Endocrinol Metab. 2001;86(5):1930–5.
172. Combs TP, Wagner JA, Berger J, Doebber T, Wang WJ, Zhang BB, et al. Induction of adipocyte complement-related protein of 30 kilodaltons by PPARγ agonists: a potential mechanism of insulin sensitization. Endocrinology. 2002;143:998–1007.
173. Steffes MW, Gross MD, Schreiner PJ, Yu X, Hilner JE, Gingerich R, et al. Serum adiponectin in young adults—interactions with central adiposity, circulating levels of glucose, and insulin resistance: the CARDIA study. Ann Epidemiol. 2004;14(7):492–8.
174. Oh DK, Ciaraldi T, Henry RR. Adiponectin in health and disease. Diabetes Obes Metab. 2007;9(3):282–9.
175. Wang Y, Wang X, Lau WB, Yuan Y, Booth D, Li J-J, et al. Adiponectin inhibits tumor necrosis factor-α-induced vascular inflammatory response via caveolin-mediated ceramidase recruitment and activation. Circ Res. 2014;114(5):792–805.

176. Zoico E, Garbin U, Olioso D, Mazzali G, Fratta Pasini AM, Di Francesco V, et al. The effects of adiponectin on interleukin-6 and MCP-1 secretion in lipopolysaccharide-treated 3T3-L1 adipocytes: role of the NF-kappaB pathway. Int J Mol Med. 2009;24(6):847–51.

177. Salvator H, Grassin-Delyle S, Brollo M, Couderc L-J, Abrial C, Victoni T, et al. Adiponectin inhibits the production of TNF-α, IL-6 and chemokines by human lung macrophages. Front Pharmacol. 2021;12:718929.

178. Ukkola O, Santaniemi M. Adiponectin: a link between excess adiposity and associated comorbidities? J Mol Med. 2002;80(11):696–702.

179. Ohashi K, Parker JL, Ouchi N, Higuchi A, Vita JA, Gokce N, et al. Adiponectin promotes macrophage polarization toward an anti-inflammatory phenotype. J Biol Chem. 2010;285(9):6153–60.

180. Surendar J, Frohberger SJ, Karunakaran I, Schmitt V, Stamminger W, Neumann A-L, et al. Adiponectin limits IFN-γ and IL-17 producing CD4 T cells in obesity by restraining cell intrinsic glycolysis. Front Immunol. 2019;10:2555.

181. Steppan CM, Bailey ST, Bhat S, Brown EJ, Banerjee RR, Wright CM, et al. The hormone resistin links obesity to diabetes. Nature. 2001;409(6818):307–12.

182. Adeghate E. An update on the biology and physiology of resistin. Cell Mol Life Sci. 2004;61(19–20):2485–96.

183. Stumvoll M, Häring H. Resistin and adiponectin—of mice and men. Obes Res. 2002;10(11):1197–9.

184. McTernan PG, McTernan CL, Chetty R, Jenner K, Fisher FM, Lauer MN, et al. Increased resistin gene and protein expression in human abdominal adipose tissue. J Clin Endocrinol Metab. 2002;87(5):2407.

185. Banerjee RR, Lazar MA. Dimerization of resistin and resistin-like molecules is determined by a single cysteine. J Biol Chem. 2001;276(28):25970–3.

186. Blagoev B, Kratchmarova I, Nielsen MM, Fernandez MM, Voldby J, Andersen JS, et al. Inhibition of adipocyte differentiation by resistin-like molecule alpha. Biochemical characterization of its oligomeric nature. J Biol Chem. 2002;277(44):42011–6.

187. Patel SD, Rajala MW, Rossetti L, Scherer PE, Shapiro L. Disulfide-dependent multimeric assembly of resistin family hormones. Science. 2004;304(5674):1154–8.

188. Ghosh S, Singh AK, Aruna B, Mukhopadhyay S, Ehtesham NZ. The genomic organization of mouse resistin reveals major differences from the human resistin: functional implications. Gene. 2003;305(1):27–34.

189. Kim KH, Lee K, Moon YS, Sul HS. A cysteine-rich adipose tissue-specific secretory factor inhibits adipocyte differentiation. J Biol Chem. 2001;276(14):11252–6.

190. Patel L, Buckels AC, Kinghorn IJ, Murdock PR, Holbrook JD, Plumpton C, et al. Resistin is expressed in human macrophages and directly regulated by PPAR gamma activators. Biochem Biophys Res Commun. 2003;300(2):472–6.

191. Pektaş M, Kurt AH, Ün İ, Tiftik RN, Büyükafşar K. Effects of 17β-estradiol and progesterone on the production of adipokines in differentiating 3T3-L1 adipocytes: role of rho-kinase. Cytokine. 2015;72(2):130–4.

192. Lee JH, Bullen JW, Stoyneva VL, Mantzoros CS. Circulating resistin in lean, obese, and insulin-resistant mouse models: lack of association with insulinemia and glycemia. Am J Physiol Endocrinol Metab. 2005;288(3):E625–32.

193. Levy JR, Davenport B, Clore JN, Stevens W. Lipid metabolism and resistin gene expression in insulin-resistant Fischer 344 rats. Am J Physiol Endocrinol Metab. 2002;282(3):E626–33.

194. Degawa-Yamauchi M, Bovenkerk JE, Juliar BE, Watson W, Kerr K, Jones R, et al. Serum resistin (FIZZ3) protein is increased in obese humans. J Clin Endocrinol Metab. 2003;88(11):5452–5.

195. Xu H, Barnes GT, Yang Q, Tan G, Yang D, Chou CJ, et al. Chronic inflammation in fat plays a crucial role in the development of obesity-related insulin resistance. J Clin Invest. 2003;112(12):1821–30.

196. Vendrell J, Broch M, Vilarrasa N, Molina A, Gómez JM, Gutiérrez C, et al. Resistin, adiponectin, ghrelin, leptin, and proinflammatory cytokines: relationships in obesity. Obes Res. 2004;12(6):962–71.
197. Olefsky JM, Glass CK. Macrophages, inflammation, and insulin resistance. Annu Rev Physiol. 2010;72:219–46.
198. Milan G, Granzotto M, Scarda A, Calcagno A, Pagano C, Federspil G, et al. Resistin and adiponectin expression in visceral fat of obese rats: effect of weight loss. Obes Res. 2002;10(11):1095–103.
199. Silswal N, Singh AK, Aruna B, Mukhopadhyay S, Ghosh S, Ehtesham NZ. Human resistin stimulates the pro-inflammatory cytokines TNF-alpha and IL-12 in macrophages by NF-kappaB-dependent pathway. Biochem Biophys Res Commun. 2005;334(4):1092–101.
200. Kaser S, Kaser A, Sandhofer A, Ebenbichler CF, Tilg H, Patsch JR. Resistin messenger-RNA expression is increased by proinflammatory cytokines in vitro. Biochem Biophys Res Commun. 2003;309(2):286–90.
201. Fasshauer M, Klein J, Neumann S, Eszlinger M, Paschke R. Tumor necrosis factor alpha is a negative regulator of resistin gene expression and secretion in 3T3-L1 adipocytes. Biochem Biophys Res Commun. 2001;288(4):1027–31.
202. Lehrke M, Reilly MP, Millington SC, Iqbal N, Rader DJ, Lazar MA. An inflammatory cascade leading to hyperresistinemia in humans. PLoS Med. 2004;1(2):e45.
203. Reilly MP, Lehrke M, Wolfe ML, Rohatgi A, Lazar MA, Rader DJ. Resistin is an inflammatory marker of atherosclerosis in humans. Circulation. 2005;111(7):932–9.
204. Malyszko J, Malyszko JS, Pawlak K, Mysliwiec M. Resistin, a new adipokine, is related to inflammation and renal function in kidney allograft recipients. Transplant Proc. 2006;38(10):3434–6.
205. Nagaev I, Bokarewa M, Tarkowski A, Smith U. Human resistin is a systemic immune-derived proinflammatory cytokine targeting both leukocytes and adipocytes. PLoS One. 2006;1:e31.
206. Tarkowski A, Bjersing J, Shestakov A, Bokarewa MI. Resistin competes with lipopolysaccharide for binding to toll-like receptor 4. J Cell Mol Med. 2010;14(6B):1419–31.
207. Cuesta N, Fernández-Veledo S, Punzón C, Moreno C, Barrocal B, Sreeramkumar V, et al. Opposing actions of TLR2 and TLR4 in adipocyte differentiation and mature-onset obesity. Int J Mol Sci. 2022;23(24):15682.
208. Kusminski CM, da Silva NF, Creely SJ, Fisher FM, Harte AL, Baker AR, et al. The in vitro effects of resistin on the innate immune signaling pathway in isolated human subcutaneous adipocytes. J Clin Endocrinol Metab. 2007;92(1):270–6.
209. Old LJ. Tumor necrosis factor (TNF). Science. 1985;230(4726):630–2.
210. Bodmer J-L, Schneider P, Tschopp J. The molecular architecture of the TNF superfamily. Trends Biochem Sci. 2002;27(1):19–26.
211. Gahring LC, Carlson NG, Kulmar RA, Rogers SW. Neuronal expression of tumor necrosis factor alpha in the murine brain. Neuroimmunomodulation. 1996;3(5):289–303.
212. Kriegler M, Perez C, DeFay K, Albert I, Lu SD. A novel form of TNF/cachectin is a cell surface cytotoxic transmembrane protein: ramifications for the complex physiology of TNF. Cell. 1988;53(1):45–53.
213. Robache-Gallea S, Morand V, Bruneau JM, Schoot B, Tagat E, Réalo E, et al. In vitro processing of human tumor necrosis factor-alpha. J Biol Chem. 1995;270(40):23688–92.
214. Wajant H, Pfizenmaier K, Scheurich P. Tumor necrosis factor signaling. Cell Death Differ. 2003;10(1):45–65.
215. Torti FM, Dieckmann B, Beutler B, Cerami A, Ringold GM. A macrophage factor inhibits adipocyte gene expression: an in vitro model of cachexia. Science. 1985;229(4716):867–9.
216. Beutler B, Cerami A. Cachectin (tumor necrosis factor): a macrophage hormone governing cellular metabolism and inflammatory response. Endocr Rev. 1988;9(1):57–66.
217. Morin CL, Eckel RH, Marcel T, Pagliassotti MJ. High fat diets elevate adipose tissue-derived tumor necrosis factor-alpha activity. Endocrinology. 1997;138(11):4665–71.

218. Kern PA, Saghizadeh M, Ong JM, Bosch RJ, Deem R, Simsolo RB. The expression of tumor necrosis factor in human adipose tissue. Regulation by obesity, weight loss, and relationship to lipoprotein lipase. J Clin Invest. 1995;95(5):2111–9.

219. Spiegelman BM. PPAR-gamma: adipogenic regulator and thiazolidinedione receptor. Diabetes. 1998;47(4):507–14.

220. Zhang B, Berger J, Hu E, Szalkowski D, White-Carrington S, Spiegelman BM, et al. Negative regulation of peroxisome proliferator-activated receptor-gamma gene expression contributes to the antiadipogenic effects of tumor necrosis factor-alpha. Mol Endocrinol. 1996;10(11):1457–66.

221. Moller DE. Potential role of TNF-alpha in the pathogenesis of insulin resistance and type 2 diabetes. Trends Endocrinol Metab. 2000;11(6):212–7.

222. Ferguson-Smith AC, Chen YF, Newman MS, May LT, Sehgal PB, Ruddle FH. Regional localization of the interferon-beta 2/B-cell stimulatory factor 2/hepatocyte stimulating factor gene to human chromosome 7p15-p21. Genomics. 1988;2(3):203–8.

223. Hammacher A, Ward LD, Weinstock J, Treutlein H, Yasukawa K, Simpson RJ. Structure-function analysis of human IL-6: identification of two distinct regions that are important for receptor binding. Protein Sci. 1994;3(12):2280–93.

224. Ghosh S, Ashcraft K. An IL-6 link between obesity and cancer. Front Biosci (Elite Ed). 2013;5(2):461–78.

225. Taga T, Hibi M, Hirata Y, Yamasaki K, Yasukawa K, Matsuda T, et al. Interleukin-6 triggers the association of its receptor with a possible signal transducer, gp130. Cell. 1989;58(3):573–81.

226. Schwantner A, Dingley AJ, Ozbek S, Rose-John S, Grötzinger J. Direct determination of the interleukin-6 binding epitope of the interleukin-6 receptor by NMR spectroscopy. J Biol Chem. 2004;279(1):571–6.

227. Mihara M, Hashizume M, Yoshida H, Suzuki M, Shiina M. IL-6/IL-6 receptor system and its role in physiological and pathological conditions. Clin Sci (Lond). 2012;122(4):143–59.

228. Fried SK, Bunkin DA, Greenberg AS. Omental and subcutaneous adipose tissues of obese subjects release interleukin-6: depot difference and regulation by glucocorticoid. J Clin Endocrinol Metab. 1998;83(3):847–50.

229. Mohamed-Ali V, Flower L, Sethi J, Hotamisligil G, Gray R, Humphries SE, et al. Beta-adrenergic regulation of IL-6 release from adipose tissue: in vivo and in vitro studies. J Clin Endocrinol Metab. 2001;86(12):5864–9.

230. Vicennati V, Vottero A, Friedman C, Papanicolaou DA. Hormonal regulation of interleukin-6 production in human adipocytes. Int J Obes Relat Metab Disord. 2002;26(7):905–11.

231. Fain JN, Madan AK, Hiler ML, Cheema P, Bahouth SW. Comparison of the release of adipokines by adipose tissue, adipose tissue matrix, and adipocytes from visceral and subcutaneous abdominal adipose tissues of obese humans. Endocrinology. 2004;145(5):2273–82.

232. Pou KM, Massaro JM, Hoffmann U, Vasan RS, Maurovich-Horvat P, Larson MG, et al. Visceral and subcutaneous adipose tissue volumes are cross-sectionally related to markers of inflammation and oxidative stress: the Framingham heart study. Circulation. 2007;116(11):1234–41.

233. Fontana L, Eagon JC, Trujillo ME, Scherer PE, Klein S. Visceral fat adipokine secretion is associated with systemic inflammation in obese humans. Diabetes. 2007;56(4):1010–3.

234. Mohamed-Ali V, Goodrick S, Rawesh A, Katz DR, Miles JM, Yudkin JS, et al. Subcutaneous adipose tissue releases interleukin-6, but not tumor necrosis factor-alpha, in vivo. J Clin Endocrinol Metab. 1997;82(12):4196–200.

235. Vgontzas AN, Papanicolaou DA, Bixler EO, Kales A, Tyson K, Chrousos GP. Elevation of plasma cytokines in disorders of excessive daytime sleepiness: role of sleep disturbance and obesity. J Clin Endocrinol Metab. 1997;82(5):1313–6.

236. Gnacińska M, Małgorzewicz S, Lysiak-Szydłowska W, Sworczak K. The serum profile of adipokines in overweight patients with metabolic syndrome. Endokrynol Pol. 2010;61(1):36–41.

237. Bastard JP, Jardel C, Bruckert E, Blondy P, Capeau J, Laville M, et al. Elevated levels of interleukin 6 are reduced in serum and subcutaneous adipose tissue of obese women after weight loss. J Clin Endocrinol Metab. 2000;85(9):3338–42.

238. Kern PA, Ranganathan S, Li C, Wood L, Ranganathan G. Adipose tissue tumor necrosis factor and interleukin-6 expression in human obesity and insulin resistance. Am J Physiol Endocrinol Metab. 2001;280(5):E745–51.

239. Wallenius V, Wallenius K, Ahrén B, Rudling M, Carlsten H, Dickson SL, et al. Interleukin-6-deficient mice develop mature-onset obesity. Nat Med. 2002;8(1):75–9.

240. Di Gregorio GB, Hensley L, Lu T, Ranganathan G, Kern PA. Lipid and carbohydrate metabolism in mice with a targeted mutation in the IL-6 gene: absence of development of age-related obesity. Am J Physiol Endocrinol Metab. 2004;287(1):E182–7.

241. Eder K, Baffy N, Falus A, Fulop AK. The major inflammatory mediator interleukin-6 and obesity. Inflamm Res. 2009;58(11):727–36.

242. Desai A, Jung M-Y, Olivera A, Gilfillan AM, Prussin C, Kirshenbaum AS, et al. IL-6 promotes an increase in human mast cell numbers and reactivity through suppression of suppressor of cytokine signaling 3. J Allergy Clin Immunol. 2016;137(6):1863–1871.e6.

243. Puigserver P, Wu Z, Park CW, Graves R, Wright M, Spiegelman BM. A cold-inducible coactivator of nuclear receptors linked to adaptive thermogenesis. Cell. 1998;92(6):829–39.

244. Roca-Rivada A, Castelao C, Senin LL, Landrove MO, Baltar J, Crujeiras AB, et al. FNDC5/irisin is not only a myokine but also an adipokine. PLoS One. 2013;8(4):e60563.

245. Baar K, Wende AR, Jones TE, Marison M, Nolte LA, Chen M, et al. Adaptations of skeletal muscle to exercise: rapid increase in the transcriptional coactivator PGC-1. FASEB J. 2002;16(14):1879–86.

246. Handschin C, Spiegelman BM. The role of exercise and PGC1alpha in inflammation and chronic disease. Nature. 2008;454(7203):463–9.

247. Boström P, Wu J, Jedrychowski MP, Korde A, Ye L, Lo JC, et al. A PGC1-α-dependent myokine that drives brown-fat-like development of white fat and thermogenesis. Nature. 2012;481:463–8.

248. Spiegelman BM. Banting lecture 2012: regulation of adipogenesis: toward new therapeutics for metabolic disease. Diabetes. 2013;62:1774–82.

249. Huh JY, Panagiotou G, Mougios V, Brinkoetter M, Vamvini MT, Schneider BE, et al. FNDC5 and irisin in humans: I. predictors of circulating concentrations in serum and plasma and II. mRNA expression and circulating concentrations in response to weight loss and exercise. Metabolism. 2012;61(12):1725–38.

250. Stengel A, Hofmann T, Goebel-Stengel M, Elbelt U, Kobelt P, Klapp BF. Circulating levels of irisin in patients with anorexia nervosa and different stages of obesity-correlation with body mass index. Peptides. 2013;39(1):125–30.

251. Moreno-Navarrete JM, Ortega F, Serrano M, Guerra E, Pardo G, Tinahones F, et al. Irisin is expressed and produced by human muscle and adipose tissue in association with obesity and insulin resistance. J Clin Endocrinol Metab. 2013;98(4):E769–78.

252. Crujeiras AB, Pardo M, Roca-Rivada A, Navas-Carretero S, Zulet MA, Martínez JA, et al. Longitudinal variation of circulating irisin after an energy restriction-induced weight loss and following weight regain in obese men and women. Am J Hum Biol. 2014;26(2):198–207.

253. Pardo M, Crujeiras AB, Amil M, Aguera Z, Jiménez-Murcia S, Baños R, et al. Association of irisin with fat mass, resting energy expenditure, and daily activity in conditions of extreme body mass index. Int J Endocrinol. 2014;2014:857270.

254. Li M, Yang M, Zhou X, Fang X, Hu W, Zhu W, et al. Elevated circulating levels of irisin and the effect of metformin treatment in women with polycystic ovary syndrome. J Clin Endocrinol Metab. 2015;100(4):1485–93.

255. Roberts MD, Bayless DS, Company JM, Jenkins NT, Padilla J, Childs TE, et al. Elevated skeletal muscle irisin precursor FNDC5 mRNA in obese OLETF rats. Metabolism. 2013;62(8):1052–6.

256. Højlund K, Boström P. Irisin in obesity and type 2 diabetes. J Diabetes Complicat. 2013;27(4):303–4.
257. Lopez-Legarrea P, de la Iglesia R, Crujeiras AB, Pardo M, Casanueva FF, Zulet MA, et al. Higher baseline irisin concentrations are associated with greater reductions in glycemia and insulinemia after weight loss in obese subjects. Nutr Diabetes. 2014;4(2):e110.
258. Choi ES, Kim MK, Song MK, Kim JM, Kim ES, Chung WJ, et al. Association between serum irisin levels and non-alcoholic fatty liver disease in health screen examinees. PLoS One. 2014;9(10):e110680.
259. Wrann CD, White JP, Salogiannnis J, Laznik-Bogoslavski D, Wu J, Ma D, et al. Exercise induces hippocampal BDNF through a PGC-1α/FNDC5 pathway. Cell Metab. 2013;18(5):649–59.
260. Kraemer RR, Shockett P, Webb ND, Shah U, Castracane VD. A transient elevated irisin blood concentration in response to prolonged, moderate aerobic exercise in young men and women. Horm Metab Res. 2014;46(2):150–4.
261. Norheim F, Langleite TM, Hjorth M, Holen T, Kielland A, Stadheim HK, et al. The effects of acute and chronic exercise on PGC-1α, irisin and browning of subcutaneous adipose tissue in humans. FEBS J. 2014;281(3):739–49.
262. Hofmann T, Elbelt U, Ahnis A, Kobelt P, Rose M, Stengel A. Irisin levels are not affected by physical activity in patients with anorexia nervosa. Front Endocrinol (Lausanne). 2014;4:202.
263. Hofmann T, Elbelt U, Stengel A. Irisin as a muscle-derived hormone stimulating thermogenesis—a critical update. Peptides. 2014;54:89–100.
264. Lee P, Linderman JD, Smith S, Brychta RJ, Wang J, Idelson C, et al. Irisin and FGF21 are cold-induced endocrine activators of brown fat function in humans. Cell Metab. 2014;19(2):302–9.
265. Daskalopoulou SS, Cooke AB, Gomez Y-H, Mutter AF, Filippaios A, Mesfum ET, et al. Plasma irisin levels progressively increase in response to increasing exercise workloads in young, healthy, active subjects. Eur J Endocrinol. 2014;171(3):343–52.
266. Huh JY, Mougios V, Kabasakalis A, Fatouros I, Siopi A, Douroudos II, et al. Exercise-induced irisin secretion is independent of age or fitness level and increased irisin may directly modulate muscle metabolism through AMPK activation. J Clin Endocrinol Metab. 2014;99(11):E2154.
267. Huh JY, Dincer F, Mesfum E, Mantzoros CS. Irisin stimulates muscle growth-related genes and regulates adipocyte differentiation and metabolism in humans. Int J Obes (Lond). 2014;38(12):1538.
268. Ajoolabady A, Liu S, Klionsky DJ, Lip GYH, Tuomilehto J, Kavalakatt S, et al. ER stress in obesity pathogenesis and management. Trends Pharmacol Sci. 2022;43(2):97–109.
269. Ozcan U, Cao Q, Yilmaz E, Lee A-H, Iwakoshi NN, Ozdelen E, et al. Endoplasmic reticulum stress links obesity, insulin action, and type 2 diabetes. Science. 2004;306(5695):457–61.
270. Nakatani Y, Kaneto H, Kawamori D, Yoshiuchi K, Hatazaki M, Matsuoka T, et al. Involvement of endoplasmic reticulum stress in insulin resistance and diabetes. J Biol Chem. 2005;280(1):847–51.
271. Sharma NK, Das SK, Mondal AK, Hackney OG, Chu WS, Kern PA, et al. Endoplasmic reticulum stress markers are associated with obesity in nondiabetic subjects. J Clin Endocrinol Metab. 2008;93(11):4532–41.
272. Hummasti S, Hotamisligil GS. Endoplasmic reticulum stress and inflammation in obesity and diabetes. Circ Res. 2010;107(5):579–91.
273. Milanski M, Degasperi G, Coope A, Morari J, Denis R, Cintra DE, et al. Saturated fatty acids produce an inflammatory response predominantly through the activation of TLR4 signaling in hypothalamus: implications for the pathogenesis of obesity. J Neurosci. 2009;29(2):359–70.
274. Shi H, Kokoeva MV, Inouye K, Tzameli I, Yin H, Flier JS. TLR4 links innate immunity and fatty acid-induced insulin resistance. J Clin Invest. 2006;116(11):3015–25.
275. Gough NR. UPR to TLR connection. Sci Signal. 2010;3:119.

276. Blaak EE, van Baak MA, Kemerink GJ, Pakbiers MT, Heidendal GA, Saris WH. Beta-adrenergic stimulation and abdominal subcutaneous fat blood flow in lean, obese, and reduced-obese subjects. Metabolism. 1995;44(2):183–7.

277. Jansson PA, Larsson A, Lönnroth PN. Relationship between blood pressure, metabolic variables and blood flow in obese subjects with or without non-insulin-dependent diabetes mellitus. Eur J Clin Investig. 1998;28(10):813–8.

278. Kabon B, Nagele A, Reddy D, Eagon C, Fleshman JW, Sessler DI, et al. Obesity decreases perioperative tissue oxygenation. Anesthesiology. 2004;100(2):274–80.

279. Pasarica M, Sereda OR, Redman LM, Albarado DC, Hymel DT, Roan LE, et al. Reduced adipose tissue oxygenation in human obesity: evidence for rarefaction, macrophage chemotaxis, and inflammation without an angiogenic response. Diabetes. 2009;58(3):718–25.

280. O'Rourke RW, White AE, Metcalf MD, Olivas AS, Mitra P, Larison WG, et al. Hypoxia-induced inflammatory cytokine secretion in human adipose tissue stromovascular cells. Diabetologia. 2011;54(6):1480–90.

281. Spencer M, Unal R, Zhu B, Rasouli N, McGehee RE, Peterson CA, et al. Adipose tissue extracellular matrix and vascular abnormalities in obesity and insulin resistance. J Clin Endocrinol Metab. 2011;96(12):E1990–8.

282. Trayhurn P. Hypoxia and adipose tissue function and dysfunction in obesity. Physiol Rev. 2013;93(1):1–21.

283. Carrière A, Carmona M-C, Fernandez Y, Rigoulet M, Wenger RH, Pénicaud L, et al. Mitochondrial reactive oxygen species control the transcription factor CHOP-10/GADD153 and adipocyte differentiation: a mechanism for hypoxia-dependent effect. J Biol Chem. 2004;279(39):40462–9.

284. Cummins EP, Taylor CT. Hypoxia-responsive transcription factors. Pflugers Arch. 2005;450(6):363–71.

285. Kenneth NS, Rocha S. Regulation of gene expression by hypoxia. Biochem J. 2008;414(1):19–29.

286. Brahimi-Horn MC, Pouysségur J. Oxygen, a source of life and stress. FEBS Lett. 2007;581(19):3582–91.

287. Semenza GL. HIF-1 and mechanisms of hypoxia sensing. Curr Opin Cell Biol. 2001;13(2):167–71.

288. Graham AM, Presnell JS. Hypoxia inducible factor (HIF) transcription factor family expansion, diversification, divergence and selection in eukaryotes. PLoS One. 2017;12(6):e0179545.

289. Semenza GL. Targeting HIF-1 for cancer therapy. Nat Rev Cancer. 2003;3(10):721–32.

290. Arany Z, Huang LE, Eckner R, Bhattacharya S, Jiang C, Goldberg MA, et al. An essential role for p300/CBP in the cellular response to hypoxia. Proc Natl Acad Sci U S A. 1996;93(23):12969–73.

291. Ema M, Hirota K, Mimura J, Abe H, Yodoi J, Sogawa K, et al. Molecular mechanisms of transcription activation by HLF and HIF1alpha in response to hypoxia: their stabilization and redox signal-induced interaction with CBP/p300. EMBO J. 1999;18(7):1905–14.

292. Crandall DL, Hausman GJ, Kral JG. A review of the microcirculation of adipose tissue: anatomic, metabolic, and angiogenic perspectives. Microcirculation. 1997;4(2):211–32.

293. Hausman GJ, Richardson RL. Adipose tissue angiogenesis. J Anim Sci. 2004;82(3):925–34.

294. Ye J, Gao Z, Yin J, He Q. Hypoxia is a potential risk factor for chronic inflammation and adiponectin reduction in adipose tissue of Ob/Ob and dietary obese mice. Am J Physiol Endocrinol Metab. 2007;293(4):E1118–28.

295. Ozmen F, Ozmen MM, Gelecek S, Bilgic İ, Moran M, Sahin TT. STEAP4 and HIF-1α gene expressions in visceral and subcutaneous adipose tissue of the morbidly obese patients. Mol Immunol. 2016;73:53–9.

296. Zhang X, Lam KSL, Ye H, Chung SK, Zhou M, Wang Y, et al. Adipose tissue-specific inhibition of hypoxia-inducible factor 1{alpha} induces obesity and glucose intolerance by impeding energy expenditure in mice. J Biol Chem. 2010;285(43):32869–77.

297. Cancello R, Henegar C, Viguerie N, Taleb S, Poitou C, Rouault C, et al. Reduction of macrophage infiltration and chemoattractant gene expression changes in white adipose tissue of morbidly obese subjects after surgery-induced weight loss. Diabetes. 2005;54(8):2277–86.
298. Koumenis C, Naczki C, Koritzinsky M, Rastani S, Diehl A, Sonenberg N, et al. Regulation of protein synthesis by hypoxia via activation of the endoplasmic reticulum kinase PERK and phosphorylation of the translation initiation factor eIF2alpha. Mol Cell Biol. 2002;22(21):7405–16.
299. Hosogai N, Fukuhara A, Oshima K, Miyata Y, Tanaka S, Segawa K, et al. Adipose tissue hypoxia in obesity and its impact on adipocytokine dysregulation. Diabetes. 2007;56(4):901–11.
300. Rausch ME, Weisberg S, Vardhana P, Tortoriello DV. Obesity in C57BL/6J mice is characterized by adipose tissue hypoxia and cytotoxic T-cell infiltration. Int J Obes. 2008;32(3):451–63.
301. Chen B, Lam KSL, Wang Y, Wu D, Lam MC, Shen J, et al. Hypoxia dysregulates the production of adiponectin and plasminogen activator inhibitor-1 independent of reactive oxygen species in adipocytes. Biochem Biophys Res Commun. 2006;341(2):549–56.
302. Segawa K, Fukuhara A, Hosogai N, Morita K, Okuno Y, Tanaka M, et al. Visfatin in adipocytes is upregulated by hypoxia through HIF1alpha-dependent mechanism. Biochem Biophys Res Commun. 2006;349(3):875–82.
303. Glassford AJ, Yue P, Sheikh AY, Chun HJ, Zarafshar S, Chan DA, et al. HIF-1 regulates hypoxia- and insulin-induced expression of apelin in adipocytes. Am J Physiol Endocrinol Metab. 2007;293(6):E1590–6.
304. He Q, Gao Z, Yin J, Zhang J, Yun Z, Ye J. Regulation of HIF-1{alpha} activity in adipose tissue by obesity-associated factors: adipogenesis, insulin, and hypoxia. Am J Physiol Endocrinol Metab. 2011;300(5):E877–85.
305. Kim KH, Song MJ, Chung J, Park H, Kim JB. Hypoxia inhibits adipocyte differentiation in a HDAC-independent manner. Biochem Biophys Res Commun. 2005;333(4):1178–84.
306. Zhou S, Lechpammer S, Greenberger JS, Glowacki J. Hypoxia inhibition of adipocytogenesis in human bone marrow stromal cells requires transforming growth factor-beta/Smad3 signaling. J Biol Chem. 2005;280(24):22688–96.
307. Lin Q, Lee Y-J, Yun Z. Differentiation arrest by hypoxia. J Biol Chem. 2006;281(41):30678–83.
308. Yin X, Lanza IR, Swain JM, Sarr MG, Nair KS, Jensen MD. Adipocyte mitochondrial function is reduced in human obesity independent of fat cell size. J Clin Endocrinol Metab. 2014;99(2):E209–16.
309. Putti R, Sica R, Migliaccio V, Lionetti L. Diet impact on mitochondrial bioenergetics and dynamics. Front Physiol. 2015;6:109.
310. Heinonen S, Buzkova J, Muniandy M, Kaksonen R, Ollikainen M, Ismail K, et al. Impaired mitochondrial biogenesis in adipose tissue in acquired obesity. Diabetes. 2015;64(9):3135–45.
311. Bournat JC, Brown CW. Mitochondrial dysfunction in obesity. Curr Opin Endocrinol Diabetes Obes. 2010;17(5):446–52.
312. Liesa M, Shirihai OS. Mitochondrial dynamics in the regulation of nutrient utilization and energy expenditure. Cell Metab. 2013;17(4):491–506.
313. Rambold AS, Kostelecky B, Elia N, Lippincott-Schwartz J. Tubular network formation protects mitochondria from autophagosomal degradation during nutrient starvation. Proc Natl Acad Sci U S A. 2011;108(25):10190–5.
314. Khraiwesh H, López-Domínguez JA, López-Lluch G, Navas P, de Cabo R, Ramsey JJ, et al. Alterations of ultrastructural and fission/fusion markers in hepatocyte mitochondria from mice following calorie restriction with different dietary fats. J Gerontol A Biol Sci Med Sci. 2013;68(9):1023–34.
315. Woo CY, Jang JE, Lee SE, Koh EH, Lee KU. Mitochondrial dysfunction in adipocytes as a primary cause of adipose tissue inflammation. Diabetes Metab J. 2019;43(3):247–56.
316. Kusminski CM, Scherer PE. Mitochondrial dysfunction in white adipose tissue. Trends Endocrinol Metab. 2012;23(9):435–43.

317. Jheng H-F, Huang S-H, Kuo H-M, Hughes MW, Tsai Y-S. Molecular insight and pharmacological approaches targeting mitochondrial dynamics in skeletal muscle during obesity. Ann N Y Acad Sci. 2015;1350:82–94.
318. Lahera V, de Las HN, López-Farré A, Manucha W, Ferder L. Role of mitochondrial dysfunction in hypertension and obesity. Curr Hypertens Rep. 2017;19(2):11.
319. Rong JX, Qiu Y, Hansen MK, Zhu L, Zhang V, Xie M, et al. Adipose mitochondrial biogenesis is suppressed in db/db and high-fat diet-fed mice and improved by rosiglitazone. Diabetes. 2007;56(7):1751–60.
320. Choo H-J, Kim J-H, Kwon O-B, Lee CS, Mun JY, Han SS, et al. Mitochondria are impaired in the adipocytes of type 2 diabetic mice. Diabetologia. 2006;49(4):784–91.
321. Koh EH, Park J-Y, Park H-S, Jeon MJ, Ryu JW, Kim M, et al. Essential role of mitochondrial function in adiponectin synthesis in adipocytes. Diabetes. 2007;56(12):2973–81.
322. Vaamonde-García C, Riveiro-Naveira RR, Valcárcel-Ares MN, Hermida-Carballo L, Blanco FJ, López-Armada MJ. Mitochondrial dysfunction increases inflammatory responsiveness to cytokines in normal human chondrocytes. Arthritis Rheum. 2012;64(9):2927–36.
323. McLaughlin T, Ackerman SE, Shen L, Engleman E. Role of innate and adaptive immunity in obesity-associated metabolic disease. J Clin Invest. 2017;127(1):5–13.
324. Curat CA, Miranville A, Sengenès C, Diehl M, Tonus C, Busse R, et al. From blood monocytes to adipose tissue-resident macrophages: induction of diapedesis by human mature adipocytes. Diabetes. 2004;53(5):1285–92.
325. Cinti S, Mitchell G, Barbatelli G, Murano I, Ceresi E, Faloia E, et al. Adipocyte death defines macrophage localization and function in adipose tissue of obese mice and humans. J Lipid Res. 2005;46(11):2347–55.
326. Curat CA, Wegner V, Sengenès C, Miranville A, Tonus C, Busse R, et al. Macrophages in human visceral adipose tissue: increased accumulation in obesity and a source of resistin and visfatin. Diabetologia. 2006;49(4):744–7.
327. Harman-Boehm I, Blüher M, Redel H, Sion-Vardy N, Ovadia S, Avinoach E, et al. Macrophage infiltration into omental versus subcutaneous fat across different populations: effect of regional adiposity and the comorbidities of obesity. J Clin Endocrinol Metab. 2007;92(6):2240–7.
328. Bourlier V, Zakaroff-Girard A, Miranville A, De Barros S, Maumus M, Sengenes C, et al. Remodeling phenotype of human subcutaneous adipose tissue macrophages. Circulation. 2008;117(6):806–15.
329. Bassols J, Ortega FJ, Moreno-Navarrete JM, Peral B, Ricart W, Fernández-Real J-M. Study of the proinflammatory role of human differentiated omental adipocytes. J Cell Biochem. 2009;107(6):1107–17.
330. Weisberg SP, McCann D, Desai M, Rosenbaum M, Leibel RL, Ferrante AW. Obesity is associated with macrophage accumulation in adipose tissue. J Clin Invest. 2003;112(12):1796–808.
331. Clément K, Viguerie N, Poitou C, Carette C, Pelloux V, Curat CA, et al. Weight loss regulates inflammation-related genes in white adipose tissue of obese subjects. FASEB J. 2004;18(14):1657–69.
332. Lumeng CN, Bodzin JL, Saltiel AR. Obesity induces a phenotypic switch in adipose tissue macrophage polarization. J Clin Invest. 2007;117(1):175–84.
333. Castoldi A, Naffah de Souza C, Câmara NOS, Moraes-Vieira PM. The macrophage switch in obesity development. Front Immunol. 2015;6:637.
334. Boulenouar S, Michelet X, Duquette D, Alvarez D, Hogan AE, Dold C, et al. Adipose type one innate lymphoid cells regulate macrophage homeostasis through targeted cytotoxicity. Immunity. 2017;46(2):273–86.
335. Zheng C, Yang Q, Xu C, Shou P, Cao J, Jiang M, et al. CD11b regulates obesity-induced insulin resistance via limiting alternative activation and proliferation of adipose tissue macrophages. Proc Natl Acad Sci U S A. 2015;112(52):E7239–48.
336. Spite M, Hellmann J, Tang Y, Mathis SP, Kosuri M, Bhatnagar A, et al. Deficiency of the leukotriene B4 receptor, BLT-1, protects against systemic insulin resistance in diet-induced obesity. J Immunol. 2011;187(4):1942–9.

337. Nagareddy PR, Kraakman M, Masters SL, Stirzaker RA, Gorman DJ, Grant RW, et al. Adipose tissue macrophages promote myelopoiesis and monocytosis in obesity. Cell Metab. 2014;19(5):821–35.
338. Talukdar S, Oh DY, Bandyopadhyay G, Li D, Xu J, McNelis J, et al. Neutrophils mediate insulin resistance in mice fed a high-fat diet through secreted elastase. Nat Med. 2012;18(9):1407–12.
339. Elgazar-Carmon V, Rudich A, Hadad N, Levy R. Neutrophils transiently infiltrate intra-abdominal fat early in the course of high-fat feeding. J Lipid Res. 2008;49(9):1894–903.
340. Watanabe Y, Nagai Y, Honda H, Okamoto N, Yanagibashi T, Ogasawara M, et al. Bidirectional crosstalk between neutrophils and adipocytes promotes adipose tissue inflammation. FASEB J. 2019;33(11):11821–35.
341. Shortman K, Naik SH. Steady-state and inflammatory dendritic-cell development. Nat Rev Immunol. 2007;7(1):19–30.
342. Steinman RM, Banchereau J. Taking dendritic cells into medicine. Nature. 2007;449(7161):419–26.
343. Steinman RM. Dendritic cells and vaccines. Proc (Bayl Univ Med Cent). 2008;21(1):3–8.
344. Soedono S, Cho KW. Adipose tissue dendritic cells: critical regulators of obesity-induced inflammation and insulin resistance. Int J Mol Sci. 2021;22(16):8666.
345. Bertola A, Ciucci T, Rousseau D, Bourlier V, Duffaut C, Bonnafous S, et al. Identification of adipose tissue dendritic cells correlated with obesity-associated insulin-resistance and inducing Th17 responses in mice and patients. Diabetes. 2012;61(9):2238–47.
346. Stefanovic-Racic M, Yang X, Turner MS, Mantell BS, Stolz DB, Sumpter TL, et al. Dendritic cells promote macrophage infiltration and comprise a substantial proportion of obesity-associated increases in CD11c+ cells in adipose tissue and liver. Diabetes. 2012;61(9):2330–9.
347. Cho KW, Zamarron BF, Muir LA, Singer K, Porsche CE, DelProposto JB, et al. Adipose tissue dendritic cells are independent contributors to obesity-induced inflammation and insulin resistance. J Immunol. 2016;197(9):3650–61.
348. Żelechowska P, Agier J, Kozłowska E, Brzezińska-Błaszczyk E. Mast cells participate in chronic low-grade inflammation within adipose tissue. Obes Rev. 2018;19(5):686–97.
349. Wang J, Shi G-P. Mast cell stabilization: novel medication for obesity and diabetes. Diabetes Metab Res Rev. 2011;27(8):919–24.
350. Liu J, Divoux A, Sun J, Zhang J, Clément K, Glickman JN, et al. Genetic deficiency and pharmacological stabilization of mast cells reduce diet-induced obesity and diabetes in mice. Nat Med. 2009;15(8):940–5.
351. Carballo I, Alonso-Sampedro M, Gonzalez-Conde E, Sanchez-Castro J, Vidal C, Gude F, et al. Factors influencing Total serum IgE in adults: the role of obesity and related metabolic disorders. Int Arch Allergy Immunol. 2021;182(3):220–8.
352. Exley MA, Hand L, O'Shea D, Lynch L. Interplay between the immune system and adipose tissue in obesity. J Endocrinol. 2014;223(2):R41–8.
353. Vazquez MI, Catalan-Dibene J, Zlotnik A. B cells responses and cytokine production are regulated by their immune microenvironment. Cytokine. 2015;74(2):318–26.
354. Winer DA, Winer S, Chng MHY, Shen L, Engleman EG. B lymphocytes in obesity-related adipose tissue inflammation and insulin resistance. Cell Mol Life Sci. 2014;71(6):1033–43.
355. Trottier MD, Naaz A, Li Y, Fraker PJ. Enhancement of hematopoiesis and lymphopoiesis in diet-induced obese mice. Proc Natl Acad Sci U S A. 2012;109(20):7622–9.
356. Winer DA, Winer S, Shen L, Wadia PP, Yantha J, Paltser G, et al. B cells promote insulin resistance through modulation of T cells and production of pathogenic IgG antibodies. Nat Med. 2011;17(5):610–7.
357. Nishimura S, Manabe I, Nagasaki M, Eto K, Yamashita H, Ohsugi M, et al. CD8+ effector T cells contribute to macrophage recruitment and adipose tissue inflammation in obesity. Nat Med. 2009;15(8):914–20.
358. Winer S, Paltser G, Chan Y, Tsui H, Engleman E, Winer D, et al. Obesity predisposes to Th17 bias. Eur J Immunol. 2009;39(9):2629–35.

Chapter 3
Inflammation and Diabetes Mellitus

Sooyoung Lim, Sudipa Sarkar, and Rexford S. Ahima

Abbreviations

ADA	American Diabetes Association
APC	Antigen-presenting cell
AT	Adipose tissue
BMI	Body mass index
CAA	Serum amyloid A
CANTOS	Canakinumab Anti-Inflammatory Thrombosis Outcomes Study
CCL	Chemokine (C-C motif) ligand
CI	Confidence interval
CRP	C-reactive protein
CTLA4	Cytotoxic T lymphocyte-associated protein 4
CVD	Cardiovascular disease
CXCL	Chemokine (C-X-C motif) ligand
DAISY	Diabetes Autoimmunity Study in the Young
DEFEND	Durable Response Therapy Evaluation for Early or New-Onset Type 1 Diabetes
DIPP	Diabetes Prediction and Prevention study
EBV	Epstein-Barr virus
FDA	Food and Drug Administration
FFA	Free fatty acid
GLP-1	Glucagon-like peptide 1

S. Lim · S. Sarkar (✉) · R. S. Ahima
Division of Endocrinology, Diabetes, and Metabolism, Johns Hopkins University, Baltimore, MD, USA
e-mail: slim46@jhu.edu; ssarka19@jhmi.edu; ahima@jhmi.edu

© The Author(s), under exclusive license to Springer Nature Switzerland AG 2023
D. Avtanski, L. Poretsky (eds.), *Obesity, Diabetes and Inflammation*, Contemporary Endocrinology, https://doi.org/10.1007/978-3-031-39721-9_3

GLP-1RA   GLP-1 receptor agonist
GPR120   G-coupled receptor 120
HbA1c   Hemoglobin A1c
HFD   High-fat diet
HLA   Human leukocyte antigen
ICI   Immune checkpoint inhibitors
IL   Interleukin
MHC   Major histocompatibility complex
MoBa   Mother and Child Cohort study
NAFLD   Non-alcoholic fatty liver disease
NASH   Non-alcoholic steatohepatitis
NOD   Non-obese diabetic mouse model
OGTT   Oral glucose tolerance test
PD-1   Programmed cell dead 1
PD-L1   Programmed cell death ligand 1
PTPN22   Protein tyrosine phosphatase non-receptor type 22
ROS   Reactive oxygen species
sCD163   Serum cluster of differentiation protein 163
SCFA   Short-chain fatty acid
SGLT2   Sodium-glucose co-transporter 2
T1D   Type 1 diabetes
T2D   Type 2 diabetes
TEDDY   The Environmental Determinants of Diabetes in the Young
TNFα   Tumor-necrosis factor α
UI   Uncertainty interval

Introduction

The American Diabetes Association (ADA)'s criteria for diagnosing diabetes are as follows: (1) Fasting plasma glucose $\geq$126 mg/dL or (2) 2-h plasma glucose $\geq$200 mg/dL after a 75-g oral glucose tolerance test (OGTT) or (3) Hemoglobin A1c (HbA1c) $\geq$ 6.5% or (4) A random plasma glucose $\geq$200 mg/dL with symptoms consistent with hyperglycemia [1].

The most widely accepted model of the pathogenesis of T1D was first proposed by George Eisenbarth in 1986, which describes the process in three stages. In stage 1, an unknown trigger event occurs, which initiates an autoimmune and inflammatory response toward the pancreatic βcells in genetically susceptible individuals. In this stage, affected individuals have two or more positive autoantibodies to the beta cells (GAD65, IAA, IA-2, ZnT2, or Tspan7) but are able to maintain normoglycemia. In stage 2, individuals develop dysglycemia due to inadequate insulin production from autoimmune destruction of the β-cell and continued β-cell dysfunction. In stage 3, individuals develop hyperglycemia due to insulin deficiency necessitating insulin therapy [2, 3]. Ninety percent of patients with typical clinical presentations of T1D have combinations of positive autoantibodies, which are thought to be markers and not pathogenic per se. In genetically susceptible individuals, having two or more of these markers was associated with a 60–80% chance of T1D development over the next 10–15 years [4, 5]. However, it is also important to note that not everyone progresses to stage 3, and many patients have detectable autoantibodies without ever acquiring insulin dependence.

Unlike T1D, T2D, a chronic progressive disease, is not associated with autoimmunity against the β-cells. T2D is characterized by insulin resistance and β-cell dysfunction, eventually resulting in hyperglycemia [6]. In T2D, the β-cells cannot continue to sustain an appropriate amount of insulin in the setting of insulin resistance, leading to decreased insulin secretion and hyperglycemia [7]. In individuals with normoglycemia, there is a reciprocal relationship between insulin action and insulin secretion, in which if insulin action decreases, as is seen in insulin resistance, insulin secretion increases. However, in patients with impaired glucose tolerance or T2D, insulin secretion is inadequate in the setting of a decrease in insulin action [8, 9].

Epidemiology and Risk Factors

T2D accounts for up to 95% of diabetes cases [10]. It is a heterogeneous disease that in 2019 was found to affect over 400 million people internationally, most of whom were residents of low- and middle-income countries [10–12]. Moreover, the number of individuals affected by diabetes is projected to exceed 780 million by 2045 [12]. The peak incidence of T2D is in the sixth decade of life [13], although the prevalence of T2D has been increasing among adolescents [14]. The incidence of T2D has also been increasing, with an age-standardized incidence rate of 228.5 (95% uncertainty interval (UI) 213.7–244.3) in 1990, to 279.1 (95% UI 256.6–304.3) in 2007 [15].

Risk factors for T2D include the following: elevated body mass index (BMI), unhealthy diet, a sedentary lifestyle, and family history [16]. Both overweight state and obesity are associated with T2D. The strengths of these associations were demonstrated in one meta-analysis of 18 prospective cohort studies, which included men and women ages 18–80 in regions including Europe, the USA, and Asia-Pacific. In comparison to normal weight (BMI 18–24.9 kg/m^2), overweight state (BMI 25–29.9 kg/m^2 or nearest to this range) had a relative risk of 2.99 (95% confidence interval (CI) 2.42–3.71) for T2D, and obesity (BMI $\geq$ 30 kg/m^2 or nearest to this range) had a relative risk of 7.19 (95% CI 5.74–9.00) [17].

T1D is defined by clinical features and the presence of autoimmune destruction of the pancreatic β-cells leading to insulin deficiency. Classically, patients with T1D present in their childhood with several days to weeks of polyuria, polydipsia, hyperglycemia, fatigue, and weight loss in a catabolic state. Diabetic ketoacidosis is the second most common presentation and is more often seen in younger children less than 6 years old and those from underserved populations. Historically, T1D has been associated with a lean body habitus and a younger age of onset. However, increasingly obese body habitus and diagnosis at an older age, such as after the fifth decade in patients' lives are being observed. In general, older individuals tend to have a slower disease progression and are often misdiagnosed as having T2D [18].

The incidence of T1D has been steadily increasing worldwide, though regional differences persist. In pediatric populations, the incidence of T1D is estimated to be between 1 and 3 per 100,000 per year in Asia, 10 and 20 per 100,000 in South European countries and the US, and 30 and 60 per 100,000 in Scandinavia [19]. Overall, the incidence has been steadily increasing by about 3–4% per year in the past 30 years, with the rate of increase most pronounced in previously low-incidence countries. This increase is seen within a generation and is thus thought to be driven by non-genetic factors such as environmental exposures.

The specific triggers that initiate the inflammatory response cascade toward the β-cells are still to be elucidated. However, multiple longitudinal cohort studies have identified possible candidates, including infection, dietary changes, and alteration in the microbiota [20]. Some studies support viral infection as a trigger. Coxsackievirus and adenovirus receptors unique to β-cells are found in secretory granules and may contribute to β-cell vulnerability to viral infection during insulin secretion [21]. The Diabetes Autoimmunity Study in the Young (DAISY) showed that enterovirus infection was associated with earlier disease onset in high-risk children [22]. Rotavirus, parechovirus, scaffold virus, severe influenza, and cytomegalovirus have also been implicated in the development of islet autoimmunity, although the results have been mixed overall [23–26]. More recently, SARS-CoV-2 has been suggested as a possible trigger as an increase in the incidence of new-onset T1D was observed during the COVID-19 pandemic. In the pediatric population, the hazard ratio for risk of being diagnosed with T1D in those with SARS-CoV-2 compared to those without SARS-CoV-2 infection or those infected with other respiratory viruses ranged between 1.31 and 2.66 [27, 28]. The mechanisms behind these observations are speculative at this time, although immune dysregulation, impaired glucose homeostasis, increased insulin resistance, and activation of the renin-angiotensin-aldosterone system have been suggested as contributors [29].

Specific dietary exposures such as gluten and sugar have been studied with mixed results. While the Diabetes Prediction and Prevention (DIPP) study and Danish National Birth Cohort study showed an association between gluten intake and the incidence of islet autoimmunity and T1D, the DAISY and the Norwegian Mother and Child Cohort study (MoBa) study did not [30–33]. Dietary sugar was also proposed to contribute to T1D development as its consumption has steadily increased over the past several decades. Increased dietary sugar intake can worsen pancreatic β-cell stress from increased insulin demand. In the DAISY, dietary sugar was associated with the progression though not with the initial development of T1D.

Multiple studies have found altered intestinal microbiota in patients with T1D, suggesting a role for the shift in gut microbiota, specifically the resultant decrease in anti-inflammatory short-chain fatty acids (SCFAs), in the pathogenesis of T1D. Compared to controls, patients with T1D or islet autoimmunity tend to have a greater proportion of *Bacteroides* species and fewer bacteria that produce SCFAs, such as *Bifidobacteria* [34–37]. This shift results in a decrease in butyrate, an SCFA associated with various anti-inflammatory effects [38, 39]. In a larger study within The Environmental Determinants of Diabetes in the Young (TEDDY) that evaluated 783 mostly White, non-Hispanic children, the microbiomes of control children contained more genes related to the biosynthesis of SCFA compared to those who developed T1D or islet autoimmunity, although the differences were modest [40]. Mariño et al. [41] found that when non-obese diabetic (NOD) mice (a murine model of T1D) were fed with a diet that increased blood and fecal concentrations of SCFAs, the mice were protected against progression to diabetes. However, increasing blood and fecal SCFA concentrations have shown mixed results in human studies. For instance, a 6-week human pilot study found that high-amylose maize-resistant starch modified with acetate and butyrate supplements given to patients with long-standing T1D increased plasma and fecal SCFA and that plasma SCFA concentration was associated with better glycemic control [42]. However, another small randomized controlled trial that tested an oral butyrate supplement in patients with longstanding T1D did not show changes in autoimmunity, glucose metabolism, or β-cell function [43].

Genetics

Family history contributes significantly to the development of T2D, as having an affected parent increases an individual's risk of having T2D by up to 40% [44]. The genetics of T2D has been and continues to be extensively studied. Genome-wide association studies among different populations worldwide have demonstrated numerous significant genome-wide common variants (minor allele frequency > 5%) associations with T2D [45, 46]. Lower frequency variants contribute less to the risk of T2D [46].

More than 40 genetic loci have been related to T1D risk, many of which are linked to autoimmune and inflammatory disorders. These include HLA, preproinsulin, PTPN22, CTLA-4, IL2 interferon-induced helicase, lectin-like gene, and ERBB3e [47]. The strongest associations of risk of T1D are seen with specific alleles of genes for HLA, which are genes within the MHC expressed by cells used by the immune system to differentiate self from non-self.

Certain HLA class II DR and DQ haplotypes can increase or decrease susceptibility to developing T1D. For instance, in Caucasian families, DRB1*04:05-DQA1*03:01-DQB1*03:02 has an odds ratio (OR) of 11.37, while DRB1*14:01-DQA101:01-DQB105:03 has an OR of 0.02 for T1D [48]. In addition to specific haplotypes, specific heterozygous genotypes such as DR3/DR4 (DRB1*03:01-DQA1*05:01-DQB1*02:01/DRB1*04:01-DQA1*03:01-DQB1*03:01) can further amplify the risk of T1D, even compared to individual haplotype risks combined. DR3/DR4 has also been associated with earlier onset T1D as well as a higher frequency of islet cell antibodies, which suggests specific genotypes may not only confer the risk of developing T1D but also be associated with the severity [49, 50]. However, it is important to note that even a high-risk genotype such as heterozygous DR3/4 only accounts for about 40% of T1D susceptibility [47].

HLA class I molecules are also associated with T1D, although to a lesser extent. For example, after accounting for linkage disequilibrium (i.e., finding specific alleles together more frequently than expected), HLA-B*39:06 was found to increase susceptibility to developing T1D (OR 10.31). In contrast, HLA-B*57:01 was found to be protective (OR 0.19) [51]. Polymorphisms of genes involved in T cell downregulation, such as CTLA4 (cytotoxic T-lymphocyte-associated protein 4) and PTPN22 (protein tyrosine phosphatase non-receptor type 22), have ORs ranging between 0.5 and 3 [52–56]. Polymorphisms of CTLA4 and PTPN22 are also implicated in other autoimmune diseases.

Inflammation, the Immune System, and Diabetes

Inflammation is a key process in the development of diabetes. In the current model of T1D pathogenesis, antigen-presenting cells (APCs) present β-cell peptides to CD4+ T cells, which then activate CD8+ cytotoxic T cells to target and destroy pancreatic β-cells expressing self-antigens on major histocompatibility complex class I (MHC class I) molecules. Local production of pro-inflammatory cytokines and chemokines from other immune cells amplifies this process by recruiting and activating more immune cells and increasing β-cell expression of MHC class I antigens. Regulatory T cells, whose function is to suppress the immune response and maintain self-tolerance become less effective, and B cells contribute further by producing autoantibodies against β-cells [57]. In support of this idea, examining the pancreas from organ donors with recent-onset T1D or islet autoimmunity shows patchy immune cell infiltrations within and around the pancreatic islets, a process called insulitis [58]. Insulitis is seen mainly in insulin-containing islets. Predominant immune cells found in insulitis are cytotoxic CD8+ T cells, followed by CD4+ T cells and B cells (CD20+). Other immune cells, such as neutrophils, mast cells, and natural killer cells, are present in varying degrees [59]. In those with recent-onset T1D, HLA class I and II molecule over-expression is seen in insulitis lesions [60, 61]. Due to these findings and other observations, T1D is thought to be driven by T cell-mediated autoimmune β-cell destruction. While this view still holds, increasing evidence suggests the pathogenesis of T1D is much more complex and involves multiple players, such as environmental factors, genetic susceptibilities, B cells, cytokines, and pancreatic β-cells.

While considered pathognomonic, insulitis is observed in vastly differing degrees depending on the patient's age of onset and disease duration. In a meta-analysis by In't Veld et al. [62] that included studies published since the year 1902 and which contained 151 cases of insulitis, young patients (≤ 14 years old) with shorter duration of disease (≤ 1 month) had the highest proportion of insulitis (73%) compared to young patients with longer (> 1 year) duration of disease (4%). In older patients, insulitis was much less prevalent: for those between 15 and 40 years old at the age of onset and disease duration of <1 month, only 29% had insulitis. Moreover, patients who develop T1D at an older age may have up to 60% of their islets still containing β-cells with a positive insulin stain [63]. These observations suggest that not only β-cell loss but also residual β-cell dysfunction causes T1D in older patients.

In T2D, inflammation is present at multiple levels. Insulitis is a hallmark of T1D, but it is also present in T2D [64]. As noted above, obesity is associated with T2D. Inflammation in multiple organ systems, including adipose tissue (AT), skeletal muscle, liver, and pancreatic islets, is a major characteristic of obesity [65]. In both animal and human studies, macrophage infiltration is seen in AT inflammation. Macrophages particularly congregate around dead adipocytes, create crown-like structures, and are thought to contribute to insulin resistance. According to the traditional view, obesity associates with a change in macrophages from the anti-inflammatory M2 to the pro-inflammatory M1 phenotype. However, recent evidence suggests that macrophages may have more complex roles in AT, including influencing adipocyte progenitor proliferation and homeostasis [65–67]. For example, both lean and obese mice with partially depleted M2 phenotype macrophages in AT displayed an increase in insulin sensitivity and adipogenic markers expression [67]. In addition to macrophages, the $CD8^+$ to $CD4^+$ T cell ratio increases in obesity [65].

Additional factors, including glucotoxicity, lipotoxicity, oxidative stress, and amyloid deposition, contribute to the β-cell dysfunction, in part via inflammatory processes [64]. Lipotoxicity occurs when chronically elevated free fatty acid (FFA) levels cause β-cell dysfunction [68]. In a study using a β-cell line with knocked-down G-protein coupled receptor 120 (GPR120) (a FFA receptor associated with lowering inflammation), exposure to palmitic acid resulted in a decrease in *insulin* and an increase in the pro-inflammatory chemokine (C-X-C motif) ligand (CXCL1) 1 and chemokine (C-C motif) ligand (CCL) (*ccl2*) chemokines gene expression. Using a GPR120 agonist increased the gene expression of *insulin* and decreased those of cxcl1 and ccl2 [69].

Glucotoxicity negatively impacts β-cells through inflammation. Pancreatic islets incubated in a high-glucose (33 mM) medium resulted in over two-fold increase in interleukin (IL) 1β (IL-1β) production and almost two-fold upregulation of the NF-κB activity, compared to cells grown in a low-glucose (33 mM) medium. NF-κB is a nuclear transcription factor that is involved in islet cell apoptosis. For islets incubated in elevated glucose, exposure to IL-1 receptor antagonist prevented the increase in NF-κB activity, and the β-cell apoptosis was suppressed. Moreover, islets grown in elevated glucose had a diminished ability to secrete insulin in response to acute exposure to glucose, reflecting a decrease in β-cell function. The decreased response was partly ameliorated by exposure to an IL-1 receptor antagonist [70]. This study demonstrated how elevated glucose, via the inflammatory cytokine IL-1β, leads to β-cell dysfunction and death.

Inflammation contributes to insulin resistance, and insulin resistance, in turn, leads to inflammation. Immune cells in adipose tissue (AT), including macrophages, $CD4^+$ T cells, and $CD8^+$ effector T cells, contribute to insulin resistance in obesity [65]. High-fat diet (HFD)-fed mice treated with CD8 antibody showed fewer $CD8^+$ T cells and pro-inflammatory M1 macrophages in the epididymal AT compared to control normal diet-fed mice [71]. At the same time, the number of CD4$^+$ T cells or anti-inflammatory M2 macrophages was not impacted. CD8 antibody treatment also decreased the epididymal AT expression of the pro-inflammatory cytokines IL-6 and tumor-necrosis factor α (TNF-α) and improved insulin resistance and glucose intolerance, as measured by the insulin tolerance test and OGTT [71].

T2D is associated with non-alcoholic fatty liver disease (NAFLD) [72]. NAFLD includes a spectrum of liver diseases, ranging from hepatic steatosis to non-alcoholic steatohepatitis (NASH). Obesity leads to hepatic inflammation and a rise in hepatic macrophages, increasing pro-inflammatory cytokines and resulting in insulin resistance [73]. Insulin resistance also contributes to the development of NASH [74].

The Role of Cytokines in the Development of Diabetes

Various cytokines have been implicated in the pathogenesis of T1D. However, targeting a specific cytokine to prevent or slow down the development of T1D in humans had mixed or negative results. This may be because most cytokines have both pro- and anti-inflammatory roles, which can change depending on the context, the complex dynamic between different cytokines, changes in β-cell cytokine receptor expression patterns, or underrecognized disease heterogeneity in selected trial patients. Here we discuss a few cytokines that appear promising as therapeutic targets.

IL-2 promotes the growth and differentiation of CD4+ T cells. A low dose of IL-2 has been shown to promote the differentiation of CD4+ T cells to Treg cells, which can then decrease the autoimmune response. In mice, low-dose IL-2 given intraperitoneally prevented T1D [75], and in human studies, it increased the circulation frequency of Treg [76, 77]. However, whether this could translate to β-cell preservation in humans is still to be investigated.

TNFα is a proinflammatory cytokine that has been shown to promote the development of autoimmune diabetes in mice. Blockade of TNFα delayed disease onset in NOD mice in an age-dependent manner [78]. In humans, TNFα receptor blockade with etanercept showed improvement in glycemic control and C-peptide secretion [79]. Treatment with golimumab, an IgG antibody against TNFα, helped to preserve endogenous insulin production in children and young adults with newly diagnosed T1D [80].

IL-21 is involved in the trafficking of CD8+ T cells to pancreatic islets. A phase 2 trial of adults recently diagnosed with T1D combination therapy with IL-21 blockade and a GLP-1 receptor agonist (thought to decrease β-cell stress and prevent apoptosis) preserved C-peptide, compared to placebo. A similar effect was not seen with IL-21 blockade monotherapy [81].

Multiple other cytokines have been investigated, and there are many ongoing clinical trials (reviewed extensively elsewhere [82, 83]).

Immune Checkpoint Inhibitor-Induced Diabetes

Immune checkpoint inhibitors (ICI) are monoclonal antibodies against programmed cell death 1 (PD-1), programmed cell death ligand 1 (PD-L1), or CTLA-4. Cancer cells express PD-L1, which binds to the receptor PD-1 on T cells to avoid T cell activation. CTLA-4 receptors on T cells function in a similar manner. By blocking this interaction, ICI reactivates T-cell recognition of tumor cells. However, as a result, ICI can also cause collateral damage to normal organs, including the pancreas, which can lead to ICI-induced diabetes (ICI-DM). The prevalence of ICI-DM is reported to be between 0.2 and 2%, with the number of cases increasing each year [84, 85]. According to a 2021 systemic review of 200 cases by Lo Preiato et al. [86], the majority of cases occurred in patients treated with anti-PD1 monotherapy (68.5%), followed by PD-L1 (7%) and CTLA-4 (0.5%). The remaining cases (23.5%) occurred in combination or sequential therapy with CTLA-1 and anti-PD1. The median time to onset was about 9 weeks or 3.5 cycles of ICI, and diabetic ketoacidosis was the initial presentation for more than half of the patients. Unlike other ICI-induced adverse reactions, ICI-DM could not be ameliorated by steroid treatment. Almost all patients required treatment with daily multi-dose insulin injections, indicating irreversible damage to pancreatic function [86, 87]. While ICI-DM shares many similarities with T1D, considerable differences have also been observed. It tends to present in a more rapid timeline, and diabetic ketoacidosis, as the initial presentation, was higher than in T1D. Also, of the 75.5% of cases tested for GAD65 antibodies, only 43% had positive titers, which is lower than what is typically observed in T1D. Those with a positive antibody had a shorter time to disease onset than those without (7 vs. 13 weeks). Of the 39% of cases where HLA haplotypes were tested, 51.3% had the DR4 phenotype, and 14.1% had the DR9 phenotype, which is overall higher than what is seen in T1D [86, 87]. Lastly, the risk of ICI-DM increases with older age and with the presence of preexisting non-T1D [88].

Treatment

Metformin

Along with lifestyle interventions, metformin is a treatment option for T2D [89]. Metformin is a biguanide that was developed in 1922 but was not used for treating diabetes in humans until the 1950s [90]. Metformin decreases hepatic glucose output, and one mechanism by which it does so may be via its inhibition of hepatocyte mitochondrial respiration, with a decrease in ATP and increase in AMP, and also lowering glucose output. Moreover, greater levels of AMP inhibit gluconeogenesis via the inhibition of fructose-1,6-bisphosphatase, an enzyme involved in gluconeogenesis [91].

The anti-inflammatory effects of metformin on AT, the cardiovascular system, and the immune system have been studied by several investigators [92–95]. In rats exposed to palmitic acid to induce inflammation, metformin lowered perivascular AT levels of IL-6, TNFα, and CCL2 [96].

Glucagon-Like Peptide-1 (GLP-1) Receptor Agonists

Glucagon-like peptide 1 (GLP-1) is an incretin hormone that upregulates insulin secretion in nutrient intake. In 2005, exenatide became the first Food and Drug Administration (FDA) approved GLP-1 receptor agonist (GLP-1RA) for the treatment of T2D [97]. Currently, both short-acting and long-acting GLP-1RAs are approved for the treatment of T2D. In addition to increasing insulin secretion in hyperglycemia, GLP-1RAs decrease glucagon secretion, slow gastric emptying, and result in weight loss [98]. Moreover, some of the GLP-1RAs have been approved by the FDA specifically for weight loss (liraglutide, semaglutide), cardiovascular risk reduction in patients with T2D, and cardiovascular disease (CVD) (liraglutide, dulaglutide, semaglutide) or T2D and multiple cardiovascular risk factors (dulaglutide).

In both pre-clinical and clinical studies, GLP-1 RAs have been shown to decrease markers of systemic and local inflammation. In one study [99], mice were fed HFD as a model of human obesity and treated with either placebo or the GLP-1 RA liraglutide for 1 week at the end of the HFD period. Although no change in weight was detected before and after treatment with liraglutide, decreases in cardiac TNFα and NF-κB levels were observed. In one clinical study [100], 24 participants with obesity and T2D were randomized to either a placebo or the GLP-1 RA exenatide treatment (10 µg twice daily for 12 weeks). At the end of the study period, no significant change in body weight was detected in either treatment group. However, exenatide treatment resulted in multiple anti-inflammatory changes (decreases in reactive oxygen species (ROS) in mononuclear cells), decreases in the expression of proinflammatory mediators (JNK1, TLR4, TLR2, and SOCS3 in mononuclear cells), and decreases in plasma proinflammatory cytokines (MCP-1, MMP-9, and IL-6) and the cytokine-like protein serum amyloid A (SAA) [100]. Similarly, in another study [101], 10 participants with T2D received liraglutide for 8 weeks. Compared to age- and sex-matched control participants, participants with T2D had greater levels of inflammatory marker serum soluble CD163 (sCD163), a marker of proinflammatory macrophages. Liraglutide decreased sCD163 (220 ng/mL–171 ng/mL, $p < 0.001$) in patients with T2D. In addition, liraglutide decreased TNFα, IL-1β, and IL-6 levels in peripheral blood mononuclear cells.

Sodium-Glucose Co-Transporter 2 Inhibitors

Sodium-glucose cotransporter-2 inhibitors (SGLT2 inhibitors) lower the renal glucose threshold by preventing the reuptake of filtered glucose by SGLT2 in the proximal convoluted tubule. The FDA approved four SGLT2 inhibitors for people with T2D: empagliflozin, canagliflozin, dapagliflozin, and ertugliflozin. The SGLT2 inhibitors lower HbA1c by 0.6–1% compared with the placebo [102]. In addition to glucose lowering, these agents have been approved to reduce the risk of major adverse cardiovascular events (canagliflozin), cardiovascular death (empagliflozin), and heart failure (dapagliflozin) in patients with T2D and CVD.

The use of SGLT2 inhibitors is associated with natriuresis, reduced plasma volume, and lower blood pressure. In addition, in preclinical studies, SGLT2 inhibitors have been found to reduce AT inflammation [103–105]. In one study of mice either administered HFD only or HFD and empagliflozin, high-dose empagliflozin administration (10 mg/kg body weight) was associated with a 49% decrease in M1 proinflammatory macrophages in AT ($p < 0.01$, compared to the HFD-fed only group) and an increase in M2 anti-inflammatory macrophages [104].

The effect of SGLT2 inhibitors on inflammation in human AT has also been studied. In one study [106], epicardial and subcutaneous AT samples from patients undergoing coronary artery bypass graft surgery were exposed to either dapagliflozin or control. Compared to the control, dapagliflozin increased AT glucose uptake and decreased adipokine secretion of CXCL8, CCL2, and CCL5 in the insulin-resistant epicardial AT. In a randomized, placebo-controlled trial of patients with T2D and coronary artery disease (EMPA-CARD) [107], the effect of empagliflozin on markers of systemic inflammation was also studied. Changes in the plasma proinflammatory cytokine levels from baseline to 26 weeks were studied and compared between the placebo ($n = 39$) and treatment group ($n = 43$). The adjusted mean difference between the two groups was -1.06 for IL-6 (95% CI -1.80 - -1.32) ($p = 0.0006$), which demonstrated that empagliflozin significantly decreased IL-6 production compared to placebo.

Immune-Based Therapies

While the mainstay treatment for T1D remains insulin, multiple clinical trials have sought to target the immune system to either prevent the progression of T1D or to reverse the process. In addition to anti-cytokine therapies mentioned above, T cell modulation, B cell depletion, and antigen-based treatments have also been tested with variable success.

One of the first immune-based therapies tested in T1D was cyclosporin, a calcineurin inhibitor that inhibits the synthesis of IL-2 (a key cytokine for T cell proliferation and differentiation). In the 1980s, Feutren et al. [108] conducted a double-blind trial of 122 patients with recent onset T1D and showed that the cyclosporin group had significantly higher rates of remission, defined as fasting blood glucose <7.8 mmol/L, postprandial blood glucose <11.1 mmol/L, and HbA1C $\leq$ 7.5% off of insulin, compared to the placebo group, at 9 months of treatment (24.1% vs. 5.8%). However, cyclosporin was unable to induce durable disease remission, and the dose required for remission was high, which resulted in significant toxicity and thus limited its clinical use [109]. These early studies highlighted the importance of T cells in T1D pathogenesis and opened a path for other T cell therapies.

More recently, anti-CD3 monoclonal antibodies (teplizumab and otelixizumab) have shown promising results (Table 3.1). The mechanism of anti-CD3 therapy is thought to be related to the enhancement of regulatory T-cell activity and, therefore, self-tolerance. Teplizumab has been evaluated in recent-onset T1D patients and individuals at high risk of developing T1D. It has shown improvement in β-cell preservation and delay in the onset of T1D. Sherry et al. [115] investigated teplizumab in a phase 3 randomized controlled study involving 516 patients aged 8–35 years with new-onset (defined as <12 weeks) T1D [115]. In this study, the group that received a 14-day course of teplizumab had reduced loss of C-peptide, as measured by C-peptide mean area under the curve, compared to the placebo group, which received a placebo at baseline and week 26, at 2 years, suggesting enhanced preservation of β-cell function [115, 116]. However, teplizumab did not decrease exogenous insulin use (< 0.5 U/kg per day) or reverse diabetes, possibly due to a lack of initial β-cell mass [115]. As a follow-up, a phase 2 randomized controlled study involving 76 participants at high risk but without overt T1D investigated the role of teplizumab in delaying the onset of the disease. The participants were relatives of patients with T1D and had stage 2 type 1 diabetes, defined as having two or more pancreatic autoantibodies and evidence of dysglycemia after an oral glucose tolerance test. They were treated with a single 14-day course of teplizumab. The primary end-point of the study was the elapsed time from randomization to the clinical diagnosis of diabetes. In this study, 43% of the teplizumab group and 72% of the placebo group developed T1D during a median follow-up of 745 days. The median time to diagnosis of T1D was delayed by 2 years in the teplizumab group compared to the placebo (48.4 vs. 24.4 months) [117]. As a result, teplizumab was approved by the FDA in November 2022 for patients with stage 2 T1D aged 8 or older to delay the onset of stage 3 T1D. Teplizumab is the first drug to be approved for such use. In both studies, the most common adverse events with teplizumab were lymphopenia and rash. However, the proportion of patients with infection did not differ between the groups, and both lymphopenia and rash spontaneously resolved [116, 117]. An ongoing clinical trial investigates teplizumab in children and adolescents with recent-onset T1D [118].

Otelixizumab, another anti-CD3 antibody, has also shown improved β-cell preservation in phase 1 and 2 trials involving patients with recent-onset T1D [119–121]. However, the high total dose of otelixizumab (48–64 mg) used in the phase 2 trial was associated with 75% of the participants developing acute mononucleosis-like symptoms from Epstein–Barr (EBV) reactivation [120]. Phase 3 trials for adults and adolescents (Durable Response Therapy Evaluation for Early or Non-Onset Type 1

Table 3.1 Overview of immune-based therapies that have been studied in individuals with type 1 diabetes or at risk of developing type 1 diabetes

Trial Drug	Target/ mechanism	Trial type and study population	Intervention	Primary outcome	Notable adverse events	Ongoing clinical trial
Teplizumab	T-cell (anti-CD3)	Phase 3 RCT [110] Recent onset T1D (n = 516) Ages 8–25	14-day infusion course at baseline and week 26	Less C-peptide loss at 2 years; No difference in exogenous insulin use	Lymphopenia Rash	Teplizumab in children and adolescents with recent onset type 1 diabetes (NCT04598893)
		Phase 2 RCT [111] Stage 2 T1DM (*n* = 76) Ages 8–49	14-day course at baseline	2-year delay in diagnosis of T1DM		
Abatacept	T-cell co-stimulation (CTLA4-Ig)	Phase 2 RCT [112] Recent onset T1D (*n* = 112) Ages 6–45	Day 1, 14, 28 then monthly infusion over 2 years	Higher stimulated C-peptide level at 2 years; Estimated 9.6-month delay in β-cell decline	No significant difference between treatment and placebo group	Abatacept in prevention of diabetes in relatives at risk for type 1 diabetes (NCT01773707).
GAD-alum	Antigen-based therapy	Phase 2 RCT [113] Recent onset T1D (*n* = 109) Ages 12–24	Monthly intra-lymphatic injection of GAD-alum for 3 doses + vitamin D supplementation	No difference in stimulated serum C-peptide at 15 months; In subgroup analysis, HLA DR3-DQ2 patients had higher C-peptide AUC at 15 months	No significant difference between treatment and placebo groups	GAD-alum plus vitamin D in recent onset T1D and HLA DR3-DQ2 (NCT05018585)
Golimumab	B cell (anti-TNFα)	Phase 2 RCT [114] Recent onset T1D (n = 84) Age 6–21	Every 2 weeks subcutaneous injection for 52 weeks	Higher mean stimulated C-peptide level at 52 weeks; Less exogenous insulin use	Higher incidence of non-severe hypoglycemia	None

TNFα tumor necrosis factor-α, *RCT* randomized controlled trial, T1D, type 1 diabetes, *GAD-alum* aluminum-formulated glutamic acid decarboxylase therapy

Diabetes (DEFEND)-1 and DEFEND-2) thus used a much lower total dose of ote-lixizumab (3.1 mg). They failed to reach primary endpoints, including C-peptide preservation [122, 123]. Currently, there is no ongoing trial involving otelixizumab.

The binding of the T cell receptor CD28 with its ligands CD80 and CD86 on APCs induces a strong activation signal for T cells or co-stimulation. Abatacept, or CTLA4-Ig, blocks CD28 from binding to CD80/86 [124, 125]. Orban et al. [126] conducted a randomized controlled trial testing abatacept vs. placebo in 112 patients aged 6–45 years with recently (< 100 days) diagnosed T1D. The medication was administered on days 1, 14, and 28 and then monthly for a total of 27 infusions over 2 years. At 2 years, the abatacept group had a 59% higher stimulated C-peptide level compared to the placebo group, with an estimated 9.6-month delay in the decline of β-cell function. The mixed effect model showed that the rate of β-cell function decline was similar between the abatacept and placebo groups during the 2 years [126]. However, at the 1-year post-treatment follow-up, the abatacept group had a higher stimulated C-peptide level at 0.217 nmol/L (95% CI 0.168–0.268), com-pared to 0.141 nmol/L (95% CI 0.071–0.215) in the placebo group. This result dem-onstrated that the difference in β-cell preservation persisted after treatment cessation [127]. A clinical trial of abatacept involving the prevention of diabetes in relatives at risk for type 1 diabetes is ongoing [128].

The Canakinumab Anti-inflammatory Thrombosis Outcomes Study (CANTOS) [129] randomized participants with a history of myocardial infarction and elevated C-reactive protein (CRP) to either canakinumab (a monoclonal antibody against IL-1β), or placebo. The objective was to determine whether canakinumab lowered the primary outcome of nonfatal myocardial infarction, nonfatal stroke, or cardio-vascular death. Canakinumab reduced the primary outcome by 15%, and as such, it highlighted the importance of targeting inflammation to reduce cardiovascular risk. Given that the role of IL-1β has been studied (as noted above), one study investi-gated the effect of canakinumab on the incidence of new-onset diabetes within the CANTOS. Although increasing CRP was associated with incident diabetes, canakinumab was not found to be associated with incident diabetes, compared to placebo [130]. However, the clinical evidence regarding IL-1β and diabetes is mixed, as some studies have demonstrated improvement in glycemia in patients with T2D on IL-1 blocking treatment [131, 132].

Systemic Inflammation and Diabetes

Individuals with T1D or T2D and/or obesity are at increased risk of severe illness and/or death from COVID-19 caused by the coronavirus SARS-CoV-2. The causes of these associations have been investigated and continue to be investigated, and inflammation plays a crucial role. Serum IL-6 has been noted to be an independent predictor of the severity of disease and mortality in patients with COVID-19 [133]. It has been hypothesized that the inflammatory response in the setting of COVID-19, with increased levels of pro-inflammatory cytokines, including IL-6, increases insulin resistance in the skeletal muscles and liver, leading to worse hyperglycemia in the context of diabetes and, in turn, contributing to vascular endothelial injury. Such injury could add to the risk of thromboembolic events and cardiovascular death [29]. Another potential explanation for the link between diabetes and worse outcomes with COVID-19 is that individuals with T2D have significantly less natural killer cell activity than those without diabetes or prediabetes. Moreover, greater HbA1c levels in those with T2D are associated with lower natural killer cell activity levels [29, 134].

The relationship between adverse outcomes and T2D is not limited only to COVID-19 but is also seen in the setting of other viral illnesses, including influenza. Among older adults hospitalized with influenza, those with diabetes were more likely to experience severe influenza-associated outcomes, including intensive care unit admission (relative risk 1.84, 95% CI 1.67–2.04), mechanical ventilation (relative risk 1.95, 95% CI 1.74–2.20), and death during hospitalization (relative risk 1.48, 95% CI 1.23–1.80) [135]. In a study using an in vitro model of the respiratory barrier, exposure to glycemic variability was associated with increased endothelial cell expression of TNF-α and IL-6, after primary influenza A infection, compared to exposure to constant glucose levels [136].

Conclusions

Inflammation is central to the pathogenesis of diabetes. Inflammation, in conjunction with genetics and environmental risk factors, leads to the development of T1D, although the exact triggers that initiate the inflammatory process continue to be investigated. Moreover, inflammation contributes to the β-cell dysfunction seen in T2D. Also, in T2D, inflammation is present in multiple organs, including the islets, AT, and the liver. Some of the current pharmacotherapies for T2D, including GLP-1 RAs and SGLT2 inhibitors, have anti-inflammatory effects identified in pre-clinical and clinical studies. Inflammation remains a promising therapeutic target for preventing the development of T1D in high-risk individuals.

References

1. American Diabetes Association professional practice committee. 2. Classification and diagnosis of diabetes: standards of medical care in diabetes—2022. Diabetes Care. 2021;45(Supplement_1):S17–38.
2. Eisenbarth GS, Type I. Diabetes Mellitus. N Engl J Med. 1986;314(21):1360–8.
3. Insel RA, Dunne JL, Atkinson MA, Chiang JL, Dabelea D, Gottlieb PA, et al. Staging presymptomatic type 1 diabetes: a scientific statement of JDRF, the Endocrine Society, and the American Diabetes Association. Diabetes Care. 2015;38(10):1964–74.

4. Ziegler AG, Rewers M, Simell O, Simell T, Lempainen J, Steck A, et al. Seroconversion to multiple islet autoantibodies and risk of progression to diabetes in children. JAMA. 2013;309(23):2473–9.

5. Krischer JP, Lynch KF, Schatz DA, Ilonen J, Lernmark Å, Hagopian WA, et al. The 6 year incidence of diabetes-associated autoantibodies in genetically at-risk children: the TEDDY study. Diabetologia. 2015;58(5):980–7.

6. Kahn SE. The relative contributions of insulin resistance and beta-cell dysfunction to the pathophysiology of type 2 diabetes. Diabetologia. 2003;46(1):3–19.

7. Ling C, Bacos K, Rönn T. Epigenetics of type 2 diabetes mellitus and weight change—a tool for precision medicine? Nat Rev Endocrinol. 2022;18(7):433–48.

8. Stumvoll M, Tataranni PA, Stefan N, Vozarova B, Bogardus C. Glucose Allostasis. Diabetes. 2003;52(4):903–9.

9. Stumvoll M, Goldstein BJ, van Haeften TW. Type 2 diabetes: principles of pathogenesis and therapy. Lancet. 2005;365(9467):1333–46.

10. Dennis JM, Shields BM, Henley WE, Jones AG, Hattersley AT. Disease progression and treatment response in data-driven subgroups of type 2 diabetes compared with models based on simple clinical features: an analysis using clinical trial data. Lancet Diabetes Endocrinol. 2019;7(6):442–51.

11. Safiri S, Karamzad N, Kaufman JS, Bell AW, Nejadghaderi SA, Sullman MJM, et al. Prevalence, deaths and disability-adjusted-life-years (DALYs) due to type 2 diabetes and its attributable risk factors in 204 countries and territories, 1990–2019: results from the Global Burden of Disease Study 2019. Front Endocrinol. 2022;13:838027. https://doi.org/10.3389/fendo.2022.838027.

12. Home, Resources, diabetes L with, Acknowledgement, FAQs, Contact, et al. IDF Diabetes Atlas | Tenth Edition [Internet]. [cited 2022 Nov 15]. https://diabetesatlas.org/

13. Khan MAB, Hashim MJ, King JK, Govender RD, Mustafa H, Al KJ. Epidemiology of Type 2 diabetes—global burden of disease and forecasted trends. J Epidemiol Glob Health. 2020;10(1):107–11.

14. Viner R, White B, Christie D. Type 2 diabetes in adolescents: a severe phenotype posing major clinical challenges and public health burden. Lancet. 2017;389(10085):2252–60.

15. Lin X, Xu Y, Pan X, Xu J, Ding Y, Sun X, et al. Global, regional, and national burden and trend of diabetes in 195 countries and territories: an analysis from 1990 to 2025. Sci Rep. 2020;10(1):14790.

16. Zheng Y, Ley SH, Hu FB. Global aetiology and epidemiology of type 2 diabetes mellitus and its complications. Nat Rev Endocrinol. 2018;14(2):88–98.

17. Abdullah A, Peeters A, de Courten M, Stoelwinder J. The magnitude of association between overweight and obesity and the risk of diabetes: a meta-analysis of prospective cohort studies. Diabetes Res Clin Pract. 2010;89(3):309–19.

18. Adult-Onset Type 1 Diabetes: Current Understanding and Challenges | Diabetes Care | American Diabetes Association [Internet]. [cited 2022 Nov 28]. https://diabetesjournals.org/care/article/44/11/2449/138477/Adult-Onset-Type-1-Diabetes-Current-Understanding

19. Patterson CC, Harjutsalo V, Rosenbauer J, Neu A, Cinek O, Skrivarhaug T, et al. Trends and cyclical variation in the incidence of childhood type 1 diabetes in 26 European centres in the 25 year period 1989–2013: a multicentre prospective registration study. Diabetologia. 2019;62(3):408–17.

20. Norris JM, Johnson RK, Stene LC. Type 1 diabetes—early life origins and changing epidemiology. Lancet Diabetes Endocrinol. 2020;8(3):226–38.

21. Richardson SJ, Morgan NG. Enteroviral infections in the pathogenesis of type 1 diabetes: new insights for therapeutic intervention. Curr Opin Pharmacol. 2018;43:11–9.

22. Enterovirus Infection and Progression From Islet Autoimmunity to Type 1 Diabetes | Diabetes | American Diabetes Association [Internet]. [cited 2022 Nov 28]. https://diabetesjournals.org/diabetes/article/59/12/3174/26597/Enterovirus-Infection-and-Progression-From-Islet

23. Roep BO. A viral link for type 1 diabetes. Nat Med. 2019;25(12):1816–8.

24. Honeyman MC, Coulson BS, Stone NL, Gellert SA, Goldwater PN, Steele CE, et al. Association between rotavirus infection and pancreatic islet autoimmunity in children at risk of developing type 1 diabetes. Diabetes. 2000;49(8):1319–24.
25. Perrett KP, Jachno K, Nolan TM, Harrison LC. Association of Rotavirus Vaccination with the incidence of type 1 diabetes in children. JAMA Pediatr. 2019;173(3):280–2.
26. Hiemstra HS, Schloot NC, van Veelen PA, Willemen SJM, Franken KLMC, van Rood JJ, et al. Cytomegalovirus in autoimmunity: T cell crossreactivity to viral antigen and autoantigen glutamic acid decarboxylase. Proc Natl Acad Sci. 2001;98(7):3988–91.
27. Kendall EK, Olaker VR, Kaelber DC, Xu R, Davis PB. Association of SARS-CoV-2 infection with new-onset Type 1 diabetes among pediatric patients from 2020 to 2021. JAMA Netw Open. 2022;5(9):e2233014.
28. Barrett CE. Risk for newly diagnosed diabetes 30 days after SARS-CoV-2 infection among persons aged 18 years — United States, March 1, 2020–June 28, 2021. MMWR Morb Mortal Wkly Rep. 2022;71:59–65. https://www.cdc.gov/mmwr/volumes/71/wr/mm7102e2.htm.
29. Lim S, Bae JH, Kwon HS, Nauck MA. COVID-19 and diabetes mellitus: from pathophysiology to clinical management. Nat Rev Endocrinol. 2021;17(1):11–30.
30. Hakola L, Miettinen ME, Syrjälä E, Åkerlund M, Takkinen HM, Korhonen TE, et al. Association of cereal, gluten, and dietary fiber intake with islet autoimmunity and Type 1 diabetes. JAMA Pediatr. 2019;173(10):953–60.
31. Antvorskov JC, Halldorsson TI, Josefsen K, Svensson J, Granström C, Roep BO, et al. Association between maternal gluten intake and type 1 diabetes in offspring: national prospective cohort study in Denmark. BMJ. 2018;362:k3547.
32. Lund-Blix NA, Tapia G, Mårild K, Brantsaeter AL, Njølstad PR, Joner G, et al. Maternal and child gluten intake and association with type 1 diabetes: the Norwegian mother and child cohort study. PLoS Med. 2020;17(3):e1003032.
33. Lund-Blix NA, Dong F, Mårild K, Seifert J, Barón AE, Waugh KC, et al. Gluten intake and risk of islet autoimmunity and progression to Type 1 diabetes in children at increased risk of the disease: the diabetes autoimmunity study in the young (DAISY). Diabetes Care. 2019;42(5):789–96.
34. de Goffau MC, Luopajärvi K, Knip M, Ilonen J, Ruohtula T, Härkönen T, et al. Fecal microbiota composition differs between children with β-cell autoimmunity and those without. Diabetes. 2013;62(4):1238–44.
35. Davis-Richardson AG, Ardissone AN, Dias R, Simell V, Leonard MT, Kemppainen KM, et al. Bacteroides dorei dominates gut microbiome prior to autoimmunity in Finnish children at high risk for type 1 diabetes. Front Microbiol. 2014;5:1. https://doi.org/10.3389/fmicb.2014.00678.
36. Mejía-León ME, Petrosino JF, Ajami NJ, Domínguez-Bello MG, de la Barca AMC. Fecal microbiota imbalance in Mexican children with type 1 diabetes. Sci Rep. 2014;4(1):3814.
37. Endesfelder D, Engel M, Davis-Richardson AG, Ardissone AN, Achenbach P, Hummel S, et al. Towards a functional hypothesis relating anti-islet cell autoimmunity to the dietary impact on microbial communities and butyrate production. Microbiome. 2016;4(1):17.
38. Cleophas MCP, Ratter JM, Bekkering S, Quintin J, Schraa K, Stroes ES, et al. Effects of oral butyrate supplementation on inflammatory potential of circulating peripheral blood mononuclear cells in healthy and obese males. Sci Rep. 2019;9(1):775.
39. He J, Zhang P, Shen L, Niu L, Tan Y, Chen L, et al. Short-chain fatty acids and their association with Signalling pathways in inflammation, glucose and lipid metabolism. Int J Mol Sci. 2020;21(17):6356.
40. Vatanen T, Franzosa EA, Schwager R, Tripathi S, Arthur TD, Vehik K, et al. The human gut microbiome in early-onset type 1 diabetes from the TEDDY study. Nature. 2018;562(7728):589–94.
41. Mariño E, Richards JL, McLeod KH, Stanley D, Yap YA, Knight J, et al. Gut microbial metabolites limit the frequency of autoimmune T cells and protect against type 1 diabetes. Nat Immunol. 2017;18(5):552–62.

42. Bell KJ, Saad S, Tillett BJ, McGuire HM, Bordbar S, Yap YA, et al. Metabolite-based dietary supplementation in human type 1 diabetes is associated with microbiota and immune modulation. Microbiome. 2022;10(1):9.
43. de Groot PF, Nikolic T, Imangaliyev S, Bekkering S, Duinkerken G, Keij FM, et al. Oral butyrate does not affect innate immunity and islet autoimmunity in individuals with long-standing type 1 diabetes: a randomised controlled trial. Diabetologia. 2020;63(3):597–610.
44. Toniolo A, Cassani G, Puggioni A, Rossi A, Colombo A, Onodera T, et al. The diabetes pandemic and associated infections: suggestions for clinical microbiology. Rev Med Microbiol. 2019;30(1):1–17.
45. Voight BF, Scott LJ, Steinthorsdottir V, Morris AP, Dina C, Welch RP, et al. Twelve type 2 diabetes susceptibility loci identified through large-scale association analysis. Nat Genet. 2010;42(7):579–89.
46. Fuchsberger C, Flannick J, Teslovich TM, Mahajan A, Agarwala V, Gaulton KJ, et al. The genetic architecture of type 2 diabetes. Nature. 2016;536(7614):41–7.
47. Noble JA. Immunogenetics of type 1 diabetes: a comprehensive review. J Autoimmun. 2015;64:101–12.
48. Erlich H, Valdes AM, Noble J, Carlson JA, Varney M, Concannon P, et al. HLA DR-DQ haplotypes and genotypes and type 1 diabetes risk: analysis of the Type 1 diabetes genetics consortium families. Diabetes. 2008;57(4):1084–92.
49. Awa WL, Boehm BO, Kapellen T, Rami B, Rupprath P, Marg W, et al. HLA-DR genotypes influence age at disease onset in children and juveniles with type 1 diabetes mellitus. Eur J Endocrinol. 2010;163(1):97–104.
50. Caillat-Zucman S, Garchon HJ, Timsit J, Assan R, Boitard C, Djilali-Saiah I, et al. Age-dependent HLA genetic heterogeneity of type 1 insulin-dependent diabetes mellitus. J Clin Invest. 1992;90(6):2242–50.
51. Noble JA, Valdes AM, Varney MD, Carlson JA, Moonsamy P, Fear AL, et al. HLA class I and genetic susceptibility to Type 1 diabetes: results from the Type 1 diabetes genetics consortium. Diabetes. 2010;59(11):2972–9.
52. Wang J, Liu L, Ma J, Sun F, Zhao Z, Gu M. Common variants on cytotoxic T lymphocyte Antigen-4 polymorphisms contributes to Type 1 diabetes susceptibility: evidence based on 58 studies. PLoS One. 2014;9(1):e85982.
53. Bottini N, Musumeci L, Alonso A, Rahmouni S, Nika K, Rostamkhani M, et al. A functional variant of lymphoid tyrosine phosphatase is associated with type I diabetes. Nat Genet. 2004;36(4):337–8.
54. Zheng W, She JX. Genetic association between a lymphoid tyrosine phosphatase (PTPN22) and Type 1 diabetes. Diabetes. 2005;54(3):906–8.
55. Giza S, Goulas A, Gbandi E, Effraimidou S, Papadopoulou-Alataki E, Eboriadou M, et al. The role of PTPN22 C1858T gene polymorphism in diabetes mellitus Type 1: first evaluation in Greek children and adolescents. Biomed Res Int. 2013;2013:721604.
56. Steck A, Baschal E, Jasinski J, Boehm B, Bottini N, Concannon P, et al. rs2476601 T allele (R620W) defines high-risk PTPN22 type I diabetes-associated haplotypes with preliminary evidence for an additional protective haplotype. Genes Immun. 2009;10(Suppl 1):S21–6.
57. DiMeglio LA, Evans-Molina C, Oram RA. Type 1 diabetes. Lancet. 2018;391(10138):2449–62.
58. Veld PI, De Munck N, Van Belle K, Buelens N, Ling Z, Weets I, et al. β-Cell replication is increased in donor organs from young patients after prolonged life support. Diabetes. 2010;59(7):1702–8.
59. Morgan NG, Richardson SJ. Fifty years of pancreatic islet pathology in human type 1 diabetes: insights gained and progress made. Diabetologia. 2018;61(12):2499–506.
60. Morgan NG. Bringing the human pancreas into focus: new paradigms for the understanding of Type 1 diabetes. Diabet Med. 2017;34(7):879–86.
61. Itoh N, Hanafusa T, Miyazaki A, Miyagawa J, Yamagata K, Yamamoto K, et al. Mononuclear cell infiltration and its relation to the expression of major histocompatibility complex anti-

gens and adhesion molecules in pancreas biopsy specimens from newly diagnosed insulin-dependent diabetes mellitus patients. J Clin Invest. 1993;92(5):2313–22.

62. In't Veld P. Insulitis in human type 1 diabetes. Islets. 2011;3(4):131–8.

63. Ii DJK. Extent of beta cell destruction is important but insufficient to predict the onset of Type 1 diabetes mellitus. PLoS One. 2008;3(1):e1374.

64. Donath MY, Shoelson SE. Type 2 diabetes as an inflammatory disease. Nat Rev Immunol. 2011;11(2):98–107.

65. Wu H, Ballantyne CM. Metabolic inflammation and insulin resistance in obesity. Circ Res. 2020;126(11):1549–64.

66. Hill DA, Lim HW, Kim YH, Ho WY, Foong YH, Nelson VL, et al. Distinct macrophage populations direct inflammatory versus physiological changes in adipose tissue. Proc Natl Acad Sci. 2018;115(22):E5096–105.

67. Nawaz A, Aminuddin A, Kado T, Takikawa A, Yamamoto S, Tsuneyama K, et al. CD206+ M2-like macrophages regulate systemic glucose metabolism by inhibiting proliferation of adipocyte progenitors. Nat Commun. 2017;8(1):1–16.

68. Oh YS, Bae GD, Baek DJ, Park EY, Jun HS. Fatty acid-induced lipotoxicity in pancreatic Beta-cells during development of Type 2 diabetes. Front Endocrinol. 2018;9:384.

69. Wang Y, Xie T, Zhang D, Leung PS. GPR120 protects lipotoxicity-induced pancreatic β-cell dysfunction through regulation of PDX1 expression and inhibition of islet inflammation. Clin Sci. 2019;133(1):101–16.

70. Maedler K, Sergeev P, Ris F, Oberholzer J, Joller-Jemelka HI, Spinas GA, et al. Glucose-induced β cell production of IL-1β contributes to glucotoxicity in human pancreatic islets. J Clin Invest. 2002;110(6):851–60.

71. Nishimura S, Manabe I, Nagasaki M, Eto K, Yamashita H, Ohsugi M, et al. CD8+ effector T cells contribute to macrophage recruitment and adipose tissue inflammation in obesity. Nat Med. 2009;15(8):914–20.

72. Muthiah M, Ng CH, Chan KE, Fu CE, Lim WH, Tan DJH, et al. Type 2 diabetes mellitus in metabolic-associated fatty liver disease vs. type 2 diabetes mellitus non-alcoholic fatty liver disease: a longitudinal cohort analysis. Ann Hepatol. 2023;28(1):100762.

73. McNelis JC, Olefsky JM. Macrophages, immunity, and metabolic disease. Immunity. 2014;41(1):36–48.

74. Kitade H, Chen G, Ni Y, Ota T. Nonalcoholic fatty liver disease and insulin resistance: new insights and potential new treatments. Nutrients. 2017;9(4):387.

75. Grinberg-Bleyer Y, Baeyens A, You S, Elhage R, Fourcade G, Gregoire S, et al. IL-2 reverses established type 1 diabetes in NOD mice by a local effect on pancreatic regulatory T cells. J Exp Med. 2010;207(9):1871–8.

76. Rosenzwajg M, Churlaud G, Mallone R, Six A, Derian N, Chaara W, et al. Low-dose interleukin-2 fosters a dose-dependent regulatory T cell tuned milieu in T1D patients. J Autoimmun. 2015;58:48–58.

77. Hartemann A, Bensimon G, Payan CA, Jacqueminet S, Bourron O, Nicolas N, et al. Low-dose interleukin 2 in patients with type 1 diabetes: a phase 1/2 randomised, double-blind, placebo-controlled trial. Lancet Diabetes Endocrinol. 2013;1(4):295–305.

78. Yang XD, Tisch R, Singer SM, Cao ZA, Liblau RS, Schreiber RD, et al. Effect of tumor necrosis factor alpha on insulin-dependent diabetes mellitus in NOD mice. I. the early development of autoimmunity and the diabetogenic process. J Exp Med. 1994;180(3):995–1004.

79. Mastrandrea L, Yu J, Behrens T, Buchlis J, Albini C, Fourtner S, et al. Etanercept treatment in children with new-onset Type 1 diabetes: pilot randomized, placebo-controlled, double-blind study. Diabetes Care. 2009;32(7):1244–9.

80. Quattrin T, Haller MJ, Steck AK, Felner EI, Li Y, Xia Y, et al. Golimumab and Beta-cell function in youth with new-onset Type 1 diabetes. N Engl J Med. 2020;383(21):2007–17.

81. Von HM, Bain SC, Bode B, Clausen JO, Coppieters K, Gaysina L, et al. Anti-interleukin-21 antibody and liraglutide for the preservation of β-cell function in adults with recent-onset type

1 diabetes: a randomised, double-blind, placebo-controlled, phase 2 trial. Lancet Diabetes Endocrinol. 2021;9(4):212–24.

82. Lu J, Liu J, Li L, Lan Y, Liang Y. Cytokines in type 1 diabetes: mechanisms of action and immunotherapeutic targets. Clin Transl Immunol. 2020;9(3):e1122. https://doi.org/10.1002/cti2.1122.

83. Atkinson MA, Roep BO, Posgai A, Wheeler DCS, Peakman M. The challenge of modulating β-cell autoimmunity in type 1 diabetes. Lancet Diabetes Endocrinol. 2019;7(1):52–64.

84. Kotwal A, Haddox C, Block M, Kudva YC. Immune checkpoint inhibitors: an emerging cause of insulin-dependent diabetes. BMJ Open Diabetes Res Care. 2022;7(1):e000591. https://drc.bmj.com/content/7/1/e000591.

85. Tsang VHM, McGrath RT, Clifton-Bligh RJ, Scolyer RA, Jakrot V, Guminski AD, et al. Checkpoint inhibitor–associated autoimmune diabetes is distinct from type 1 diabetes. J Clin Endocrinol Metab. 2019;104(11):5499–506.

86. Lo Preiato V, Salvagni S, Ricci C, Ardizzoni A, Pagotto U, Pelusi C. Diabetes mellitus induced by immune checkpoint inhibitors: type 1 diabetes variant or new clinical entity? Review of the literature. Rev Endocr Metab Disord. 2021;22(2):337–49.

87. Zhang R, Cai XL, Liu L, Han XY, Ji LN. Type 1 diabetes induced by immune checkpoint inhibitors. Chin Med J. 2020;133(21):2595–8.

88. Chen X, Affinati AH, Lee Y, Turcu AF, Henry NL, Schiopu E, et al. Immune checkpoint inhibitors and risk of Type 1 diabetes. Diabetes Care. 2022;45(5):1170–6.

89. ElSayed NA, Aleppo G, Aroda VR, Bannuru RR, Brown FM, Bruemmer D, et al. 9. Pharmacologic approaches to glycemic treatment: standards of care in diabetes—2023. Diabetes Care. 2022;46(Supplement_1):S140–57.

90. Bailey CJ. Metformin: historical overview. Diabetologia. 2017;60(9):1566–76.

91. Rena G, Pearson ER, Sakamoto K. Molecular mechanism of action of metformin: old or new insights? Diabetologia. 2013;56(9):1898–906.

92. Kristófi R, Eriksson JW. Metformin as an anti-inflammatory agent: a short review. J Endocrinol. 2021;251(2):R11–22.

93. Li X, Li J, Wang L, Li A, Qiu Z, Wen QL, et al. The role of metformin and resveratrol in the prevention of hypoxia-inducible factor 1α accumulation and fibrosis in hypoxic adipose tissue. Br J Pharmacol. 2016;173(12):2001–15.

94. Ye J, Zhu N, Sun R, Liao W, Fan S, Shi F, et al. Metformin inhibits chemokine expression through the AMPK/NF-κB signaling pathway. J Interf Cytokine Res. 2018;38(9):363–9.

95. Mummidi S, Das NA, Carpenter AJ, Kandikattu H, Krenz M, Siebenlist U, et al. Metformin inhibits aldosterone-induced cardiac fibroblast activation, migration and proliferation in vitro, and reverses aldosterone+salt-induced cardiac fibrosis in vivo. J Mol Cell Cardiol. 2016;98:95–102.

96. Sun Y, Li J, Xiao N, Wang M, Kou J, Qi L, et al. Pharmacological activation of AMPK ameliorates perivascular adipose/endothelial dysfunction in a manner interdependent on AMPK and SIRT1. Pharmacol Res. 2014;89:19–28.

97. Byetta (exenatide) injection. :34.

98. GLP-1 receptor agonists in the treatment of type 2 diabetes—state-of-the-art-ScienceDirect [Internet]. [cited 2022 Nov 19]. https://www.sciencedirect.com/science/article/pii/S2212877820301769.

99. Noyan-Ashraf MH, Shikatani EA, Schuiki I, Mukovozov I, Wu J, Li RK, et al. A glucagon-like Peptide-1 analog reverses the molecular pathology and cardiac dysfunction of a mouse model of obesity. Circulation. 2013;127(1):74–85.

100. Chaudhuri A, Ghanim H, Vora M, Sia CL, Korzeniewski K, Dhindsa S, et al. Exenatide exerts a potent antiinflammatory effect. J Clin Endocrinol Metab. 2012;97(1):198–207.

101. Hogan AE, Gaoatswe G, Lynch L, Corrigan MA, Woods C, O'Connell J, et al. Glucagon-like peptide 1 analogue therapy directly modulates innate immune-mediated inflammation in individuals with type 2 diabetes mellitus. Diabetologia. 2014;57(4):781–4.

102. Cowie MR, Fisher M. SGLT2 inhibitors: mechanisms of cardiovascular benefit beyond gly-caemic control. Nat Rev Cardiol. 2020;17(12):761–72.
103. Trnovska J, Svoboda P, Pelantova H, Kuzma M, Kratochvilova H, Kasperova BJ, et al. Complex positive effects of SGLT-2 inhibitor Empagliflozin in the liver, kidney and adipose tissue of hereditary hypertriglyceridemic rats: possible contribution of attenuation of cell senescence and oxidative stress. Int J Mol Sci. 2021;22(19):10606.
104. Xu L, Nagata N, Nagashimada M, Zhuge F, Ni Y, Chen G, et al. SGLT2 inhibition by empa-gliflozin promotes fat utilization and browning and attenuates inflammation and insulin resistance by polarizing M2 macrophages in diet-induced obese mice. EBioMedicine. 2017;20:137–49.
105. Aragón-Herrera A, Moraña-Fernández S, Otero-Santiago M, Anido-Varela L, Campos-Toimil M, García-Seara J, et al. The lipidomic and inflammatory profiles of visceral and subcutaneous adipose tissues are distinctly regulated by the SGLT2 inhibitor empagliflozin in Zucker diabetic fatty rats. Biomed Pharmacother. 2023;161:114535.
106. Díaz-Rodríguez E, Agra RM, Fernández ÁL, Adrio B, García-Caballero T, González-Juanatey JR, et al. Effects of dapagliflozin on human epicardial adipose tissue: modulation of insulin resistance, inflammatory chemokine production, and differentiation ability. Cardiovasc Res. 2018;114(2):336–46.
107. Gohari S, Reshadmanesh T, Khodabandehloo H, Karbalaee-Hasani A, Ahangar H, Arsang-Jang S, et al. The effect of EMPAgliflozin on markers of inflammation in patients with con-comitant type 2 diabetes mellitus and coronary artery disease: the EMPA-CARD randomized controlled trial. Diabetol Metab Syndr. 2022;14(1):170.
108. Feutren G, Assan R, Karsenty G, Rostu HD, Sirmai J, Papoz L, et al. Cyclosporin increases the rate and length of remissions in insulin-dependent diabetes of recent onset: results of a multicentre double-blind trial. Lancet. 1986;328(8499):119–24.
109. Filippo GD, Carel JC, Boitard C, Bougnères PF. Long-term results of early cyclosporin ther-apy in juvenile IDDM. Diabetes. 1996;45(1):101–4.
110. Hagopian W, et al. Teplizumab preserves C-peptide in recent-onset type 1 diabetes: two-year results from the randomized, placebo-controlled Protégé trial. Diabetes. 2013;62(11):3901–8. https://doi.org/10.2337/db13-0236.
111. Herold KC, et al. An anti-CD3 antibody, Teplizumab, in relatives at risk for Type 1 diabetes. N Engl J Med. 2019;381(7):603–13. https://doi.org/10.1056/NEJMoa1902226.
112. Orban T, et al. Co-stimulation modulation with abatacept in patients with recent-onset type 1 diabetes: a randomised, double-blind, placebo-controlled trial. Lancet. 2011;378(9789):412–9. https://doi.org/10.1016/S0140-6736(11)60886-6.
113. Ludvigsson J, Sumnik Z, Pelikanova T, et al. Intralymphatic glutamic acid decarboxylase with vitamin D supplementation in recent-onset Type 1 diabetes: a double-blind, random-ized, placebo-controlled phase IIb trial. Diabetes Care. 2021;44(7):1604–12. https://doi.org/10.2337/dc21-0318.
114. Quattrin T, et al. Golimumab and Beta-cell function in youth with new-onset type 1 diabetes. N Engl J Med. 2020;383(21):2007–17. https://doi.org/10.1056/NEJMoa2006136.
115. Sherry N, Hagopian W, Ludvigsson J, Jain SM, Wahlen J, Ferry RJ, et al. Teplizumab for treatment of type 1 diabetes (Protégé study): 1-year results from a randomised, placebo-controlled trial. Lancet. 2011;378(9790):487–97.
116. Hagopian W, Ferry RJ Jr, Sherry N, Carlin D, Bonvini E, Johnson S, et al. Teplizumab pre-serves C-peptide in recent-onset type 1 diabetes: two-year results from the randomized, placebo-controlled protégé trial. Diabetes. 2013;62(11):3901–8.
117. Herold KC, Bundy BN, Long SA, Bluestone JA, DiMeglio LA, Dufort MJ, et al. An anti-CD3 antibody, teplizumab, in relatives at risk for type 1 diabetes. N Engl J Med. 2019;381(7):603–13.
118. Provention Bio, Inc. A Multicenter, Multinational Extension of Study PRV-031-001 to evalu-ate the long-term safety of teplizumab (PRV-031), a humanized, FcR non-binding, anti-CD3 monoclonal antibody, in children and adolescents with recent-onset type 1 diabetes mellitus

[Internet]. clinicaltrials.gov; 2022 Aug [cited 2022 Nov 28]. Report No.: NCT04598893. https://clinicaltrials.gov/ct2/show/NCT04598893.

119. Herold KC, Hagopian W, Auger JA, Poumian-Ruiz E, Taylor L, Donaldson D, et al. Anti-CD3 monoclonal antibody in new-onset type 1 diabetes mellitus. N Engl J Med. 2002;346(22):1692–8.

120. Keymeulen B, Vandemeulebroucke E, Ziegler AG, Mathieu C, Kaufman L, Hale G, et al. Insulin needs after CD3-antibody therapy in new-onset type 1 diabetes. N Engl J Med. 2005;352(25):2598–608.

121. Keymeulen B, Walter M, Mathieu C, Kaufman L, Gorus F, Hilbrands R, et al. Four-year metabolic outcome of a randomised controlled CD3-antibody trial in recent-onset type 1 diabetic patients depends on their age and baseline residual beta cell mass. Diabetologia. 2010;53(4):614–23.

122. Aronson R, Gottlieb PA, Christiansen JS, Donner TW, Bosi E, Bode BW, et al. Low-dose Otelixizumab anti-CD3 monoclonal antibody DEFEND-1 study: results of the randomized phase III study in recent-onset human type 1 diabetes. Diabetes Care. 2014;37(10):2746–54.

123. Ambery P, Donner TW, Biswas N, Donaldson J, Parkin J, Dayan CM. Efficacy and safety of low-dose otelixizumab anti-CD3 monoclonal antibody in preserving C-peptide secretion in adolescent type 1 diabetes: DEFEND-2, a randomized, placebo-controlled, double-blind, multi-Centre study. Diabet Med. 2014;31(4):399–402.

124. Bluestone JA, Clair EWS, Turka LA. CTLA4Ig: bridging the basic immunology with clinical application. Immunity. 2006;24(3):233–8.

125. Rachid O, Osman A, Abdi R, Haik Y. CTLA4-Ig (abatacept): a promising investigational drug for use in type 1 diabetes. Expert Opin Investig Drugs. 2020;29(3):221–36.

126. Orban T, Bundy B, Becker DJ, DiMeglio LA, Gitelman SE, Goland R, et al. Co-stimulation modulation with Abatacept in patients with recent-onset Type 1 diabetes: a randomised double-masked controlled trial. Lancet. 2011;378(9789):412–9.

127. Orban T, Bundy B, Becker DJ, DiMeglio LA, Gitelman SE, Goland R, et al. Costimulation modulation with abatacept in patients with recent-onset Type 1 diabetes: follow-up 1 year after cessation of treatment. Diabetes Care. 2014;37(4):1069–75.

128. National Institute of Diabetes and Digestive and Kidney Diseases (NIDDK). CTLA4-Ig (Abatacept)for Prevention of Abnormal Glucose Tolerance and Diabetes in Relatives At - Risk for Type 1 Diabetes [Internet]. clinicaltrials.gov; 2022 Apr [cited 2023 Apr 20]. Report No.: NCT01773707. https://clinicaltrials.gov/ct2/show/NCT01773707

129. Ridker PM, Everett BM, Thuren T, MacFadyen JG, Chang WH, Ballantyne C, et al. Antiinflammatory therapy with canakinumab for atherosclerotic disease. N Engl J Med. 2017;377(12):1119–31.

130. Verma S, Mathew V, Farkouh ME. Targeting inflammation in the prevention and treatment of type 2 diabetes: insights from CANTOS∗. J Am Coll Cardiol. 2018;71(21):2402–4.

131. Larsen CM, Faulenbach M, Vaag A, Vølund A, Ehses JA, Seifert B, et al. Interleukin-1–receptor antagonist in Type 2 diabetes mellitus. N Engl J Med. 2007;356(15):1517–26.

132. Sloan-Lancaster J, Abu-Raddad E, Polzer J, Miller JW, Scherer JC, De Gaetano A, et al. Double-blind, randomized study evaluating the glycemic and anti-inflammatory effects of subcutaneous LY2189102, a neutralizing IL-1β antibody, in patients with Type 2 diabetes. Diabetes Care. 2013;36(8):2239–46.

133. Del Valle DM, Kim-Schulze S, Huang HH, Beckmann ND, Nirenberg S, Wang B, et al. An inflammatory cytokine signature predicts COVID-19 severity and survival. Nat Med. 2020;26(10):1636–43.

134. Kim JH, Park K, Lee SB, Kang S, Park JS, Ahn CW, et al. Relationship between natural killer cell activity and glucose control in patients with type 2 diabetes and prediabetes. J Diabetes Investig. 2019 Sep;10(5):1223–8.

135. Owusu D, Rolfes MA, Arriola CS, Daily Kirley P, Alden NB, Meek J, et al. Rates of severe influenza-associated outcomes among older adults Living with diabetes—Influenza hospitalization surveillance network (FluSurv-NET), 2012–2017. Open Forum Infect Dis. 2022;9(5):ofac131.
136. Marshall RJ, Armart P, Hulme KD, Chew KY, Brown AC, Hansbro PM, et al. Glycemic variability in diabetes increases the severity of influenza. MBio. 2020;11(2):e02841–19.

Chapter 4
Diabetes, Obesity, and Oxidative Stress

Nadezda Apostolova, Elena Rafailovska, Suzana Dinevska-Kjovkarovska, and Biljana Miova

Abbreviations

8-OHdG	8-hydroxy-2′-deoxyguanosine
Acetyl-CoA	Acetyl-coenzyme A
AGE	Advanced glycation end-products
ASK1	Apoptosis signaling kinase 1
ATF-6α	Activating transcription factor 6 alpha
BMI	Body mass index
C/EBP	CCAAT-enhancer-binding protein
CAT	Catalase
CHOP	CCAAT-enhancer-binding protein homologous protein
DM	Diabetes mellitus
ER	Endoplasmic reticulum
ETC	Electron transport chain

N. Apostolova
CIBERehd—Department of Pharmacology, University of Valencia, Valencia, Spain

Foundation for the Promotion of Health and Biomedical Research in the Valencian Region (FISABIO), Valencia, Spain
e-mail: nadezda.apostolova@uv.es

E. Rafailovska · S. Dinevska-Kjovkarovska
Department of Experimental Physiology and Biochemistry, Institute of Biology, Faculty of Natural Sciences and Mathematics, University "Ss Cyril and Methodius",
Skopje, Republic of North Macedonia
e-mail: elena.rafailovska@pmf.ukim.mk; suzanadk@pmf.ukim.mk

B. Miova (✉)
CIBERehd—Department of Pharmacology, University of Valencia, Valencia, Spain
e-mail: bmiova@pmf.ukim.mk

© The Author(s), under exclusive license to Springer Nature Switzerland AG 2023

D. Avtanski, L. Poretsky (eds.), *Obesity, Diabetes and Inflammation*, Contemporary Endocrinology, https://doi.org/10.1007/978-3-031-39721-9_4

FFA	Free fatty acid
FMN	Flavin mononucleotide
GAPDH	Glyceraldehyde-3-phosphate dehydrogenase
GLUT4	Glucose transporter type 4
GPx	Glutathione peroxidase
GR	Glutathione reductase
GSH	Glutathione
HbA1c	Glycosylated hemoglobin
HMOX1	heme oxygenase 1 (*s.* HO-1)
NQO1	NAD(P)H dehydrogenase quinone 1
IR	Insulin resistance
IRE1α	Inositol-requiring enzyme 1 alpha
JNK	c-Jun N-terminal kinase
MafA	Musculoaponeurotic fibrosarcoma protein A
MAPK	Mitogen-activated protein kinase
Mfn	Mitofusin
mTORC1	Mammalian (*s.* mechanistic) target of rapamycin complex 1
mtROS	Mitochondrial reactive oxygen species
NF-κB	Nuclear factor kappa B
NOX	NADPH oxidase
NQO1	NAD(P)H dehydrogenase quinone 1
OS	Oxidative stress
OXPHOS	Oxidative phosphorylation
PARP	Poly(ADP) ribose polymerase
PBMC	Peripheral blood mononuclear cells
PDX1	Pancreatic and duodenal homeobox 1
PERK	Protein kinase RNA-like endoplasmic reticulum kinase
PGC-1α	Peroxisome proliferator-activated receptor gamma coactivator 1 alpha
PI3K	Phosphatidylinositol-3 kinase
PKB	Protein kinase B
PKC	Protein kinase C
PKR	Protein kinase RNA-like
PPARγ	Peroxisome proliferator-activated receptor gamma
RNS	Reactive nitrogen species
ROS	Reactive oxygen species
SOD	Superoxide dismutase
T2DM	Type 2 diabetes mellitus
TBARS	Thiobarbituric acid reactive substances
TCA	Tricarboxylic acid
UCP2	Uncoupling protein 2
UPR	Unfolded protein response
WAT	White adipose tissue
XBP1	X-box binding protein 1

Introduction

Obesity and type 2 diabetes mellitus (T2DM) are currently the most common metabolic disorders worldwide, growing rapidly in prevalence and representing some of the major public health challenges of the twenty-first century.

A large number of epidemiological studies have provided strong evidence that the increasing prevalence of obesity is closely associated with T2DM [1–3]. These two conditions affect people of all ages and may manifest early in life, as is the case of childhood obesity. Both are influenced by a number of factors, including the shift to massive urbanization, sedentary lifestyles, and high-caloric diets [4], which is why some experts denominate this dual epidemic "diabesity" [5].

According to the World Health Organization (WHO), obesity is "abnormal or excessive fat accumulation that presents a risk to health" with a body mass index (BMI) $\geq$ 30 kg/m^2 [6], while the World Obesity Federation (WOF) considers it a progressive, relapsing, and chronic disease [7]. Rates of obesity are increasing dramatically worldwide, with 700 million persons expected to be affected by 2045, thus posing an enormous public health burden worldwide. Obesity may be an inheritable disease, and genetic variations of several genes, such as MC4R and PCSK1, have been described as risk factors for high BMI and obesity [8]. Diabetes mellitus (DM) is a chronic metabolic disorder that manifests through major defects in a complete absence of insulin synthesis, secretion, and/or activity. Type 1 DM is an autoimmune disorder that affects pancreatic β-cells and results in a deficient or complete lack of insulin synthesis/secretion. In contrast, type 2 DM is characterized by high, low, or normal insulin secretion but is manifested by a major decrease in insulin activity, including a reduced capacity of β-cells to take up glucose and regulate insulin secretion via modulation of the activity of insulin receptors [9].

As a metabolic disorder itself, obesity is an important risk factor for T2DM and accounts for 80–85% of the risk of an individual developing it. A linear relationship between BMI and T2DM has been highlighted by a number of studies [10, 11], and the risk of T2DM is known to rise when BMI exceeds 23 [12]. According to a new systematic evaluation of 18 weight-related disorders, diabetes tops the list of risks. Men and women with BMI $\geq$ 30 kg/m^2 had a seven-fold and a 12-fold increased risk of developing T2DM, respectively, compared to those in normal weight ranges (BMI $\leq$ 25 kg/m^2) [13]. Thus, even though not all people with T2DM are obese, and many obese people do not have diabetes, the majority of people with T2DM are overweight or obese.

A common denominator in the underlying pathophysiology of T2DM and obesity is insulin resistance (IR), a reduced biological response to insulin in peripheral tissues such as the liver, adipose tissue, and skeletal muscle. **Mitochondrial dysfunction, endoplasmic reticulum (ER) stress, and DNA damage, which are tightly connected with alterations in the cellular and subcellular reduction-oxidation (redox) balance/oxidative stress,** are some of the pathogenic mechanisms in both obesity and DM. The aim of this chapter is to describe the link between oxidative stress and the development of both obesity and DM.

Oxidative Stress

Oxidative stress (OS), a concept introduced into biomedical research 30 years ago, is generally defined as "an imbalance between oxidants and antioxidants in favor of the former, leading to a disruption of redox signaling and control, and/or molecular damage" [14]. Physiological OS is low-level OS and plays a role in fundamental cellular functions through redox signaling and regulation, while it also participates in cellular mechanisms of self-defense. Indeed, oxidant molecules are released by numerous cellular processes such as cell respiration (mitochondria), lipid synthesis, metal metabolism, lysosomal activity, phagocytosis, and biotransformation of xenobiotics. In contrast, supraphysiological oxidative challenge (oxidative distress) leads to severe disruption of redox signaling and produces different forms of oxidative damage in the macromolecules. OS is believed to play an important role in the normal aging process, as well as in the pathogenesis of virtually all chronic diseases, including cardiovascular disease, cancer, liver injury, neurodegenerative diseases, immune dysfunction, and DM. Although the term OS has been overused and criticized for oversimplifying understanding, it remains relevant given the implicit association of stress with adaptive responses [14].

Reactive oxygen species (ROS) are short-living products of the cellular aerobic metabolism, the majority of which are free radicals, i.e., molecules that contain one or more unpaired electrons in their outer orbital. Major ROS are superoxide anion ($\bullet O_2^-$), hydrogen peroxide (H_2O_2), and hydroxyl radical ($\bullet OH$). Nitric oxide (NO), a free radical itself, is an important signaling molecule that regulates multiple processes, including hemodynamics (as it regulates the vascular tone), the process of leukocyte adhesion, platelet aggregation, and angiogenesis. NO and $\bullet O_2^-$ can combine and produce a very reactive intermediate peroxynitrite ($\bullet ONOO^-$), which is a member of the so-called reactive nitrogen species (RNS) [15].

Excessive ROS production is neutralized by antioxidant systems, which can be classified as enzymatic and non-enzymatic. The latter includes numerous exogenous (natural or synthetic) or endogenous compounds that remove/scavenge free radicals or their precursors or act by inhibiting the formation of ROS by binding to the metal ions needed for the catalysis of ROS generation. Natural small-molecular weight antioxidants include glutathione (GSH), arginine, citrulline, taurine, creatine, uric acid, selenium, zinc, vitamin E, vitamin C, and vitamin A, among others. These antioxidant defenses are further bolstered by antioxidant enzymes, including superoxide dismutase (SOD), catalase (CAT), NAD(P)H dehydrogenase quinone 1 (NQO1), heme oxygenase (decycling) 1 (HMOX1, formerly HO-1), and the GSH system, which has several components that possess synergistic actions, such as glutathione-S-transferase, glutathione reductase (GR), and glutathione peroxidase (GPx).

Oxidative challenge triggers a stress response, implemented through molecular redox switches that initiate the activation of defense system gene expression. Major "master regulators" are Nrf2/Keap1 and NF-κB/IκB. Related responses include a variety of cellular repair and/or removal programs, such as hypoxia-induced response, the heat shock response, the unfolded protein response (UPR), and autophagy [15].

Mitochondrial reactive oxygen species (mtROS) produced by the respiratory chain during the process of oxidative phosphorylation (OXPHOS) are considered the main portion of free radicals in most cell types [16]. Shortly after cellular production of H_2O_2 in normal aerobic metabolism in intact cells was established, isolated mitochondria were identified as its major source, predominantly via one-electron reduction of molecular oxygen to $\bullet O_2^-$ (0.2–2.0% of the molecular oxygen consumed by mitochondria) and its subsequent dismutation to H_2O_2 by mitochondrial and cytosolic SOD [15] as depicted in Fig.4.1. In mitochondria isolated from rat skeletal muscle, 11 different sites at which electrons can leak to produce ROS have been described [17]; however, the sites themselves and the amounts of mtROS produced at each of these sites is a highly controversial question, and the answers depend on the experimental conditions used. Most research points to the flavin mononucleotide (FMN) site and CoQ binding site of complex I, and to the Q cycle of complex III at the electron transport chain (ETC), as the predominant sources of mitochondrial $\bullet O_2^-$ generation [18].

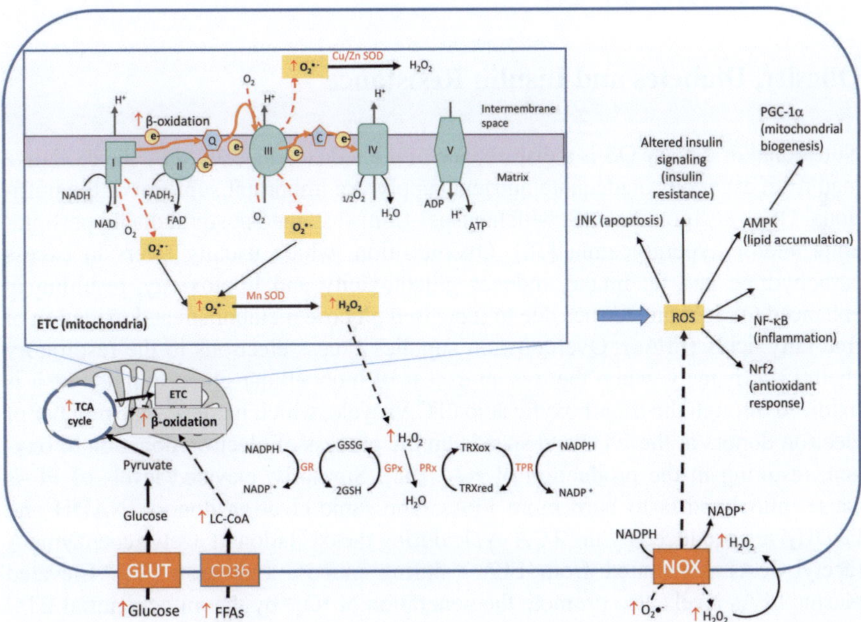

Fig. 4.1 Elevated glucose and free fatty acids (FFAs) promote the TCA cycle and β-oxidation in mitochondria. This leads to increased production of ROS through the mitochondrial electron transport chain (ETC). Moreover, the increased levels of NADPH derived from glycolysis cause an increase in the activity of NOX enzymes which contribute to ROS generation. In such conditions, the primary antioxidant cellular defense (enzymatic and non-enzymatic) is overwhelmed, and the excess amount of ROS is accumulated in the cell. Increased ROS promote antioxidant response through Nrf2 and PGC-1α pathway but also lead to insulin resistance, inflammation, and apoptosis

Besides the ETC, other sites in mitochondria may produce mtROS, specifically several enzymes [19]. Importantly, mtROS production is under direct and indirect regulation by a number of signaling pathways and processes, including Ca^{2+} influx, energy demand, redox status, hypoxia, inflammation, autophagy/mitophagy, mitochondrial biogenesis, and ER stress. In addition, other cellular compartments are also ROS producers, with NADPH oxidases (NOX) being among the most abundant sources. This plasma membrane-bound enzyme transfers electrons from NADPH to oxygen, thus generating $\bullet O_2^-$, which is, in turn, converted to H_2O_2 by SOD. Although the list of ROS sources is large and continues to grow, we need to bear in mind that when, how, and how much ROS are produced is highly determined by the context and cell type.

From a metabolic point of view, produced free radicals inhibit glyceraldehyde-3-phosphate dehydrogenase (GAPDH) and thereby redirect upstream metabolites into four alternative pathways: (1) glucose is shifted to the polyol pathway; (2) fructose-6-phosphate is shifted to the hexosamine pathway; (3) triose phosphates produce methylglyoxal, the main precursor of advanced glycation end-products (AGE); and (iv) dihydroxyacetone phosphate is converted to diacylglycerol, which activates the protein kinase C (PKC) pathway [20].

Obesity, Diabetes and Insulin Resistance

Nutritional or dietary OS is a disturbance of the redox state caused by the oxidative load from excess or inadequate nutrient supply. An important subform of the nutritional OS is postprandial OS, which ensues from sustained postprandial hyperlipidemia and/or hyperglycemia [16]. Overnutrition, which usually refers to excess carbohydrate and fat intake, induces glucotoxicity and lipotoxicity, resulting in enhanced OS in many tissues due to increased glucose metabolism and oxidation of free fatty acids (FFAs). Overnutrition supplies excess electrons to the respiratory chain [21]; namely, when there is an excess of intracellular glucose, much of it is oxidized through the tricarboxylic acid (TCA) cycle, which increases the number of electron donors at the ETC and speeds up the process of electron donation to oxygen, resulting in the production of $\bullet O_2^-$ [22]. Similarly, elevated levels of FFAs cause mitochondria to burn more FFAs. The same electron donors (NADH and $FADH_2$) are produced by the TCA cycle during the oxidation of acetyl-coenzyme A (acetyl-CoA) (generated from FFAs) during glucose oxidation [22]. Elevated plasma FFAs levels also promote the generation of $\bullet O_2^-$ by the mitochondrial ETC and stimulate the production of reactive intermediates through PKC-dependent activation of NOX, as seen in cultured vascular cells [23]. The presence of obesity considerably increases the amount of ROS involved in diabetes and its consequences [24].

The accumulation of AGEs, PKC activation, activation of the polyol pathway, and the hexosamine pathway are all thought to play a role in the tissue damage that occurs in diabetes [25]; however, it seems that all hyperglycemia-induced mechanisms are primarily activated by the overproduction of mtROS [22]. The increase in intracellular oxidative stress can promote PKCβ activation, and this alteration in PKCβ countenance is crucial for high-fat diet-induced obesity [26]. Numerous enzymatic cascades, including NOX, NO synthase, and xanthine oxidase, are activated by glucose metabolism, suggesting that glucose can directly increase ROS overproduction and activate these pathways [27].

Although many cell types are affected by overnutrition in relation to OS, for the sake of this chapter, two cell types will be mainly addressed: pancreatic β-cells and adipocytes. Abundant evidence from animal and epidemiological studies has shown that the nutritional environment in early life negatively impacts long-term β-cell function and increases the risk of diabetes, particularly in genetically susceptible individuals [28–30]. Pancreatic β-cells are particularly sensitive to prolonged elevations in circulating glucose and/or saturated FFAs. Thus, glucotoxicity and lipotoxicity are the major contributors to β-cell dysfunction in obesity and T2DM [22]. Specifically, β-cells undergoing glucolipotoxicity manifest pathological alterations, including decreased insulin content and glucose-stimulated insulin secretion [31]. Among other effects, this occurs through the diminished activity of two key transcriptional factors, musculoaponeurotic fibrosarcoma protein A (MafA) and pancreatic and duodenal homeobox 1 (PDX1), which bind to the promoter region of the insulin gene [32, 33].

Conversely, many studies have shown that β-cells are especially susceptible to redox imbalance, as they exhibit a relatively low expression of many antioxidant enzymes, including catalase and GPx, which makes them vulnerable to ROS-induced damage [34, 35]. Related to this, overexpression of catalase or GPx can reverse the detrimental effects of glucolipotoxicity and protect the β-cells [36, 37]. OS undermines β-cell function through different mechanisms; for example, $\bullet O_2^-$-induced activation of uncoupling protein 2 (UCP2) negatively regulates insulin secretion and has been proposed as a major link between obesity, β-cell dysfunction, and T2DM [38].

OS in obesity is caused by different factors, one of which is the presence of excessive white adipose tissue. In humans, white adipose tissue, a large and active endocrine organ implicated in energy storage, can account for 2–70% of total body weight [39]. Adipocytes are essential for the organism's metabolism since they secrete hormones and cytokines that affect the body's overall energy homeostasis [40]. When an excess of nutrients is consumed, fat builds up in the visceral and subcutaneous depots, enlarging them through hypertrophy and hyperplasia [41]. The chronic overproduction of FFAs and the dietary lipid deposition in overnutrition lead to lipotoxicity in the adipose tissue and ectopic fat deposition in myocytes, heart, liver, pancreas, and others [20, 42]. In adipose tissue, obesity can induce OS mainly via the catalytic activity of NOX and/or through dysfunctional OXPHOS [43, 44]. In adipocytes, ROS are mostly produced by NOX enzymes [45]. These enzymes exist in seven different isoforms widely expressed in various tissues. Two of them, NOX4 and NOX2, are predominantly expressed in adipocytes and macrophages, respectively, and play an important role in obesity-induced OS. It is to be noted that the source of the ROS might differ in the early, intermediate, and late stages of obesity [44]. Some studies have demonstrated that, in contrast to NOX-derived ROS, which characterizes the early stages of obesity, mtROS production is related to the late stages of obesity [44]. In the early stages of obesity, NOX4 in adipocytes is actively producing ROS, which provokes the onset of IR and initiates the recruitment of immune cells in adipose tissue. In the intermediate stages of obesity, IR and inflammation in the adipose tissue are worsened by NOX2-derived ROS from infiltrating immune cells. Finally, in the late stages of obesity, inflammation and IR in adipose tissue are maintained by mtROS from adipocytes. NOXs are expressed in the pancreatic islets of both humans and mice and are associated with a higher OS in the T2DM animal model [46].

Animal models of obesity not only display accumulation of excessive fat in white adipose tissue (WAT) but also show increased lipid peroxidation in the adipocytes, with increased NOX activity and decreased mRNA expression or activity of antioxidant enzymes SOD, CAT, and GPx [47]. Moreover, as a major non-enzymatic antioxidant, GSH accumulates in hypertrophied adipose tissue as a result of decreased GPx activity and increased expression of GSH synthetase, which is a key GSH-generating enzyme [48]. Although GSH is an antioxidant, excessive GSH levels undermine insulin's action in adipocytes and may be involved in the development of IR in obesity. Conversely, insulin additionally inhibits GPx activity, which causes adipocytes to store more GSH [48]. Chronically elevated intracellular ROS levels in adipocytes following mitochondrial dysfunction lead to IR by weakening insulin signaling [49].

The abovementioned alterations have been linked not only to defects in bioenergetics and metabolism in adipose tissue but also to the secretion of adipokines (such as leptin, adiponectin, visfatin, resistin, and apelin) and many other inflammatory mediators [50]. All these factors contribute to the development of chronic low-grade inflammation, a characteristic feature of many metabolic diseases, including obesity and diabetes. ROS production is stimulated by adipokines under physiological conditions and, even more so, under pathological situations in which ROS are produced in large, supraphysiological amounts, which in turn promotes the synthesis of adipokines [51] Leptin, which acts as an adipocyte-derived hormone, is regarded as a significant contributor to the OS caused by obesity [52]. It controls energy expenditure and is well known to be a major mediator of the proinflammatory state in obese individuals [53]. Namely, when leptin levels are increased, both human endothelial cells and the endothelium of obese mice display OS [54]. For leptin-induced OS, two potential pathways have been proposed: (1) the stimulation of FFA oxidation in the mitochondria [55] and (2) increased levels of proinflammatory cytokines [56]. Leptin is considered a crucial mediator of OS in obese diabetic subjects that correlates strongly with malondialdehyde (MDA) (a product of lipid peroxidation) levels in T2DM subjects [57]. It was reported that leptin levels in diabetic patients were either the same or lower compared to non-diabetic patients, whereas they were much greater in obese patients [57, 58].

Besides pancreatic and adipose tissue, both T2DM and obesity are characterized by IR in major metabolic tissues such as skeletal muscle and liver. The two characteristics of IR are reduced insulin sensitivity and lower rates of glucose absorption and utilization [59]. As mentioned previously, during obesity and overnutrition, excess nutrients are stored as lipids in adipose tissues and ectopic fat in many organs. This process enhances ROS production and causes a state of proinflammation [60]. Namely, T2DM is characterized by elevated blood glucose levels, an effect closely related to IR [24]. T2DM patients also display elevated pancreatic triglyceride content [61, 62], which also causes IR and impaired insulin secretion [63]. Finally, obesity-induced chronic inflammation greatly contributes to the development of IR.

One of the major issues in the management of T2DM patients is that the onset of T2DM does not present with specific acute symptoms, and many adults with T2DM do not know that they have the disease. In this fundamental stage of the pathogenesis denominated prediabetes, IR persists, while individuals display glucose levels that are only slightly above the normal values [64]. The relationship between obesity and abnormal serum glycemic levels suggests that diabetes develops along a "continuum" that includes changes in insulin signaling, modifications to glucose transport, and the malfunctioning of pancreatic cells, as well as increased OS and inflammation [65].

Numerous investigations have revealed a link between ROS and insulin activity [48, 66–68]. Excessive and prolonged exposure to ROS impairs insulin action, disrupts glucose metabolism [69], and promotes protein oxidation and carbonylation [70]. One of these carbonylated proteins is the glucose transporter type 4 (GLUT4), whose carbonylation is likely to impair insulin-stimulated glucose uptake. The diminished insulin response caused by ROS affects signaling pathways, including the activation of phosphatidylinositol-3 kinase (PI3K) and protein kinase B (PKB)/ Akt, as well as the process of lipogenesis. This attenuation can be related to the activation of stress signals by OS, including nuclear factor kappa B (NF-κB), c-Jun N-terminal kinase (JNK), p38 mitogen-activated protein kinase (MAPK), and specific isoforms of PKC [66–68]. Moreover, the formation of ROS caused by insulin is mediated by NOX [21].

In addition, although GSH is a primary antioxidant, excessive GSH decreases insulin action in adipocytes [48] and may be a cause of IR in obesity. There is an overaccumulation of GSH in hypertrophied adipose tissue as a result of decreased GPx function and increased expression of GSH synthetase, a crucial GSH-generating enzyme. Insulin additionally inhibits GPx function, which causes adipocytes to store more GSH [48]. IR, in turn, plays a key role in the pathogenesis of obesity-associated cardiometabolic complications, including metabolic syndrome components, T2DM, and cardiovascular diseases.

Key Molecular Mechanisms of Obesity, IR and DM Include Mitochondrial Dysfunction, ER Stress and ROS-Induced DNA Damage, which Are Closely Connected with the Major Cellular Disturbances Caused by OS

Mitochondrial Dysfunction

Obesity and excess consumption of nutrients are associated with mitochondrial dysfunction [71]. Indeed, impaired mitochondrial oxidative metabolism has been considered a molecular hallmark of adipose tissue in obesity [72]. A decline in mitochondrial function is also frequently observed in adipose tissue from T2DM patients and animal models of diabetes [73–75]. In addition to adipose tissue, the liver and muscles are involved in high-energy processes that require large amounts of nutrients, such as glucose and lipids, and are sites of much of the mitochondrial dysfunction that characterizes obese people. The aforementioned mitochondrial dysfunction manifests in damaged mtDNA, undermined synthesis of ATP, enhanced ROS generation, presence of OS, and triggering apoptosis [76]. This enhances the process of mitophagy, which removes dysfunctional mitochondria [42]. However, a mitophagy-mediated decrease in the number of mitochondria is sometimes related to reduced energy expenditure. This can further enhance lipid accumulation in excess overnutrition, induce lipotoxicity, and trigger mitochondria-mediated cell apoptosis [77].

Numerous investigations have shown that DM (both insulin-deficient and insulin-resistant states) and obesity inevitably result in mitochondrial disturbances (Fig. 4.2). Although "mitochondrial dysfunction" is a term that is frequently used in this context, it is important to bear in mind the evidence of disturbances of many aspects, such as mitochondrial biogenesis, number, shape, and dynamics, including fusion and fission [78]. Fission, required for distribution and networking, and fusion, required for mixing the mitochondrial genome, occur under physiological conditions in the cell. Two isoforms of mitofusin, mitofusin 1 and 2 (Mfn1 and Mfn2), employed as fusion markers have been found to be diminished in obesity in both humans and rodents [79], and their expression is dramatically downregulated in adipose tissue of high-fat diet-fed mice compared to those fed a conventional diet [80]. Similar findings have been reported in obese T2DM patients [79, 81]. The generation of ROS often correlates with the structure of the mitochondrial reticulum. It is known to be fragmented by high glucose availability, which may be related to enhanced ROS signaling [82]. Individuals with obesity and/or T2DM have considerably smaller and shorter skeletal muscle mitochondria with lower mitochondrial density per unit of volume than those in lean controls, and their size corresponds to whole-body insulin sensitivity [83]. This alteration of mitochondrial size and morphology results from increased mitochondrial fission, which is linked to diminished mitochondrial mass and function and IR [84, 85]. Similarly, in blood mononuclear cells from DM patients, mitochondria have been shown to be smaller, more

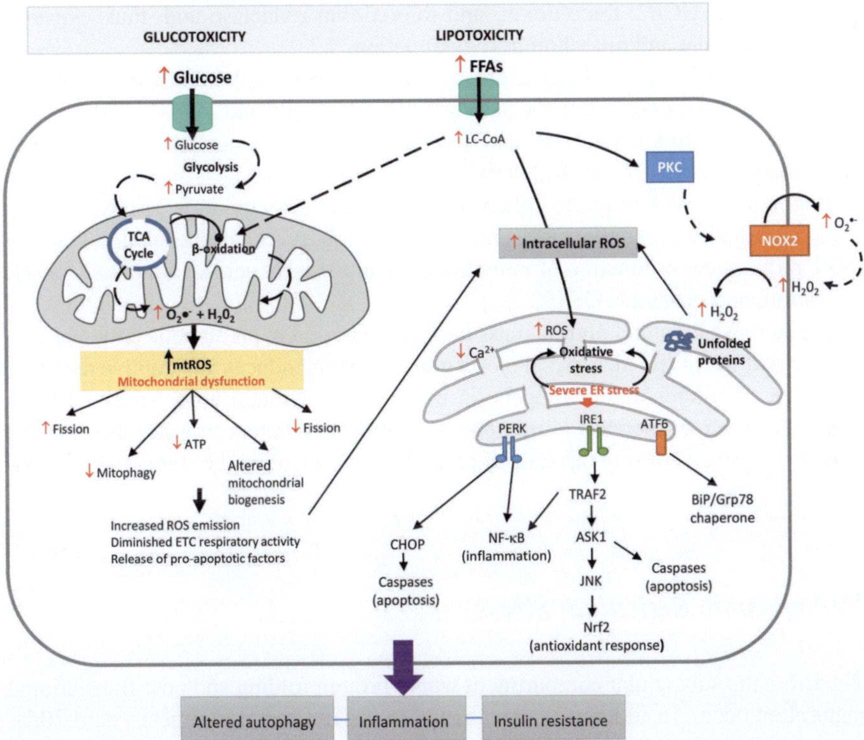

Fig. 4.2 In both obesity and T2DM, hyperglycemia and hyperlipidemia promote both mitochondrial dysfunction and ER stress. Dysfunctional mitochondria display disrupted morphology and appear swollen and fragmented compared to healthy mitochondria. These alterations coincide with an impaired respiratory capacity (e.g., decreased mitochondrial ETC complex activity) that results in diminished ATP production, increased mitochondrial ROS emissions, and the release of mitochondria-derived proapoptotic factors. The endoplasmic reticulum (ER) is a key determinant of pancreatic β-cell function or failure. Sustained/unresolved ER stress leads to proapoptotic signaling, inflammation, and activation of cell death pathways involving the PERK and IRE1 branches of the UPR. The IRE1-TRAF2-apoptosis signaling kinase 1 (ASK1) complex upregulates c-Jun N-terminal kinase (JNK) and activates several caspases and, through splicing of X-box binding protein 1 (XBP1) can activate CCAAT-enhancer-binding protein (C/EBP) homologous protein (CHOP), a proapoptotic transcription factor. In addition, the ATF6 branch activates glucose level-responsive protein Grp78/BiP, a critical ER chaperone which is promptly upregulated upon ER stress

spherical, and to occupy a less cellular area, while mitochondrial $\bullet O_2^-$ production is higher [86].

In experimental models of diabetes and obesity, mitochondrial biogenesis is reduced [87]. The peroxisome proliferator-activated receptor gamma (PPARγ) coactivator, also known as PGC-1α transcriptional coactivator, is crucial for the control of mitochondrial biogenesis [88–90]. Specifically, PGC-1α regulates the expression of genes encoding mitochondrial antioxidants, such as SOD, catalase, peroxiredoxin, UCP2, thioredoxin, and thioredoxin reductase and, thus, prevents oxidative damage and mitochondrial dysfunction.

Generally, PGC-1α is highly expressed in tissues with high-energy demands, and its defects are associated with the pathogeneses of obesity and T2DM. Additionally, there is a strong link between IR and mitochondrial dysfunction, accompanied by a large decline in PGC-1 mRNA levels [91].

In conditions of low-grade inflammation, there is dysregulation or low levels of PGC-1α, which further alters mitochondrial function, promotes the accumulation of ROS, reduces the production of mitochondrial antioxidant genes, stimulates NF-κB activation, and promotes OS [92, 93]

An increase in mitochondrial mass has been reported in prediabetic patients, suggesting that the initial increase in blood glucose levels induces an adaptive response of increased mitochondrial biogenesis in order to maintain homeostasis. This is associated with an increase in mitophagy, hinting that compromised mitochondria may be eliminated during the state of prediabetes in an attempt to reduce mitochondrial OS [64].

Endoplasmic Reticulum Stress

The ER is the subcellular compartment where protein folding and post-translational maturation occur. In addition, it plays crucial roles in lipid biosynthesis, detoxification, energy metabolism, Ca^{2+} homeostasis, and redox balance. Protein folding/maturation in the ER is highly sensitive to altered homeostasis (Ca^{2+} content, glycosylation, energy stores, redox state, metabolic and inflammatory challenges), and it is subjected to "quality control" mechanisms that ensure only properly folded proteins exit the ER [94, 95].

The processes of glucolipotoxicity are intrinsically linked to the function of the ER (Fig. 4.2). During obesity and overnutrition, there is an accumulation of high quantities of membrane fatty acids and cholesterol, which alters the membrane structure, which, together with other pathogenic factors, results in the production of unfolded/misfolded proteins and, consequently, ER stress [96]. ER stress is a fundamental molecular mechanism of glucolipotoxicity in β-cells [97] and is believed to be a major factor in the emergence of metabolic disorders linked to obesity [77].

Altered ER function triggers the unfolded protein response (UPR), an attempt to reestablish ER homeostasis. When the three branches of the UPR (inositol-requiring enzyme 1α (IRE1α), protein kinase RNA-like (PKR) endoplasmic reticulum kinase (PERK), and activating transcription factor 6α (ATF6α)) fail to correct the altered proteostasis, ER stress occurs [98, 99]. As a result, many stress pathways are activated, leading to a malfunction or cell death. GRP78/BiP is an ER chaperone protein that activates the UPR. In unstressed cells, GRP78/BiP binds to the ER luminal domains of the ER stress sensors IRE1α, PERK, and ATF-6 and maintains them in an inactivated state. During ER stress, BiP preferentially binds to unfolded and misfolded proteins and dissociates from the transmembrane sensors, facilitating their activation [100]. The activation of ER stress in hepatocytes is associated with enhanced lipid accumulation through the mammalian target of rapamycin complex 1 (mTORC1) pathway. Conversely, AMPK activation prevents excess nutrient-induced hepatic lipid accumulation by inhibiting mTORC1 signaling and ER stress response [77].

In general, an altered redox state in the ER and the cell has a direct negative impact on ER function [101]. ER stress and OS have been shown to be strongly correlated and to accentuate each other in a positive feed-forward loop, which impedes normal cell function and ultimately activates proapoptotic signaling. ER stress and OS are linked through multiple pathways, of which NOX enzymes are pivotal [102].

Functional ER is paramount for β-cells through its role in insulin synthesis, and therefore ER stress plays a fundamental part in DM pathogenesis [98]. In these cells, components of the UPR have a dual role, acting as helpful regulators under physiological circumstances or as promoters of dysfunction and cell death in response to prolonged stress [103]. Additionally, ER stress is activated in a number of other tissues when T2DM and obesity are present [103, 104]. ER stress also results in chronic inflammation, as seen in mouse adipose tissue and the liver [105, 106].

Finally, the function of ER and that of mitochondria are closely coupled and tightly regulate each other in both directions. For instance, ER stress can cause mitochondrial dysfunction and increase mitochondrial ROS production. Hepatocytes in obese animals display increased amounts of Ca^{2+} that are transported from the ER to the mitochondria through the mitochondria-associated ER membranes. This results in Ca^{2+} overload, mitochondrial malfunction, and activation of the ER stress signaling pathway [107].

ROS-Induced DNA Damage

Hyperglycemia-induced overproduction of ROS causes DNA damage, such as single-strand and double-strand breaks. Oxidative damage of macromolecules, including DNA, has been widely described for both obesity and DM in relation to altered kinetics of DNA repair factors and enhanced OS. Biochemical parameters of OS (CAT and thiobarbituric acid reactive substances (TBARS)) in peripheral blood mononuclear cells (PBMCs) from prediabetic and diabetic patients were revealed to display increased sensitivity to an ex vivo treatment with thyroid hormone T3, a molecule that accelerates oxidative metabolism and ROS production, thereby worsening diabetes. PBMCs from obese patients reacted in the same manner, except for DNA damage [108]. Serum 8-hydroxy-2′–deoxyguanosine (8-OHdG) is already increased in prediabetes, suggesting that oxidative DNA damage is present when there is even a minor elevation of blood glucose levels. The statistically significant positive correlation between serum 8-OHdG and BMI in the diabetic group indicated that obesity has an additive effect on increased blood glucose levels, thus contributing to oxidative DNA damage [108]. In diabetes, an inactive state of poly(ADP)ribose polymerase (PARP) (particularly for double-strand DNA breaks repair) is associated with persistent DNA damage signaling [109].

In mouse models of DM, hyperglycemia-coupled ROS production has been associated with a compromised DNA repair system and persistent DNA damage in the pancreas [110]. Moreover, compared to healthy controls, DNA repair capacity in T2DM patients is reported to be lower [111, 112], and DNA repair genes are downregulated [113]. Xavier et al. [114] observed induced expression of genes representing DNA repair in PBMCs of T2DM subjects with higher glycosylated hemoglobin (HbA1c) levels compared to those with lower levels of HbA1c. This effect was interpreted as a compensatory mechanism against DNA damage which is enhanced in the high-HbA1c group. Furthermore, peripheral blood leukocytes of subjects with diabetes present higher levels of DNA damage than age- and sex-matched healthy controls in male and female patients with no gender differences. Of note, DNA damage was higher in untreated patients but was not significantly different in those treated with oral antidiabetic medications (metformin and/or sulfonylureas). A correlation analysis revealed a significant association of waist circumference (central adiposity) with DNA damage index [115].

In summary, various pathophysiological metabolic factors in DM and obesity can cause DNA damage, a hallmark of both diseases. OS is probably the main mediator of DNA damage accumulation in DM and obesity and occurs both as a result of inhibited antioxidant capacity and downregulated DNA damage-repair machinery.

Conclusions

Currently, T2DM and obesity are the most common metabolic diseases worldwide. Insulin resistance, one of the main causes of disturbances of glucose homeostasis, is the main common denominator of the two diseases. Long-term exposure to high levels of blood glucose and increased fatty acid content can lead to a number of cellular and molecular changes in the body, including changes in mitochondria and overload of the electron transport chain, leading to the overproduction of ROS and mitochondrial dysfunction. Furthermore, the imbalance between the prooxidant and antioxidant defense system leads to conditions of oxidative stress, where the reactive molecules cause damage to lipids, proteins, and nucleic acids. DNA repair levels and the activity of antioxidant enzymes are reduced in DM. Insulin resistance and increased oxidative stress have also been associated with several stress response pathways, including inflammation and ER stress.

Acknowledgments The authors thank Brian Normanly for his English language editing. Conflict of Interest StatementThe authors declare the absence of any commercial or financial relationships that could be construed as a potential conflict of interest.

Funding This work was funded by the Institute of Health Carlos III in Spain (CIBER CB06/04/0071), Spanish Ministry of Science and Innovation (grant ref.

PID2021-127945OB-I00, co-funded by the European Union-FEDER 10.13039/501100011033), Generalitat Valenciana (grant ref. AICO/2021/017), and FISABIO (Foundation for the Promotion of Health and Biomedical Research in the Valencian Region, grant ref. UGP-21-236).

References

1. Bueter M, Ashrafian H, le Roux CW. Mechanisms of weight loss after gastric bypass and gastric banding. Obes Facts. 2009;2:325–31.
2. Bueter M, le Roux CW. Gastrointestinal hormones, energy balance and bariatric surgery. Int J Obes. 2011;35(3):S35–9.
3. Stefanović A, Kotur-Stevuljević J, Spasić S, Bogavac-Stanojević N, Bujisić N. The influence of obesity on the oxidative stress status and the concentration of leptin in type 2 diabetes mellitus patients. Diabetes Res Clin Pract. 2008;79:156–63.
4. Cerf ME. Beta cell physiological dynamics and dysfunctional transitions in response to islet inflammation in obesity and diabetes. Meta. 2020;10:452.
5. Kalra S, Arora S, Kapoor N. Lipokathexis: a fat paradox. J Pak Med Assoc. 2022;72:991–2.
6. Ulijaszek SJ. Obesity: preventing and managing the global epidemic. Report of a who consultation. Who technical report series 894. Pp. 252. (World Health Organization, Geneva, 2000.) SFR 56.00, ISBN 92-4-120894-5, paperback. J Biosoc Sci. 2003;35:624–5.
7. Bray GA, Kim KK, Wilding JPH. Obesity: a chronic relapsing progressive disease process. A position statement of the world obesity federation. Obes Rev. 2017;18:715–23.
8. Hofker M, Wijmenga C. A supersized list of obesity genes. Nat Genet. 2009;41:139–40.
9. Ramachandran A, Snehalatha C, Nanditha A. Classification and diagnosis of diabetes. In: Textbook of diabetes. Hoboken, NJ: Wiley; 2016. p. 23–8.
10. Schienkiewitz A, Schulze MB, Hoffmann K, Kroke A, Boeing H. Body mass index history and risk of type 2 diabetes: results from the European prospective investigation into cancer and nutrition (epic)–potsdam study. Am J Clin Nutr. 2006;84:427–33.
11. Chan JM, Rimm EB, Colditz GA, Stampfer MJ, Willett WC. Obesity, fat distribution, and weight gain as risk factors for clinical diabetes in men. Diabetes Care. 1994;17:961–9.
12. Goldiz G, Willett W, Stampfer M, Manson J, Hennekens C, Arky R, Speizer F. Weight as a risk factor for clinical diabetes in women. Am J Epidemiol. 1990;132:501–13.
13. Guh DP, Zhang W, Bansback N, Amarsi Z, Birmingham CL, Anis AH. The incidence of co-morbidities related to obesity and overweight: a systematic review and meta-analysis. BMC Public Health. 2009;9:88.
14. Sies H. Oxidative stress: introductory remarks. In: Oxidative stress. Amsterdam: Elsevier; 1985. p. 1–8.
15. Sies H. Oxidative eustress and oxidative distress: introductory remarks. In: Oxidative stress. Amsterdam: Elsevier; 2020. p. 3–12.
16. Scialò F, Fernández-Ayala DJ, Sanz A. Role of mitochondrial reverse electron transport in ROS signaling: potential roles in health and disease. Front Physiol. 2017;8:428.
17. Brand MD. Mitochondrial generation of superoxide and hydrogen peroxide as the source of mitochondrial redox signaling. Free Radic Biol Med. 2016;100:14–31.
18. Tahara EB, Navarete FDT, Kowaltowski AJ. Tissue-, substrate-, and site-specific characteristics of mitochondrial reactive oxygen species generation. Free Radic Biol Med. 2009;46:1283–97.
19. Lambert AJ, Brand MD. Reactive oxygen species production by mitochondria. Methods Mol Biol. 2009;554:165–81.

20. Eckel N, Li Y, Kuxhaus O, Stefan N, Hu FB, Schulze MB. Transition from metabolic healthy to unhealthy phenotypes and association with cardiovascular disease risk across BMI categories in 90 257 women (the nurses' health study): 30 year follow-up from a prospective cohort study. Lancet Diabet Endocrinol. 2018;6:714–24.
21. Masschelin PM, Cox AR, Chernis N, Hartig SM. The impact of oxidative stress on adipose tissue energy balance. Front Physiol. 2020;10:1638.
22. Brownlee M. The pathobiology of diabetic complications. Diabetes. 2005;54(6):1615–25.
23. Inoguchi T, Li P, Umeda F, et al. High glucose level and free fatty acid stimulate reactive oxygen species production through protein kinase C-dependent activation of NAD(P)H oxidase in cultured vascular cells. Diabetes. 2000;49:1939–45.
24. Rother KI. Diabetes treatment — bridging the divide. N Engl J Med. 2007;356:1499–501.
25. Evans JL, Goldfine ID, Maddux BA, Grodsky GM. Oxidative stress and stress-activated signaling pathways: a unifying hypothesis of type 2 diabetes. Endocr Rev. 2002;23:599–622.
26. Nijhawan P, Behl T, Arora S. Role of protein kinase C in obesity. Obes Med. 2020;18:100207.
27. Dludla P, Nkambule B, Jack B, Mkandla Z, Mutize T, Silvestri S, Orlando P, Tiano L, Louw J, Mazibuko-Mbeje S. Inflammation and oxidative stress in an obese state and the protective effects of gallic acid. Nutrients. 2018;11(1):23.
28. Glavas MM, Hui Q, Tudurí E, Erener S, Kasteel NL, Johnson JD, Kieffer TJ. Early overnutrition reduces PDX1 expression and induces β cell failure in Swiss Webster mice. Sci Rep. 2019;9(1):3619.
29. Dörner G, Plagemann A. Perinatal hyperinsulinism as possible predisposing factor for diabetes mellitus, obesity and enhanced cardiovascular risk in later life. Horm Metab Res. 1994;26:213–21.
30. Whincup P, Kaye S, Owen C, et al. Birth weight and risk of type 2 diabetes. A systematic review. JAMA. 2008;300(24):2886–97.
31. Hou N, Torii S, Saito N, Hosaka M, Takeuchi T. Reactive oxygen species-mediated pancreatic β-cell death is regulated by interactions between stress-activated protein kinases, p38 and c-Jun N-terminal kinase, and mitogen-activated protein kinase phosphatases. Endocrinology. 2008;149:1654–65.
32. Harmon JS, Stein R, Robertson RP. Oxidative stress-mediated, post-translational loss of mafa protein as a contributing mechanism to loss of insulin gene expression in glucotoxic beta cells. J Biol Chem. 2005;280:11107–13.
33. Cnop M, Abdulkarim B, Bottu G, et al. RNA sequencing identifies dysregulation of the human pancreatic islet transcriptome by the saturated fatty acid palmitate. Diabetes. 2014;63:1978–93.
34. Tiedge M, Lortz S, Drinkgern J, Lenzen S. Relation between antioxidant enzyme gene expression and antioxidative defense status of insulin-producing cells. Diabetes. 1997;46:1733–42.
35. Pi J, Bai Y, Zhang Q, et al. Reactive oxygen species as a signal in glucose-stimulated insulin secretion. Diabetes. 2007;56:1783–91.
36. Tanaka Y, Tran PO, Harmon J, Robertson RP. A role for glutathione peroxidase in protecting pancreatic β cells against oxidative stress in a model of glucose toxicity. Proc Natl Acad Sci. 2002;99:12363–8.
37. Gurgul E, Lortz S, Tiedge M, Anne J, Lenzen S. Mitochondrial catalase overexpression protects insulin-producing cells against toxicity of reactive oxygen species and proinflammatory cytokines. Diabetes. 2004;53:2271–80.
38. Zhang C-Y, Baffy G, Perret P, et al. Uncoupling protein-2 negatively regulates insulin secretion and is a major link between obesity, β cell dysfunction, and type 2 diabetes. Cell. 2001;105:745–55.
39. Rigamonti A, Brennand K, Lau F, Cowan CA. Rapid cellular turnover in adipose tissue. PLoS One. 2011;6(3):17637.
40. Frühbeck G, Gómez-Ambrosi J, Muruzábal FJ, Burrell MA. The adipocyte: a model for integration of endocrine and metabolic signaling in energy metabolism regulation. Am J Physiol Endocrinol Metab. 2001;280(6):E827–47.

41. Jo J, Gavrilova O, Pack S, Jou W, Mullen S, Sumner AE, Cushman SW, Periwal V. Hypertrophy and/or hyperplasia: dynamics of adipose tissue growth. PLoS Comput Biol. 2009;5(3):e1000324.
42. Ahmed B, Sultana R, Greene MW. Adipose tissue and insulin resistance in obese. Biomed Pharmacother. 2021;137:111315.
43. Dludla PV, Joubert E, Muller CJF, Louw J, Johnson R. Hyperglycemia-induced oxidative stress and heart disease-cardioprotective effects of rooibos flavonoids and phenylpyruvic acid-2-o-β-d-glucoside. Nutr Metab. 2017;14:45.
44. Han CY. Roles of reactive oxygen species on insulin resistance in adipose tissue. Diabetes Metab J. 2016;40:272.
45. Jankovic A, Korac A, Buzadzic B, Otasevic V, Stancic A, Daiber A, Korac B. Redox implications in adipose tissue (dys)function—a new look at old acquaintances. Redox Biol. 2015;6:19–32.
46. Li N, Li B, Brun T, Deffert-Delbouille C, Mahiout Z, Daali Y, Ma X-J, Krause K-H, Maechler P. NADPH oxidase NOX2 defines a new antagonistic role for reactive oxygen species and camp/PKA in the regulation of insulin secretion. Diabetes. 2012;61:2842–50.
47. Furukawa S, Fujita T, Shimabukuro M, Iwaki M, Yamada Y, Nakajima Y, Nakayama O, Makishima M, Matsuda M, Shimomura I. Increased oxidative stress in obesity and its impact on metabolic syndrome. J Clin Investig. 2004;114:1752–61.
48. Kobayashi H, Matsuda M, Fukuhara A, Komuro R, Shimomura I. Dysregulated glutathione metabolism links to impaired insulin action in adipocytes. Am J Physiol Endocrinol Metab. 2009;296(6):E1326–34.
49. Wang CH, Wang CC, Huang HC, Wei YH. Mitochondrial dysfunction leads to impairment of insulin sensitivity and adiponectin secretion in adipocytes. FEBS J. 2013;280:1039–50.
50. Marseglia L, Manti S, D'Angelo G, Nicotera A, Parisi E, Di Rosa G, Gitto E, Arrigo T. Oxidative stress in obesity: a critical component in human diseases. Int J Mol Sci. 2014;16:378–400.
51. Fernández-Sánchez A, Madrigal-Santillán E, Bautista M, Esquivel-Soto J, Morales-González Á, Esquivel-Chirino C, Durante-Montiel I, Sánchez-Rivera G, Valadez-Vega C, Morales-González JA. Inflammation, oxidative stress, and obesity. Int J Mol Sci. 2011;12:3117–32.
52. Korda M, Kubant R, Patton S, Malinski T. Leptin-induced endothelial dysfunction in obesity. Am J Phys Heart Circ Phys. 2008;295(4):H1514–21.
53. S-ichi Y, Edelstein D, X-liang D, Kaneda Y, Guzmán M, Brownlee M. Leptin induces mitochondrial superoxide production and monocyte chemoattractant protein-1 expression in aortic endothelial cells by increasing fatty acid oxidation via protein kinase a. J Biol Chem. 2001;276:25096–100.
54. Ajala OM, Ogunro PS, Elusanmi GF, Ogunyemi OE, Bolarinde AA. Changes in serum leptin during phases of menstrual cycle of fertile women: relationship to age groups and fertility. Int J Endocrinol Metabo. 2012;11(1):27–33.
55. Zhang H, Park Y, Wu J, Chen X, Lee S, Yang J, Dellsperger KC, Zhang C. Role of TNF-α in vascular dysfunction. Clin Sci. 2009;116:219–30.
56. Wannamethee SG, Tchernova J, Whincup P, Lowe GDO, Kelly A, Rumley A, Wallace AM, Sattar N. Plasma leptin: associations with metabolic, inflammatory and haemostatic risk factors for cardiovascular disease. Atherosclerosis. 2007;191:418–26.
57. Isaksen VT, Larsen MA, Goll R, Florholmen JR, Paulssen EJ. Hepatic steatosis, detected by hepatorenal index in ultrasonography, as a predictor of insulin resistance in obese subjects. BMC Obes. 2016;3:39.
58. Cruz MA, Cruz JF, Macena LB, Santana DS, Oliveira CC, Lima SO, Franca AV. Association of the nonalcoholic hepatic steatosis and its degrees with the values of liver enzymes and homeostasis model assessment-insulin resistance index. Gastroenterology Res. 2015;8:260–4.
59. Longo M, Zatterale F, Naderi J, Parrillo L, Formisano P, Raciti GA, Beguinot F, Miele C. Adipose tissue dysfunction as determinant of obesity-associated metabolic complications. Int J Mol Sci. 2019;20:2358.

60. Tushuizen ME, Bunck MC, Pouwels PJ, Bontemps S, van Waesberghe JH, Schindhelm RK, Mari A, Heine RJ, Diamant M. Pancreatic fat content and β-cell function in men with and without type 2 diabetes. Diabetes Care. 2007;30:2916–21.
61. van der Zijl NJ, Goossens GH, Moors CC, van Raalte DH, Muskiet MH, Pouwels PJ, Blaak EE, Diamant M. Ectopic fat storage in the pancreas, liver, and abdominal fat depots: impact on β-cell function in individuals with impaired glucose metabolism. J Clin Endocrinol Metab. 2011;96:459–67.
62. Heni M, Machann J, Staiger H, Schwenzer NF, Peter A, Schick F, Claussen CD, Stefan N, Häring H-U, Fritsche A. Pancreatic fat is negatively associated with insulin secretion in individuals with impaired fasting glucose and/or impaired glucose tolerance: a nuclear magnetic resonance study. Diabetes Metab Res Rev. 2010;26:200–5.
63. Bhansali S, Bhansali A, Walia R, Saikia UN, Dhawan V. Alterations in mitochondrial oxidative stress and mitophagy in subjects with prediabetes and type 2 diabetes mellitus. Front Endocrinol. 2017;8:347.
64. Paneni F, Costantino S, Cosentino F. Insulin resistance, diabetes, and cardiovascular risk. Curr Atheroscler Rep. 2014;13(2):1449–55.
65. Houstis N, Rosen ED, Lander ES. Reactive oxygen species have a causal role in multiple forms of insulin resistance. Nature. 2006;440:944–8.
66. Rudich A, Tirosh A, Potashnik R, Hemi R, Kanety H, Bashan N. Prolonged oxidative stress impairs insulin-induced GLUT4 translocation in 3T3-L1 adipocytes. Diabetes. 1998;47:1562–9.
67. Tirosh A, Potashnik R, Bashan N, Rudich A. Oxidative stress disrupts insulin-induced cellular redistribution of insulin receptor substrate-1 and phosphatidylinositol 3-kinase in 3T3-L1 adipocytes. J Biol Chem. 1999;274:10595–602.
68. Matsuda M, Shimomura I. Increased oxidative stress in obesity: implications for metabolic syndrome, diabetes, hypertension, dyslipidemia, atherosclerosis, and cancer. Obes Res Clin Pract. 2013;7(5):e330–41.
69. Mukai E, Fujimoto S, Inagaki N. Role of reactive oxygen species in glucose metabolism disorder in diabetic pancreatic β-cells. Biomolecules. 2022;12:1228.
70. de Mello AH, Costa AB, Engel JD, Rezin GT. Mitochondrial dysfunction in obesity. Life Sci. 2018;192:26–32.
71. Heinonen S, Buzkova J, Muniandy M, et al. Impaired mitochondrial biogenesis in adipose tissue in acquired obesity. Diabetes. 2015;64:3135–45.
72. Chattopadhyay M, Khemka VK, Chatterjee G, Ganguly A, Mukhopadhyay S, Chakrabarti S. Enhanced ROS production and oxidative damage in subcutaneous white adipose tissue mitochondria in obese and type 2 diabetes subjects. Mol Cell Biochem. 2014;399:95–103.
73. Choo H-J, Kim J-H, Kwon O-B, Lee CS, Mun JY, Han SS, Yoon Y-S, Yoon G, Choi K-M, Ko Y-G. Mitochondria are impaired in the adipocytes of type 2 diabetic mice. Diabetologia. 2006;49:784–91.
74. Laye MJ, Rector RS, Warner SO, Naples SP, Perretta AL, Uptergrove GM, Laughlin MH, Thyfault JP, Booth FW, Ibdah JA. Changes in visceral adipose tissue mitochondrial content with type 2 diabetes and daily voluntary wheel running in OLETF rats. J Physiol. 2009;587:3729–39.
75. Geto Z, Molla MD, Challa F, Belay Y, Getahun T. Mitochondrial dynamic dysfunction as a main triggering factor for inflammation associated chronic non-communicable diseases. J Inflamm Res. 2020;13:97–107.
76. McWilliams TG, Prescott AR, Montava-Garriga L, Ball G, Singh F, Barini E, Muqit MMK, Brooks SP, Ganley IG. Basal mitophagy occurs independently of PINK1 in mouse tissues of high metabolic demand. Cell Metab. 2018;27(2):439–49.
77. Sivitz WI, Yorek MA. Mitochondrial dysfunction in diabetes: from molecular mechanisms to functional significance and therapeutic opportunities. Antioxid Redox Signal. 2010;12:537–77.

78. Bach D, Pich S, Soriano FX, et al. Mitofusin-2 determines mitochondrial network architecture and mitochondrial metabolism. J Biol Chem. 2003;278:17190–7.
79. Mancini G, Pirruccio K, Yang X, Blüher M, Rodeheffer M, Horvath TL. Mitofusin 2 in mature adipocytes controls adiposity and body weight. Cell Rep. 2019;26(11):2849–58.
80. Bach D, Naon D, Pich S, et al. Expression of mfn2, the Charcot-Marie-Tooth neuropathy type 2A gene, in human skeletal muscle. Diabetes. 2005;54:2685–93.
81. Yu T, Robotham JL, Yoon Y. Increased production of reactive oxygen species in hyperglycemic conditions requires dynamic change of mitochondrial morphology. Proc Natl Acad Sci. 2006;103:2653–8.
82. Kelley DE, He J, Menshikova EV, Ritov VB. Dysfunction of mitochondria in human skeletal muscle in type 2 diabetes. Diabetes. 2002;51:2944–50.
83. Putti R, Sica R, Migliaccio V, Lionetti L. Diet impact on mitochondrial bioenergetics and dynamics. Front Physiol. 2015;6:109.
84. Jheng H-F, Tsai P-J, Guo S-M, Kuo L-H, Chang C-S, Su I-J, Chang C-R, Tsai Y-S. Mitochondrial fission contributes to mitochondrial dysfunction and insulin resistance in skeletal muscle. Mol Cell Biol. 2012;32:309–19.
85. Widlansky ME, Wang J, Shenouda SM, Hagen TM, Smith AR, Kizhakekuttu TJ, Kluge MA, Weihrauch D, Gutterman DD, Vita JA. Altered mitochondrial membrane potential, mass, and morphology in the mononuclear cells of humans with type 2 diabetes. Transl Res. 2010;156:15–25.
86. Rong JX, Qiu Y, Hansen MK, et al. Adipose mitochondrial biogenesis is suppressed in db/db and high-fat diet–fed mice and improved by rosiglitazone. Diabetes. 2007;56:1751–60.
87. Wu Z, Puigserver P, Andersson U, et al. Mechanisms controlling mitochondrial biogenesis and respiration through the thermogenic coactivator PGC-1. Cell. 1999;98:115–24.
88. De Pauw A, Tejerina S, Raes M, Keijer J, Arnould T. Mitochondrial (dys)function in adipocyte (de)differentiation and systemic metabolic alterations. Am J Pathol. 2009;175:927–39.
89. Boudina S, Graham TE. Mitochondrial function/dysfunction in white adipose tissue. Exp Physiol. 2014;99:1168–78.
90. Sergi D, Naumovski N, Heilbronn LK, Abeywardena M, O'Callaghan N, Lionetti L, Luscombe-Marsh N. Mitochondrial (dys)function and insulin resistance: from pathophysiological molecular mechanisms to the impact of diet. Front Physiol. 2019;10:532.
91. Rius-Pérez S, Torres-Cuevas I, Millán I, Ortega ÁL, Pérez S. PGC-1α, inflammation, and oxidative stress: an integrative view in metabolism. Oxidative Med Cell Longev. 2020;2020:1–20.
92. Højlund K, Mogensen M, Sahlin K, Beck-Nielsen H. Mitochondrial dysfunction in type 2 diabetes and obesity. Endocrinol Metab Clin N Am. 2008;37:713–31.
93. Park SW, Zhou Y, Lee J, Lee J, Ozcan U. Sarco(endo)plasmic reticulum Ca2+−atpase 2B is a major regulator of endoplasmic reticulum stress and glucose homeostasis in obesity. Proc Natl Acad Sci. 2010;107:19320–5.
94. Hannun YA, Obeid LM. Principles of bioactive lipid signalling: lessons from sphingolipids. Nat Rev Mol Cell Biol. 2008;9:139–50.
95. Lemmer IL, Willemsen N, Hilal N, Bartelt A. A guide to understanding endoplasmic reticulum stress in metabolic disorders. Mol Metab. 2021;47:101169.
96. Kharroubi I, Laurence L, Cardozo AK, Dogusan Z, Cnop M, Eizirik DL. Free fatty acids and cytokines induce pancreatic β-cell apoptosis by different mechanisms: role of nuclear factor-KB and endoplasmic reticulum stress. Endocrinology. 2004;145:5087–96.
97. Fernandes-da-Silva A, Miranda CS, Santana-Oliveira DA, Oliveira-Cordeiro B, Rangel-Azevedo C, Silva-Veiga FM, Martins FF, Souza-Mello V. Endoplasmic reticulum stress as the basis of obesity and metabolic diseases: focus on adipose tissue, liver, and pancreas. Eur J Nutr. 2021;60:2949–60.
98. Ron D, Walter P. Signal integration in the endoplasmic reticulum unfolded protein response. Nat Rev Mol Cell Biol. 2007;8:519–29.
99. Cao SS, Kaufman RJ. Endoplasmic reticulum stress and oxidative stress in cell fate decision and human disease. Antioxid Redox Signal. 2014;21:396–413.

100. Shrestha N, De Franco E, Arvan P, Cnop M. Pathological β-cell endoplasmic reticulum stress in type 2 diabetes: current evidence. Front Endocrinol. 2021;12:650158.
101. Vilas-Boas EA, Almeida DC, Roma LP, Ortis F, Carpinelli AR. Lipotoxicity and β-cell failure in type 2 diabetes: oxidative stress linked to NADPH oxidase and ER stress. Cell. 2021;10:3328.
102. Eizirik DL, Cardozo AK, Cnop M. The role for endoplasmic reticulum stress in diabetes mellitus. Endocr Rev. 2007;29:42–61.
103. Cnop M, Foufelle F, Velloso LA. Endoplasmic reticulum stress, obesity and diabetes. Trends Mol Med. 2012;18:59–68.
104. Kawasaki N, Asada R, Saito A, Kanemoto S, Imaizumi K. Obesity-induced endoplasmic reticulum stress causes chronic inflammation in adipose tissue. Sci Rep. 2012;2:799.
105. Umut Ö, Cao Q, Yilmaz E, Lee A-H, Iwakoshi NN, Esra Ö, Gürol T, Cem G, Glimcher LH, Hotamisligil GS. Endoplasmic reticulum stress links obesity, insulin action, and type 2 diabetes. Science. 2004;306:457–61.
106. Arruda AP, Pers BM, Parlakgül G, Güney E, Inouye K, Hotamisligil GS. Chronic enrichment of hepatic endoplasmic reticulum–mitochondria contact leads to mitochondrial dysfunction in obesity. Nat Med. 2014;20:1427–35.
107. Djelić N, Borozan S, Dimitrijević-Srećković V, Pajović N, Mirilović M, Stopper H, Stanimirović Z. Oxidative stress and DNA damage in peripheral blood mononuclear cells from normal, obese, prediabetic and diabetic persons exposed to thyroid hormone in vitro. Int J Mol Sci. 2022;23:9072.
108. Al-Aubaidy HA, Jelinek HF. Oxidative DNA damage and obesity in type 2 diabetes mellitus. Eur J Endocrinol. 2011;164:899–904.
109. Charron MJ, Bonner-Weir S. Implicating PARP and NAD+ depletion in type I diabetes. Nat Med. 1999;5(3):269–70.
110. Tay VS, Devaraj S, Koh T, Ke G, Crasta KC, Ali Y. Increased double strand breaks in diabetic β-cells with a p21 response that limits apoptosis. Sci Rep. 2019;9:1934.
111. Merecz A, Markiewicz L, Sliwinska A, Kosmalski M, Kasznicki J, Drzewoski J, Majsterek I. Analysis of oxidative DNA damage and its repair in polish patients with diabetes mellitus type 2: role in pathogenesis of diabetic neuropathy. Adv Med Sci. 2015;60:220–30.
112. Blasiak J, Arabski M, Krupa R, Wozniak K, Zadrozny M, Kasznicki J, Zurawska M, Drzewoski J. DNA damage and repair in type 2 diabetes mellitus. Mut Res. 2004;554:297–304.
113. Manoel-Caetano FS, Xavier DJ, Evangelista AF, et al. Gene expression profiles displayed by peripheral blood mononuclear cells from patients with type 2 diabetes mellitus focusing on biological processes implicated on the pathogenesis of the disease. Gene. 2012;511:151–60.
114. Xavier DJ, Takahashi P, Evangelista AF, Foss-Freitas MC, Foss MC, Donadi EA, Passos GA, Sakamoto-Hojo ET. Assessment of DNA damage and mRNA/MIRNA transcriptional expression profiles in hyperglycemic versus non-hyperglycemic patients with type 2 diabetes mellitus. Mutat Res. 2015;776:98–110.
115. Akholkar P, Gandhi A. Prevalence of obesity in diabetic and non-diabetic population. Int J Res Med Sci. 2015;3:2114–7.

Chapter 5
Advanced Glycation End Products and Diabetes

Nikola Hadzi-Petrushev, Marija Angelovski, and Mitko Mladenov

Abbreviations

AGE	Advanced glycation end-product
AGER	AGE receptor
AP1	Activator protein 1
CML	$N\varepsilon$-carboxymethyl-lysine
CVD	Cardiovascular disease
ECM	Extracellular matrix
EGFR	Epidermal growth factor receptor
EMT	Epithelial-to-mesenchymal transition
Erk1/2	Extracellular signal-regulated kinase
ET-1	Endothelin-1
FOXO	Forkhead family of transcription factors
GLP-1	Glucagon-like peptide 1
GLUT4	Glucose transporter type 4
GOLD	Glyoxal-lysine-dimer
GSH	Glutathione
IAPP	Islet amyloid peptide
IGF	Insulin-like growth factor
IL-6	Interleukin 6
IRS-1	Insulin receptor substrate 1
JAK/STAT	Janus kinase-signal transducer and activator of transcription

N. Hadzi-Petrushev (✉)
Faculty of Natural Sciences and Mathematics, Institute of Biology, Ss. Cyril and Methodius University, Skopje, Macedonia
e-mail: nikola@pmf.ukim.mk

M. Angelovski · M. Mladenov
Faculty of Natural Sciences and Mathematics, Institute of Biology, Skopje, Macedonia
e-mail: marija.angelovski@pmf.ukim.mk; mitkom@pmf.ukim.mk

© The Author(s), under exclusive license to Springer Nature Switzerland AG 2023
D. Avtanski, L. Poretsky (eds.), *Obesity, Diabetes and Inflammation*, Contemporary Endocrinology, https://doi.org/10.1007/978-3-031-39721-9_5

JNK	c-Jun N-terminal kinase
LDL	Low-density lipoprotein
LOX-1	Lectin-like oxidized low-density lipoprotein receptor 1
MAPK	Mitogen-activated protein kinase
MCP-1 (*s.* CCL2)	Monocyte chemoattractant protein 1
MG	Methylglyoxal
MMP	Matrix metalloproteinases
NF-κB	Nuclear factor kappa B
Nrf2	Nuclear factor erythroid 2-related factor 2
PAI-1	Plasminogen activator inhibitor 1
PDGF	Platelet-derived growth factor
PDX-1	Pancreatic and duodenal homeobox 1
PI3K	Phosphoinositide 3-kinase
PKB	Protein kinase B
PKC	Protein kinase C
PRRs	Pattern recognition receptors
RAGE	Receptor for advanced glycation end products
RAS	Renin–angiotensin system
ROS	Reactive oxygen species
SAPK	Stress-activated protein kinase
SIRT1	Sirtuin 1
Stab	Stabilin
TGF-β	Transforming growth factor beta
T2D	Type 2 diabetes mellitus
TLR4	Toll-like receptor 4
TNFα	Tumor necrosis factor alpha
Treg	Regulatory T cells
VEGF	Vascular endothelial growth factor

Advanced Glycation End Products: Sources, Metabolism, Interaction with Receptors

The earliest description of the interaction between glucose and amino acids, which results in the binding of sugar to the amino group of the protein, was made by French chemist Louis Camille Maillard in 1912 [1]. Many years later, the role of glycated proteins in diabetes has become a subject of great scientific interest. This spans from the simple clinical determination of glycated hemoglobin as a reliable marker for the development and management of diabetes mellitus to the comprehensive study of the implications of advanced glycation end products (AGEs) in several metabolic diseases, including diabetes mellitus.

AGEs are a chemically diverse group of oxidant compounds produced by non-enzymatic reactions (Fig. 5.1). AGEs can be produced both ex vivo and in vivo. Extensively processed foods and cigarette smoke can contain high amounts of AGEs and also provide reactive precursors for their production [2, 3]. In vivo, AGEs are

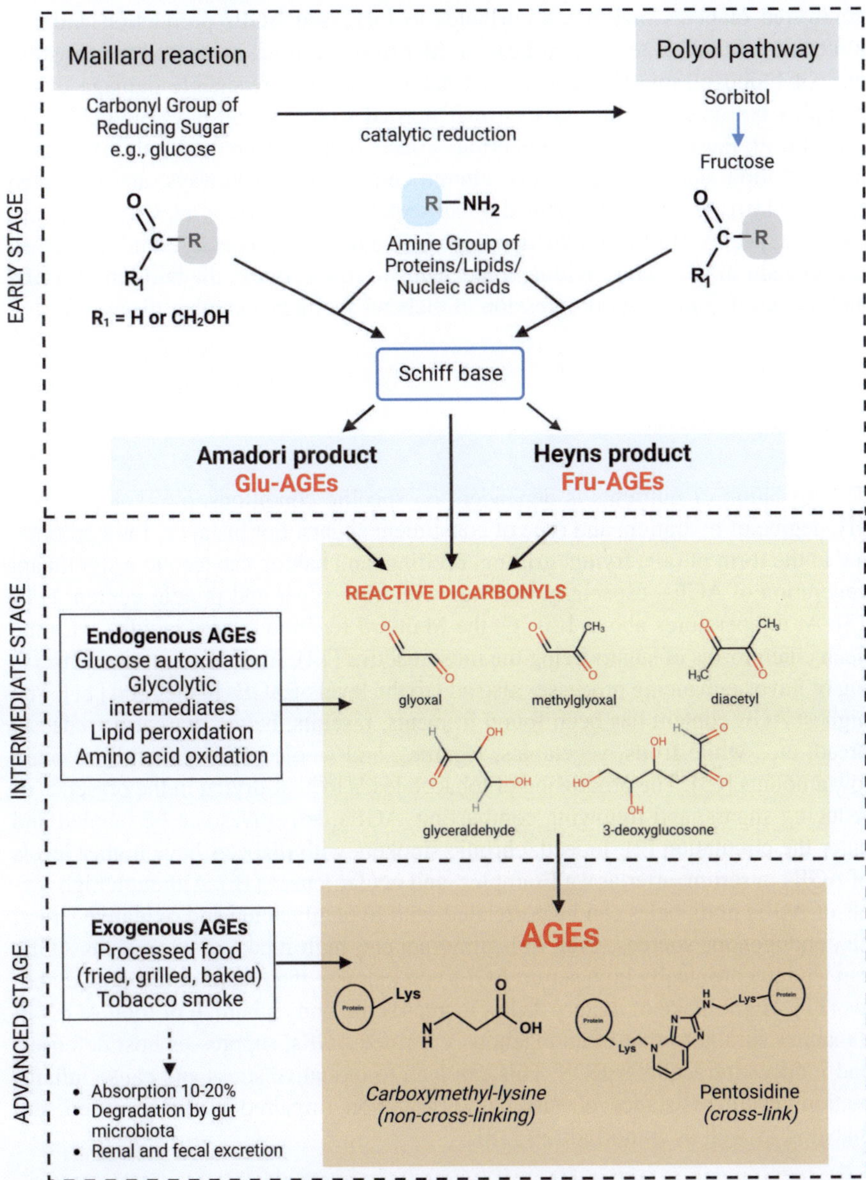

Fig. 5.1 Sources of AGEs and main steps in AGEs formation. *AGEs* advanced glycation end products, *Glu* glucose, *Fru* fructose (Created with BioRender.com)

typically formed via the condensation reaction between the carbonyl groups of reducing sugars and the amino groups of proteins but also via reactions with lipids, lipoproteins, and nucleic acids [4–6]. The process of glycoxidation is dependent on substrate availability. Thus, persistent hyperglycemia, a hallmark of poorly controlled diabetes mellitus, contributes to increased AGEs production and can affect all cellular proteins regardless of their turnover time, as well as the constituents of blood plasma [7]. The glycoxidation leads to irreversible damage of the complex biomolecules and loss of their normal structure and physiological functions [8, 9]. For proteins, the deleterious effects include decreased stability, loss of conformation and enzyme activity, altered cell signaling pathways, and disrupted turnover [10]. This is accompanied or subsequently followed by increased reactive oxygen species (ROS) production, pro-inflammatory processes, and perturbed metabolism in general, providing a mechanistic link between the buildup of AGEs and the development and progression of diabetes mellitus and other diseases [7].

Exogenous AGEs

The glycation of nutrients is dependent on specific conditions, e.g., temperature, pH, degree of hydration, and type of constituent sugars. For instance, food processing in the form of (air) frying, grilling, broiling, and baking can lead to a significant generation of AGEs, especially in foods with high sugar and protein content [11–13]. At temperatures above 120 °C, the Maillard reaction occurs rapidly, with the open chain forms of sugars being the most reactive [14]. In addition, some conserving or flavor-enhancing processes also add to the level of AGEs in the food [11]. The highest AGE content has been found in meats, biscuits, butter, margarine, cheese, bread, etc., while fruits, vegetables, legumes, and whole grains generally contain low amounts [15]. The processing of tobacco leads to heat-drying in the presence of reducing sugars, and following combustion, AGEs derivatives can be inhaled and enter the circulation [2]. Indeed, chronic smokers with diabetes have higher levels of AGEs in serum, arterial wall samples, and ocular lenses [16]. Although high levels of AGEs in diabetes can be correlated with hyperglycemia and oxidative stress, i.e., endogenous sources, even in healthy people, high intake of exogenous AGEs can lead to chronically high serum AGEs and increase the risk of developing diabetes [17]. High intake of dietary AGEs increases the body's burden of total AGEs in a manner similar to that of endogenously formed AGEs, suppresses host defenses, and induces intracellular ROS. This can lead to oxidative stress and cause inflammation, insulin resistance, obesity, cell dysfunction, impaired insulin secretion, and diabetes, as well as comorbidities [18].

Endogenous AGEs

In vivo, AGEs production is a slow process that requires supraphysiologic conditions and is usually accompanied by the generation of ROS [19]. The initial stages of the process include the production of early glycation products that progress to reactive carbonyls and AGEs. The non-enzymatic glycation, favored by hyperglycemic conditions, is the dominant process of AGE production [20]. Glycation is caused by the high reactivity of α-oxoaldehydes with the amino groups of biomolecules, such as lysine and arginine residues in proteins or guanine in nucleic acids [21]. Interestingly, fructose recommended as glucose replacement for diabetic patients has a greater ability to react with amino groups of proteins compared to glucose in vitro [22]. Usually, the carbonyl group from the reducing sugar reacts fast and reversibly with an amino group leading to the production of a Schiff base. Further, during several weeks this compound undergoes Amadori intramolecular rearrangement to a stable early glycation product [11, 23, 24]. Glycated hemoglobin and glycated serum albumin in humans are good examples of early glycation products [25]. In vivo, the polyol pathway could also be a source of reducing ketoses, leading to an early glycation product known as a Heyns product (generated by Heyns rearrangement) [26]. Regardless of the initial source, further rearrangements of the intermediates and the early glycation products lead to the generation of AGEs, along with various reactive carbonyls—glyoxal compounds and deoxyglucosones [methylglyoxal (MG), glyoxal, diacetyl, glyceraldehyde, glycol aldehyde, 1- and 3-deoxyglocosone, etc.] [11]. Additionally, in the setting of chronic hyperglycemia, autoxidation of monosaccharides, glycolysis, the metabolism of ketones, as well as the process of lipid peroxidation provide dicarbonyl compounds that act as precursors to AGEs [4, 5, 27, 28]. Similar to the Maillard reaction, the reactive dicarbonyl compounds can undergo condensation reactions with amino groups from proteins leading to the production of various final AGEs [11, 23]. Adjacent AGEs may connect with each other or with certain proteins forming protein adducts or protein cross-links [29]. AGEs are a very heterogeneous group of compounds. Prominent examples are Nε-carboxymethyl-lysine (CML), Nε-carboxyethyl-lysine, hydroimidazolone pyrraline, pentosidine, vesperlysines, lysine-arginine cross-links (glucosepane), methylglyoxal-lysine dimer, glyoxal-lysine-dimer (GOLD), glycolic acid lysine amide, and others [7, 30]. Most often determined AGEs in experimental and clinical studies are CML (usually an indicator of AGEs content in food) and pentosidine (product of reactions between ribose and arginine/lysine) as an indicator of accumulated protein damage in chronic diseases [31, 32]. The reader is directed to the reviews of Twarda-Clapa et al. [11] and Vistoli et al. [5] for comprehensive information about the mechanisms of formation and the types of AGEs.

It should be noted that AGEs production in vivo is hindered by various antioxidant mechanisms, especially by the nuclear factor erythroid 2-related factor 2-(Nrf2) regulated glyoxalase system [glyoxalase I, glyoxalase II, and reduced glutathione (GSH)] [33]. The glyoxalase system effectively catalyzes the detoxification of α-oxoaldehydes, e.g., MG to D-lactate and GSH. However, it has been found that in the setting of chronic oxidative stress, which is associated with poorly regulated diabetes, the Nrf2's activity is actually decreased [19]. For example, it is known that the level of glycated plasma proteins in healthy subjects is less than 3%, but in diabetes, it could rise to pathophysiological levels that are three times higher, leading to the promotion of oxidative stress, inflammation, and loss of protein structure and function [11] (Fig. 5.1).

Metabolism of AGEs

Dietary AGEs bound to proteins and peptides are digested in the gastric tract, followed by a different degree of proteolysis (depending on the structure and cross-linking) by trypsin in the intestines [34]. A portion of the food-derived AGEs is absorbed in the digestive tract via peptide transporters (e.g., peptidase transporter PEPT1) but also via the paracellular pathway and transcytosis or simple diffusion and made systemically available through the circulatory system [35, 36]. In humans, almost 80–90% of the dietary AGEs and precursors for AGEs are not absorbed and are subsequently available for degradation by the gut microbiota [37]. The absorbed portion remains in the body for 72 h, a time period that is sufficiently long to inflict tissue damage. This is a remarkably longer period compared to the time it takes to eliminate endogenously formed AGEs [18, 38]. The gut bacteria are able to use AGEs for their metabolism, but the presence of high levels of dietary AGEs has been shown to reduce the number and the variety of beneficial strains in the gut [12]. Hence, even the non-absorbable portion of dietary AGEs is capable of imposing damage by modifying the homeostasis of the gut microbiota and inducing inflammatory processes.

The removal of both dietary and endogenous AGEs is dependent on AGEs catabolism exerted by cellular antioxidants, turnover of macromolecules, and receptor-mediated degradation, followed by renal processing. For instance, the detoxifying enzyme cathepsin D is involved in the intracellular neutralization of AGE-modified albumin in the endosomal-lysosomal system, and the degradation products are released into the circulation [39]. Unfortunately, cross-links between AGEs and proteins are resistant to proteasomal breakdown, slowing down their turnover and delaying AGEs' detoxification [39, 40]. AGEs catabolism results in AGEs peptides filtered through the kidney glomerular membrane and then undergoing varying degrees of tubular reabsorption and excretion [34, 41]. About 30% of the consumed AGEs are excreted, with the elimination proportional to the intake but limited to a constant rate via the kidneys [42]. In diabetes, due to exposure to large amounts of circulating AGEs, the kidneys are susceptible to injury, and renal excretion could be below 5% compared to the usual 30% in healthy people [38].

Interaction of AGEs with Receptors

AGEs are ligands for pattern recognition receptors (PRRs) of the immune system. The interaction with certain receptors leads to the detoxification of AGEs and suppression of oxidative stress and inflammation, while the interaction with other receptors has opposite effects, activating processes that potentially drive the development and progression of chronic diseases. It has been shown that AGEs interact with human scavenging receptors (class A, B, E, and H), the AGE receptor (AGER) complex [oligosaccharyl transferase-48 (AGER1), 80 K-H phosphoprotein

(AGER2), galectin-3 (AGER3)], and the receptor for advanced glycation end products (RAGE) [30].

The scavenger class of receptors enables the removal of AGEs via receptor-mediated endocytosis. For instance, the class H receptors stabilin 1 (Stab1) and stabilin 2 (Stab2) are expressed in many types of cells, and they bind AGEs leading to their removal [43, 44]. However, there are also AGEs–scavenger receptor interactions that lead to negative consequences. In diabetic rats, AGEs binding to endothelium leads to increased expression of class E lectin-like oxidized low-density lipoprotein receptor 1 (LOX-1), which subsequently activates NF-κB (nuclear factor kappa B), increases ROS production, and decreases NO [45].

Another important protective mechanism against AGEs involves the antioxidant cellular receptors participating in the neutralization of the effects and subsequent degradation of AGEs—the AGER1, -R2, and -R3 receptors [43]. AGER1 and AGER2 are mainly found anchored in the endoplasmic reticulum and the plasma membrane, while AGER3 is located in the cytoplasm and also can be secreted [46, 47]. AGER1 is induced by acutely increased AGEs levels [48]. It mediates the uptake, breakdown, and the removal of AGEs, effectively preventing their accumulation. AGER1 is ubiquitously expressed and inhibits oxidative stress and inflammation by reducing: (1) the activation of NADPH oxidases; (2) the activation of NF-κB and mitogen-activated protein kinase (MAPK); (3) ROS formation; (4) the activation of the p66shc oxidative stress- and apoptosis-promoting pathway (which is activated in diabetes) [19, 49–51]. The AGER1 activity has synergistic actions with sirtuin 1 (SIRT1), which is responsible for the deacetylation and deactivation of the NF-κB signaling pathway [46]. In turn, this leads to improved insulin response and decreased inflammation. Unfortunately, chronically increased AGEs, either by high dietary intake or due to chronic diabetes, leads to the downregulation of AGER1 and SIRT1 [19, 46]. For example, in kidney disease related to diabetes, AGER1 was found to be decreased, while its overexpression led to decreased AGEs accumulation and protection against diabetic nephropathy [46, 52]. As in the case of AGER1, AGER3 expression is also increased as a result of AGEs binding [53]. This leads to endocytosis by macrophages and degradation of the AGEs. In contrast to AGER1 and -R3, AGER2 becomes phosphorylated upon AGEs binding, leading to cytokine secretion, inflammation, and altered metabolism [43].

The AGEs modulate various signaling pathways regulating the activity of factors like NF-κB, forkhead family of transcription factors (FOXO), and activator protein 1 (AP1) via binding to receptors such as RAGE, toll-like receptor 4 (TLR4), epidermal growth factor receptor (EGFR), and others, potentially leading to pathophysiological changes. For example, TLR4 was shown to be upregulated in diabetic subjects, and its interaction with AGEs, independently or cooperatively with RAGE, leads to inflammation [54]. According to some researchers, RAGE is less important for AGE-induced inflammation compared to the other PRRs [10]. However, the most often described mechanism for AGEs to exert their toxic effects is via interaction with RAGE. This receptor belongs to the immunoglobulin superfamily, has many protein isoforms, binds to an array of ligands, and is expressed in a variety of cell types (endothelial, smooth muscle cells, lung cells, neuronal cells, T cells, macrophages, endocrine cells of the pancreatic islets, etc.), in addition to being present in soluble forms [55, 56]. Similar to the case of TLR4, elevated RAGE expression has been associated with an increased risk of diabetes [57]. The soluble RAGE forms—the endogenous secretory RAGE and the proteolytically derived RAGE by the action of metalloproteases—bind AGEs without signaling consequences, thus preventing their toxic effects [58]. Similarly, the dominant-negative RAGE isoform lacks a cytosolic tail, again leading to no activation of cellular signaling pathways upon binding of AGEs. The membrane-bound functional RAGE, which is the predominant isoform, is regulated by AGEs via oxidative stress, i.e., ROS-mediated signaling [7]. The binding of AGEs to RAGE increases the expression of RAGE itself, creating a positive feedback loop, and leads to the activation of several cellular signaling pathways, including the extracellular signal-regulated kinase (Erk1/2) MAP kinase, c-Jun N-terminal kinase (JNK) MAP kinase, p38 MAP kinase, protein kinase B (PKB/Akt), p21Ras, and the Janus kinase-signal transducer and activator of transcription (JAK/STAT) pathway [59–61]. For instance, in type 2 diabetes mellitus (T2D), RAGE has the biological role of regulating increased production of pro-inflammatory cytokines, adhesion proteins, and ROS (via enzymes related to oxidative stress) and induces endothelial dysfunction [62]. RAGE expression has been shown to correlate with the level of serum AGEs, the amount of ingested AGEs, and with markers of oxidative stress, and they all are moderately elevated in uncomplicated diabetes, suggesting that the upregulation of RAGE may not be the cause but the consequence of the altered metabolic state, potentially contributing to further pathophysiological changes [63].

AGEs in Type 2 Diabetes Mellitus: Pathophysiological Mechanisms

T2D is characterized by hyperglycemia brought on by peripheral insulin resistance and insufficient β-cell insulin production. The etiology of T2D is unknown but is likely to be multifactorial. Elevated AGEs have been identified as significant contributors to the initiation and progression of pre-diabetes to diabetes [17]. This is mainly due to depleted host defenses, increased oxidative stress, and chronic inflammation corroborating the development of metabolic syndrome and T2D. AGEs are toxic to β-cells, negatively influence insulin production and secretion, and significantly contribute to the establishment of oxidative stress, inflammation, and insulin resistance in various types of cells and tissues [64–66]. The intake of AGEs from food has been associated with insulin resistance, the main underlying mechanism of T2D [67]. This relation seems to be valid for humans of any age. The high content of AGEs in processed infant food increases the predisposition for the later development of diabetes [68]. Factors like this and the increasing trend of exposure to highly processed food throughout life may partly explain the seemingly epidemic increase in diabetes [69]. Some of the AGEs-associated pathophysiological mechanisms particularly related to T2D are presented below and summarized in Fig. 5.2.

AGEs Are Toxic to β-Cells and Negatively Influence Insulin Production and Secretion

AGEs have been shown to inhibit ATP production in the mitochondria of islet cells. This was found to be due to the inhibition of cytochrome-c oxidase, mainly via elevated expression of inducible nitric oxide synthase (iNOS). Consequently, the blocked function of the ATP-sensitive potassium channels leads to the diminished

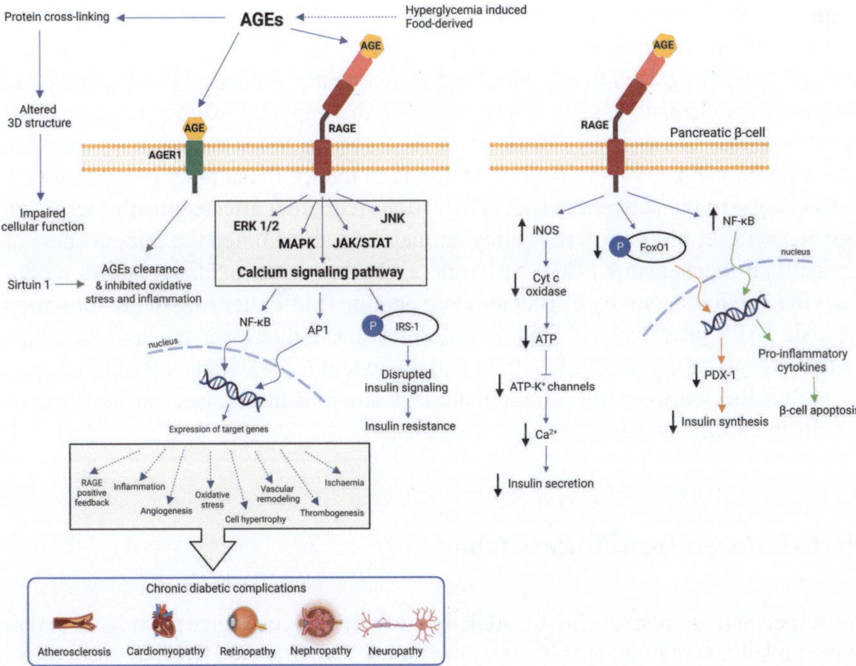

Fig. 5.2 Overview of the mechanisms linked to the deleterious effects of AGEs via interaction with AGER/RAGE receptors and by direct modification of proteins. AGEs have an important role in the pathophysiological mechanisms related to type 2 diabetes mellitus and diabetes-associated complications. *AGEs* advanced glycation end products, *AGER1* AGE receptor 1, *RAGE* receptor for advanced glycation end products, *Erk1/2 MAP kinase* extracellular signal-regulated kinase, *JNK MAP kinase* c-Jun N-terminal kinase, *JAK/STAT* Janus kinase-signal transducer and activator of transcription, *MAPK* mitogen-activated protein kinase, *NF-kB* nuclear factor kappa-light-chain-enhancer of activated B cells, *AP1* activator protein 1, *IRS-1 (P)* insulin receptor substrate (phosphorylated), *iNOS* inducible nitric oxide synthase, *Cyt c oxidase* cytochrome-c oxidase, *ATP-K$^+$-channels* ATP-sensitive potassium channels, *FoxO1 (P)* forkhead box protein O1 (phosphorylated), *PDX-1* pancreatic and duodenal homebox-1 (Created with BioRender.com)

glucose-stimulated secretion of insulin [64]. Beta cells exposed to AGEs have been shown to have reduced antioxidant capacity, specifically decreased manganese superoxide dismutase (MnSOD) activity, which would corroborate the impaired mitochondrial function [70]. Beta cell membrane depolarization may also be affected by disrupted regulation of the calcium channels dependent on SIRT1, which in T2D is suppressed by AGEs [71]. The compromised insulin release could be further aggravated by decreased insulin synthesis. AGEs mediate decreased phosphorylation of the transcription factor FOXO1, which in turn decreases the availability of the transcription factor pancreatic and duodenal homeobox 1 (PDX-1) needed for insulin transcription [72].

The persistently increased AGEs levels lead to chronic NF-κB-mediated inflammation and oxidative stress in β-cells [73]. This is potentiated by AGEs-associated upregulation of RAGE and increased β-cell apoptosis [74]. The increased ROS production and the damage of the islet cells activate the NLRP3 inflammasome, which significantly contributes to the inflammatory state [75]. AGE-induced chemotaxis and pro-inflammatory cytokine secretion lead to the recruitment of T cells and antigen-presenting cells in the islets and consequently decreased proliferation and increased apoptosis of β-cells, complementing the impaired insulin secretion. This could be partly achieved by the ability of AGEs to modulate the cytokine secretion profile in human $CD4^+$ T cells via RAGE and to reduce the number of regulatory T cells (Tregs) in the pancreatic islets [76]. High AGEs diet affected insulin secretion and caused islet infiltration in healthy animals and also limited the effectiveness of antioxidant mechanisms [76]. Furthermore, the increased oxidative stress modulates the amyloidogenicity of islet amyloid peptide (IAPP), leading to the formation of toxic IAPP intermediates [77]. RAGE binds these intermediates, and the transmitted signals promote cellular stress and dysfunction [78]. Hence, RAGE appears to be the link between the accumulation of amyloid aggregates and the loss of β-cells in chronic diabetes.

AGE-Induced Insulin Resistance

Most mechanisms responsible for AGE-induced insulin resistance are related to disrupted insulin signaling. RAGE signaling induces MAPK via JNK and phosphorylates the insulin receptor substrate 1 (IRS-1), leading to insulin resistance [79]. Additionally, the activated p38 and protein kinase C (PKC) also phosphorylate the IRS-1 and reduce the expression of the insulin receptor. For example, glycated albumin acting via RAGE was found to increase the release of pro-inflammatory cytokines as well as to affect the protein kinase C alpha (PKCα) pathway causing inhibition of insulin signaling and insulin-induced glucose metabolism [80]. Insulin resistance in the muscles was associated with STAT3 activation, which is responsible for the ubiquitination of IRS-1 [81]. In hepatocytes, AGEs were found to be responsible for inducing insulin resistance by IRS-1 phosphorylation at the serine-307 moiety [82]. Additionally, the AGEs–RAGE interaction leads to increased degradation of Iκβ proteins, increasing the NF-κB transcriptional activity and the expression of pro-inflammatory cytokines, thus contributing toward insulin resistance by decreasing glucose transporter type 4 (GLUT4) expression [83]. Both in vitro and in vivo studies have confirmed that high AGEs repress GLUT4 expression in adipocytes and myocytes via a mechanism that involves endoplasmic reticulum stress and inflammation [83, 84]. The changes in insulin resistance in target tissues may also be related to inflammatory events, i.e., AGEs-related differentiation and proliferation of immune cells that release pro-inflammatory mediators in a paracrine fashion and an increase in anti-inflammatory Tregs when AGEs intake is restricted [63]. This is supported by studies showing that adipose tissue in obese subjects contains large numbers of macrophages. AGEs can modulate the release of cytokines from macrophages and T cells, thus inducing inflammation and reducing insulin sensitivity [63, 85, 86]. Lastly, the glycose-lowering potential of insulin can also be affected by its direct glycation. In cultured cells under hyperglycemia as well as in vivo, glycation sites have been found in insulin, and its modification negatively affected its action on glucose uptake [80]. Glycated insulin was found to comprise 9% of total blood plasma insulin in T2D patients [87]. The role of AGEs in insulin resistance has been confirmed in studies showing that administration of MG induced insulin resistance, while administration of antiglycation agents (e.g., pyridoxamine) improved insulin resistance in diabetic rats [88, 89]. The supportive findings are not limited to experimental animals—4 months of dietary AGEs restriction in T2D humans was shown to increase AGER1 and SIRT1 and lower RAGE, TNFα, and plasma insulin [67] (Fig. 5.2).

AGEs and Chronic Diabetic Complications

The prevalence of T2D is increasing, making it a global epidemic requiring immediate attention [90]. Regardless of the age of patients, diabetes mellitus is currently the main contributor to significant comorbidities [63]. Chronic hyperglycemia only partially accounts for the emergence of late diabetic complications, and these cannot be completely prevented or healed by establishing strict glycemic control [91]. Thus, additional pathophysiological pathways related to the AGEs-RAGE axis are considered (Fig. 5.2). Diabetic patients were shown to have increased levels of CML, pentosidine, MG-derived hydroimidazolone, and glucosepane in serum or tissues, and their accumulation was linked to the development of diabetic complications [80, 92]. The extensive study of this matter has led to defining a state of sustained cellular dysfunction known as "metabolic memory," established due to the activation of the AGEs-RAGE axis [93, 94]. The term "memory" stems from the realization that the consequences of AGEs-RAGE axis activation remain even after establishing normoglycemia. This means that the vicious cycle of chronic inflammation and oxidative stress persists throughout the organism and essentially contributes to the development of long-term diabetic complications [7, 95, 96].

Uncertainty surrounds the exact mechanisms behind metabolic memory. It could arise due to epigenetic modifications related to the activation of the AGEs-RAGE axis, in addition to interactions with diabetogenic factors like inappropriate diet, hyperglycemia, and oxidative stress [93, 97]. The epigenetic modifications could be responsible for the expression of genes coding products involved in the pathogenesis of diabetic complications and, in this way, provide the connection between AGEs, diabetes, and diabetic complications. For example, AGE-induced histone alterations have been associated with the upregulation of the pro-inflammatory NF-κB-p65 gene expression in diabetic complications [98]. Also, in transgenerational studies in mice, the exposure to MG led to a significantly earlier onset of insulin resistance after the fifth generation compared to the controls, suggesting potential epigenetic changes [99]. The epigenetic aspect may also aid the explanation for the lack of effectiveness of the intensive control of hyperglycemia in reducing the consequences of AGEs on complications in diabetes.

AGEs have been associated with various diabetic complications: neurodegenerative diseases and diabetic neuropathy [100, 101], decreased bone strength and quality [102], erectile dysfunction and infertility [103, 104], hepatotoxicity and nonalcoholic fatty liver disease [105], polycystic ovarian syndrome [106], periodontitis [107], chronic subclinical inflammation [108], and increased risk of cancer [109]. Particular attention will be given below to the accumulating evidence about the involvement of AGEs in diabetic cardiovascular disease and diabetic kidney disease.

AGEs in Diabetic Cardiovascular Diseases

Cardiovascular disease (CVD) is the leading cause of death in diabetic patients. AGEs are associated with an increased incidence of CVD in T2D, and their levels positively correlate with pathophysiological cardiovascular changes [110]. AGEs have a prominent role in cardiomyopathy and atherosclerosis. The diabetes-associated chronic complications are related to both structural and functional modifications within the cardiovascular system and are mediated by AGE accumulation and AGE-induced signaling [111]. Chronic problems could be classified as microvascular complications caused by damage to small blood vessels and macro-vascular complications caused by damage to the arteries. Diabetic neuropathy, diabetic kidney disease, and diabetic retinopathy are examples of microvascular consequences. Macrovascular complications from diabetes mainly include atherosclerosis of the coronary, renal, cerebral, and peripheral arteries.

Increased RAGE ligands and concomitantly upregulated RAGE have been detected in diabetic blood vessels [112]. It has been shown that AGEs bind to RAGE receptors on vessel walls causing MAPK, p38, phosphoinositide 3-kinases (PIP3K), and NF-κB-mediated increased production of pro-inflammatory cytokines and ROS [111, 113]. Oxidants derived from upregulated NADPH oxidases are significant mediators of endothelial cell dysfunction and diabetic vascular injury [114].

Additionally, the increased oxidative stress augments the oxidation of low-density lipoprotein (LDL), which in turn acts as a RAGE ligand, potentiating the AGE-induced vascular changes and significantly contributing to the pathophysiological changes characteristic of CVD [115]. In T2D, glycated LDLs evade receptor-mediated clearing, decrease NO production, and accumulate in the arterial wall leading to foam cell formation. For instance, it has been shown that modification of LDL by MG led to its increased atherogenicity in diabetic subjects [116]. The activation of the AGEs-RAGE axis in the endothelia leads to the upregulation of various pro-inflammatory factors, such as vascular cell adhesion molecules, chemokines, matrix metalloproteinases (MMPs), endothelin 1 (ET-1), plasminogen activator inhibitor 1 (PAI-1), and monocyte chemoattractant protein 1 (MCP-1 *s.* CCL2) [117–120]. This altered gene expression leads to the recruitment of inflammatory cells and impaired fibrinolysis. The endothelial dysfunction and atherosclerosis are augmented by AGE-induced decreased expression and activity of endothelial NO synthase [121]. This impairs vasodilatation and also disrupts the NO-mediated decreased platelet adhesion. The NF-κB pathway also increases secretion of vascular endothelial growth factor (VEGF), which in turn impairs the repair of endothelial lesions, stimulates the accumulation of oxidized LDL, and promotes the differentiation of monocytes to macrophages, thus inducing atherogenesis [122].

AGEs are also transferred in the subendothelium leading to changes in the structure and function of the basement membrane of arteries. AGE-related cross-links of matrix proteins like collagen, elastin, and laminin contribute to vessel wall stiffness and disrupt the interaction between the matrix and the cells [86, 123]. It has been shown that vascular calcification can be achieved via MAPK/ERK, p38, PKC, and other signaling pathways in diabetic conditions [124]. The calcification process is also augmented by ROS-induced vascular smooth muscle cell apoptosis as a consequence of the activated AGEs-RAGE axis [125]. The activation of the endothelial cells, vascular inflammation, and the remodeling of the vascular wall are characteristics of diabetes-associated vascular disease. Hence, the toxic effects of AGEs are related to pathophysiological changes in the arterial wall leading to arterial stiffness, calcification of the vascular wall, atherosclerotic plaque formation, and hypertension. Essentially, vascular inflammation is the mechanistic link between diabetes and atherosclerosis, as well as between diabetes and hypertension. Indeed, increased AGEs were linked to blood vessel thickness, leading to an increase in blood pressure [123]. The fluctuations in blood pressure related to vessel wall stiffness and vascular inflammation provide a link between the pathophysiological changes in the cardiovascular system and the microvasculature of other organs, especially the kidneys.

Diabetes has profound negative effects on the peripheral vasculature, often leading to atherosclerotic vascular disease progressing to lower-limb amputations. The AGEs-RAGE axis is responsible for impaired collateral growth of blood vessels leading to poor perfusion and potentiation of diabetes-associated peripheral artery disease [126]. Accordingly, dietary AGE restriction improved wound healing in diabetic mice [127]. It has also been shown that AGEs accumulate in the endothelial cells of the vasa nervorum, mediating vascular structure damage and ischemia/

occlusion [128]. In humans, AGEs have been identified in the vasculature and the fibers of various nerves accompanied by upregulated RAGE [129]. Hence, decreased blood flow and reduced conduction velocity in both motor and sensory nerves have been associated with the effects of AGEs [130]. Capillary lesions are also involved in the pathogenesis of diabetic retinopathy [131]. The loss of pericytes in the retina's capillaries is an early event in diabetes-associated retinopathy. The decreased pericyte survival is associated with AGEs-RAGE axis-mediated reduced protein kinase B/Akt signaling and increased ROS production [132]. This leads to loss of the blood–retina barrier and dysregulation of the flux of fluids, nutrients, and other blood elements into the retina, potentially leading to macular edema and vision loss.

AGEs have been associated with a negative impact on coronary vasculature in diabetes. Activation of RAGE expressed on endothelial cells results in endothelial dysfunction of the coronary arterioles [133]. The implication of RAGE was supported by studies on animal models, which showed that susceptibility to an injury could be reduced by the knock-out of RAGE or administration of soluble RAGE [134]. AGEs are accumulated in atherosclerotic lesions and take part in AGEs-RAGE axis-mediated MMP-9 expression and apoptosis, leading to plaque instability via renin–angiotensin system (RAS) signaling in the pathogenesis of coronary atherosclerosis in T2D [135]. This was corroborated by the finding that RAGE expression is increased in diabetes and associated with apoptosis in coronary plaques [112]. In ischemic heart disease, plaque formation in the arterial wall reduces the blood supply to the heart. RAGE has also been associated with increased vulnerability to ischemia/reperfusion injury in diabetes, leading to decreased ATP levels in the heart and increased lactate dehydrogenase release [136]. Serum AGEs levels were found to be good predictors of ischemic heart disease mortality in T2D patients [137]. This was supported by a finding that diabetic patients without coronary disease had lower serum AGEs compared to patients with diabetes with coronary artery disease [138].

Besides affecting the coronary vasculature, AGEs could also directly influence the myocardial tissue, causing both systolic and diastolic dysfunction, congestive heart failure, arrhythmias, and the development of fibrosis. In cardiomyocytes, AGEs were found to be responsible for cross-linking of proteins participating in Ca^{2+} homeostasis. The impaired function of the sarcoplasmic reticulum Ca^{2+}-ATPase pump and the upregulated ryanodine receptor lead to a disbalance of Ca^{2+} in both the systolic and diastolic phases and induce overall cardiac dysfunction [139, 140]. Glycation of myocardial matrix proteins was also shown to be responsible for increased stiffness leading to diastolic dysfunction [141]. Furthermore, studies have shown that the AGEs-RAGE axis is responsible for the activation of the STAT3 and NF-κB transduction by modulating the JAK/STAT, MAPK, p38, phosphoinositide 3-kinase (PI3K), and stress-activated protein kinase (SAPK)/JNK signaling [122, 142]. Hence, the increased production of pro-inflammatory mediators may be responsible for cardiac fibrosis. A study found that the AGEs-RAGE axis interacts with the RAS, which also helps to promote cardiac fibroblast proliferation and cardiomyocyte hypertrophy in diabetes [143]. In view of that, blocking RAGE was beneficial in preventing cardiac dysfunction and fibrosis related to T2D [144].

AGEs in Diabetic Kidney Disease

Diabetic nephropathy, the leading cause of renal failure, is characterized by decreased glomerular filtration rate and microalbuminuria [145]. Increased AGEs linked to hyperglycemia have a crucial role in the pathogenesis of diabetic kidney disease [146]. AGEs are involved in the onset of diabetic nephropathy, and recent clinical studies showed a strong correlation between AGE levels and kidney disease progression and renal outcomes in T2D [147, 148]. The kidneys receive a large proportion of cardiac output, and the peritubular capillary bed is significantly exposed to the AGEs from circulation, especially when high AGE level is present, as in diabetes. The kidneys are involved in the removal of AGEs from the blood and their transfer to the tubular lumen via active secretion. Still, the adverse effects of AGEs are not limited to the tubular region. AGEs accumulation has also been detected in the glomerulus and the basement membrane [43].

The pathophysiology of diabetic kidney disease involves AGEs and their receptors, which are linked to increased renal oxidative stress and inflammation, glomerular hypertrophy, and fibrosis. The complications are propagated by loss of podocytes, mesangial hypertrophy, and thickening of tubular basement membranes [111]. In this context, tubular epithelial cells, podocytes, mesangial cells, and glomerular endothelial cells have been shown to express RAGE, which in turn mediates the increased production of ROS and transforming growth factor beta (TGF-β), as well as the increased expression of RAGE itself [111, 149, 150]. Thus, the increased exposure of the kidney to high levels of prooxidant AGEs during the early phases of T2D leads to oxidative stress and kidney damage, i.e., interstitial fibrosis and glomerular dysfunction. NF-κB, the PI3K/PKB, and the MAPK/ERK pathways are the main targets of the AGEs-RAGE axis [151]. AGEs are also involved in the activation of angiotensin II, which induces ROS production [152], along with inflammasome activation [153]. This is complemented by the depletion of antioxidant enzymes and increased activity of NADPH oxidases, iNOS, and cyclooxygenase [154].

AGEs have been shown to increase VEGF, insulin-like growth factor 1 and 2 (IGF-1 and -2), platelet-derived growth factor (PDGF), TGF-β, interleukin 6 (IL-6), tumor necrosis factor α (TNFα), and MCP-1 expression, along with the promotion of apoptotic death in mesangial cells [111, 155, 156]. These cells are essential to the structure and function of the glomerular capillary bed; hence, the prolonged activation of the AGEs-RAGE axis leads to hyperfiltration and glomerulosclerosis, the hallmarks of early diabetes-associated kidney dysfunction. The increased MCP-1 propagates leukocyte infiltration, therefore exacerbating the inflammatory processes in the kidney. The increased TGFβ1 (as a consequence of ROS-mediated JAK-STAT signaling in podocytes, mesangial cells, and epithelial cells) is responsible for glomerular hypertrophy due to the increased expression of extracellular matrix (ECM) proteins, along with induction of epithelial-to-mesenchymal transition (EMT) [156]. Furthermore, the loss of kidney structure and function is also affected by the RAGE-induced increase of heparinase activity leading to the disintegration of the glomerular basement membrane by degradation of heparin sulfate [157]. Also, AGEs are responsible for the glycation of type IV collagen and forming cross-links with matrix proteins [158]. As a result, the loss of mesangial cells and the disintegration of the basement membrane led to glomerulosclerosis and increased vascular permeability, which in turn is linked to hyperfiltration and proteinuria.

Reduced AGE clearance is one of the earliest indicators of impaired renal function in diabetes [63]. The increased accumulation of AGEs in the renal and other tissues, accompanied by suppressed AGER1, increased ROS production, and inflammation, eventually leads to severe pathogenic consequences. In healthy rats, chronic administration of AGEs led to damage to kidney structure and function, characterized by the deposition of AGEs within the renal tissue [159]. As expected, the development of diabetes-related kidney disease has been associated with increased levels of AGEs. In support of this, subjects with T2D were shown to have increased urinary excretion rates of oxidated and glycated DNA products, while both in type 1 and 2 diabetes mellitus patients, the urinary levels of AGE-modified proteins correlated with albuminuria [160, 161]. Furthermore, in diabetic mice, AGEs restriction led to the prevention of diabetes-associated kidney disease, even in the setting of persistent hyperglycemia [162].

Therapeutic Options to Reduce AGEs in Diabetes

Different therapeutic strategies have been explored in animal models and clinical studies with varying degrees of success in the attempts to reduce AGE levels and the associated effects. Below is a brief overview of some anti-AGE therapeutic approaches for diabetes and its complications.

Dietary Intervention

The daily intake of AGEs in healthy people consuming a regular modern diet usually exceeds the amount that would not cause a transient increase in the levels of inflammatory markers [66]. It was determined that the rate of tissue AGE buildup caused by carbonyls in foods was orders of magnitude higher than the rate caused by endogenous production [63]. Thus, the simplest approach to reducing AGE effect is to lower their intake. This dietary intervention could be achieved without overall caloric restriction simply by removing the abundance of animal protein and limiting food exposure to high temperatures. Cooking using more moisture (e.g., steaming or boiling) is associated with lower levels of AGEs in the food compared to food processing involving dry heat [15, 31]. The diabetic subjects who followed a low-AGEs diet manifested lowered serum AGE levels, reduced inflammation, ameliorated oxidative stress, improved insulin resistance, and reduced vascular dysfunction [50, 67, 163]. Additionally, restricting exogenous AGEs decreased RAGE expression in both diabetic mice and humans while increasing AGER1, SIRT1, and adiponectin [50, 67, 164]. Consumption of a Mediterranean diet led to a reduction of serum AGE levels and T2D remission in newly diagnosed patients with coronary heart disease [165]. However, in some studies, dietary AGE restriction was not effective in reducing AGE content in the serum and urine of diabetic subjects [166, 167], and the systematic review of the available data showed a lack of unanimity regarding the effectiveness of dietary AGE restriction [168].

Neutralization and Signaling Interference

Considering the ability of the AGEs to alter signaling pathways related to inflammation and oxidative stress, possible intervention strategies are the rapid neutralization of AGEs or targeting of the AGEs-RAGE axis. The former could be achieved by detoxification enzymes and antioxidants. The glyoxalase system and the oxidative stress response protein DJ-1 have known roles in reversing glycation [169]. Glyoxalase is Nrf2 regulated, and targeting this transcription factor related to antioxidants has been suggested as a promising strategy against elevated AGEs [170]. Various plant polyphenols increase glyoxalase expression leading to a reduction of AGEs deposition. Trans-resveratrol (alone or in combination with hesperetin), fisetin, and cyanidin have been shown to increase the expression of glyoxalase [171–173].

Blockage of RAGE using soluble RAGE, monoclonal antibodies, and FPS-ZM1 has helped to attenuate inflammation and limit vascular and renal complications in diabetes [174–176]. Glucagon-like peptide 1 (GLP-1) has also shown promising results in reducing the expression of RAGE, along with blocking its downstream effects and reducing AGE-induced oxidative stress and cell death in diabetes [177]. DNA aptamers also seem to be a promising approach to block the AGEs-RAGE axis, as well as to aid the elimination of AGEs. Kaida et al. [178] showed that a DNA aptamer with a high affinity for AGEs inhibited glomerular hypertrophy and ECM protein accumulation, leading to decreased urinary excretion of albumin and preventing renal failure in T2D animals.

Pharmacological Agents

Several pharmaceutical agents can significantly influence AGEs. Some of them, like sevelamer carbonate, work by binding AGEs specifically in the gastrointestinal system, enabling their elimination via the feces [179]. Another group of drugs includes effective AGEs chelators both in the food and in the body, thus hindering interactions between sugars and proteins and/or scavenging ROS. In contrast, other pharmaceutical agents facilitate the breakdown of AGEs complexes. Glycation is inhibited by acetylsalicylic acid, diclofenac, anti-platelet aggregation agents like clopidogrel, and drugs stimulating the production of insulin, e.g., sulfonylurea [62, 180]. Metformin is a good example of a drug that inhibits glycation by binding AGEs and also reduces the expression of RAGE and cellular inflammation in T2D patients [181]. Aminoguanidine's action on AGEs is related to the inhibition of post-Amadori glycation intermediates. In rats, aminoguanidine treatment was associated with increased urinary excretion of AGEs accompanied by reduced tissue deposition of AGEs, protection of islet β-cells, and improved cardiovascular function [41, 182, 183]. In humans, treatment with the same drug was not particularly effective against diabetes-induced complications, and safety concerns hindered further clinical trials [184]. Benfotiamine treatment and pyridoxamine treatment have been shown to effectively scavenge AGEs, reduce oxidative stress, and maintain normal endothelial function, which in some but not all instances were beneficial for reducing diabetes-associated complications in T2D patients or animal models [185–189]. Acarbose is another example of an AGE inhibitor with chelating properties, which has been effective in reducing the levels of AGEs and their receptors in blood serum [62, 190]. Due to the interaction between the polyol pathway and the process of non-enzymatic glycation, the use of aldose reductase inhibitors has been feasible and effective in reducing the progression of diabetic cataracts and deterioration of kidney function in humans [191]. In diabetes, the use of therapeutic agents such as angiotensin-converting enzyme inhibitors, angiotensin receptor antagonists, peroxisome proliferator receptor antagonists, metal chelators, and ramipril has also been shown to manifest anti-AGE effects [192]. The drug Alagebrium (*N*-phenylthiazole bromide; ALT-711) is an example of an antiglycation agent facilitating the breakdown of AGE-protein cross-link complexes. ALT-711 improved cardiovascular and renal function in diabetic animals [193]. Unfortunately, these results were not confirmed in subsequent trials on diabetic patients [194].

Nutritional and Phytotherapeutic Options

Numerous compounds with antioxidant, anti-inflammatory, and other beneficial biological activities, in purified form or as part of plant extracts/preparations, have been investigated due to their potential to target AGEs production, AGEs-RAGE signaling, and ameliorate diabetic complications. *N*-acetylcysteine, vitamin E, taurine, alpha lipoic acid, quercetin, ascorbic acid, dimerumic acid, and other antioxidants [195–199] showed varying abilities to reduce the effects of AGEs. Nevertheless, when analyzing the relationship between AGEs and diabetes, Vlassara and Uribarri [66] concluded that reducing external AGEs as oxidants is a better strategy than supplementing antioxidants, which, based on clinical and experimental data, are insufficient compared to the degree of oxidative stress. There is a large amount of experimental data about natural-derived compounds and preparations as part of phytotherapy approaches against AGEs and hyperglycemic complications. The researchers investigated the anti-AGE effects of natural products like apigenin, flavoalkaloids, green tea polyphenols, berries, curcumin, mangiferin, ginseng, etc., many of which are reviewed in the works of Parveen et al. [200] and Vijaykrishnaraj and Wang [201]. The phytotherapeutic options have shown some promising results, offering future perspectives of natural products but also requiring further investigations to confirm their safety and effectiveness.

References

1. Maillard L. Action des acides amines sur les sucres: formation des melanoidines par voie Methodique. C R Acad Sci (Paris). 1912;154:66–8.
2. Cerami C, Founds H, Nicholl I, et al. Tobacco smoke is a source of toxic reactive glycation products. Proc Natl Acad Sci U S A. 1997;94:13915–20.
3. Garay-Sevilla ME, Rojas A, Portero-Otin M, Uribarri J. Dietary AGEs as exogenous boosters of inflammation. Nutrients. 2021;13(8):2802. https://doi.org/10.3390/NU13082802.
4. Thornalley PJ. Pharmacology of methylglyoxal: formation, modification of proteins and nucleic acids, and enzymatic detoxification—a role in pathogenesis and antiproliferative chemotherapy. Gen Pharmacol. 1996;27:565–73.
5. Vistoli G, de Maddis D, Cipak A, Zarkovic N, Carini M, Aldini G. Advanced glycoxidation and lipoxidation end products (AGEs and ALEs): an overview of their mechanisms of formation. Free Radic Res. 2013;47(Suppl 1):3–27.
6. Schalkwijk CG, Stehouwer CDA, van Hinsbergh VWM. Fructose-mediated non-enzymatic glycation: sweet coupling or bad modification. Diabetes Metab Res Rev. 2004;20:369–82.
7. Khalid M, Petroianu G, Adem A. Advanced glycation end products and diabetes mellitus: mechanisms and perspectives. Biomol Ther. 2022;12(4):542. https://doi.org/10.3390/BIOM12040542.
8. Singh R, Barden A, Mori T, Beilin L. Advanced glycation end-products: a review. Diabetologia. 2001;44:129–46.
9. Huebschmann AG, Regensteiner JG, Vlassara H, Reusch JEB. Diabetes and advanced glycoxidation end products. Diabetes Care. 2006;29:1420–32.
10. Dimitropoulos A, Rosado CJ, Thomas MC. Dicarbonyl-mediated AGEing and diabetic kidney disease. J Nephrol. 2020;33:909–15.
11. Twarda-clapa A, Olczak A, Białkowska AM, Koziołkiewicz M. Advanced glycation end-products (AGEs): formation, chemistry, classification, receptors, and diseases related to AGEs. Cells. 2022;11(8):1312. https://doi.org/10.3390/CELLS11081312.
12. Snelson M, Coughlan MT. Dietary advanced glycation end products: digestion, metabolism and modulation of gut microbial ecology. Nutrients. 2019;11(2):215. https://doi.org/10.3390/NU11020215.
13. Zamora R, Hidalgo FJ. Coordinate contribution of lipid oxidation and Maillard reaction to the nonenzymatic food browning. Crit Rev Food Sci Nutr. 2007;45:49–59. https://doi.org/10.1080/10408690590900117.
14. Laroque D, Inisan C, Berger C, Vouland É, Dufossé L, Guérard F. Kinetic study on the Maillard reaction. Consideration of sugar reactivity. Food Chem. 2008;111:1032–42.
15. Uribarri J, Woodruff S, Goodman S, Cai W, Chen X, Pyzik R, Yong A, Striker GE, Vlassara H. Advanced glycation end products in foods and a practical guide to their reduction in the diet. J Am Diet Assoc. 2010;110(6):911–16.e12. https://doi.org/10.1016/J.JADA.2010.03.018.
16. Nicholl ID, Stitt AW, Moore JE, Ritchie AJ, Archer DB, Bucala R. Increased levels of advanced glycation endproducts in the lenses and blood vessels of cigarette smokers. Mol Med. 1998;4:594.
17. Uribarri J, Cai W, Peppa M, Goodman S, Ferrucci L, Striker G, Vlassara H. Circulating glycotoxins and dietary advanced glycation endproducts: two links to inflammatory response, oxidative stress, and aging. J Gerontol A Biol Sci Med Sci. 2007;62:427–33.

18. Peppa M, Mavroeidi I. Experimental animal studies support the role of dietary advanced glycation end products in health and disease. Nutrients. 2021;13(10):3467. https://doi.org/10.3390/NU13103467.

19. Vlassara H, Striker GE. Advanced glycation endproducts in diabetes and diabetic complications. Endocrinol Metab Clin N Am. 2013;42:697–719.

20. van Nguyen C. Toxicity of the AGEs generated from the Maillard reaction: on the relationship of food-AGEs and biological-AGEs. Mol Nutr Food Res. 2006;50:1140–9.

21. Scheckhuber CQ. Studying the mechanisms and targets of glycation and advanced glycation end-products in simple eukaryotic model systems. Int J Biol Macromol. 2019;127:85–94.

22. Inoue S, Takata T, Nakazawa Y, Nakamura Y, Guo X, Yamada S, Ishigaki Y, Takeuchi M, Miyazawa K. Potential of an interorgan network mediated by toxic advanced glycation end-products in a rat model. Nutrients. 2020;13:80.

23. Tessier FJ. The Maillard reaction in the human body. The main discoveries and factors that affect glycation. Pathol Biol (Paris). 2010;58:214–9.

24. Henning C, Glomb MA. Pathways of the Maillard reaction under physiological conditions. Glycoconj J. 2016;33:499–512.

25. Anguizola J, Matsuda R, Barnaby OS, Hoy KS, Wa C, DeBolt E, Koke M, Hage DS. Review: glycation of human serum albumin. Clin Chim Acta. 2013;425:64–76.

26. Heyns K, Beilfuß W. Ketosylamine rearrangement of D-threo-pentulose (D-xylulose) with alpha-amino acids. Chem Ber. 1970;103:2873–6.

27. Thornalley PJ. Dicarbonyl intermediates in the Maillard reaction. Ann N Y Acad Sci. 2005;1043:111–7.

28. Hamada Y, Araki N, Koh N, Nakamura J, Horiuchi S, Hotta N. Rapid formation of advanced glycation end products by intermediate metabolites of glycolytic pathway and polyol pathway. Biochem Biophys Res Commun. 1996;228:539–43.

29. Gkogkolou P, Böhm M. Advanced glycation end products: key players in skin aging? Dermatoendocrinol. 2012;4(3):259–70. https://doi.org/10.4161/DERM.22028.

30. Méndez JD, Xie J, Aguilar-Hernández M, Méndez-Valenzuela V. Trends in advanced glycation end products research in diabetes mellitus and its complications. Mol Cell Biochem. 2010;341:33–41.

31. Goldberg T, Cai W, Peppa M, Dardaine V, Baliga BS, Uribarri J, Vlassara H. Advanced glycoxidation end products in commonly consumed foods. J Am Diet Assoc. 2004;104:1287–91.

32. Sell DR, Nagaraj RH, Grandhee SK, Odetti P, Lapolla A, Fogarty J, Monnier VM. Pentosidine: a molecular marker for the cumulative damage to proteins in diabetes, aging, and uremia. Diabetes Metab Rev. 1991;7:239–51.

33. Xue M, Rabbani N, Momiji H, et al. Transcriptional control of glyoxalase 1 by Nrf2 provides a stress-responsive defence against dicarbonyl glycation. Biochem J. 2012;443:213–22.

34. Liang Z, Chen X, Li L, Li B, Yang Z. The fate of dietary advanced glycation end products in the body: from oral intake to excretion. Crit Rev Food Sci Nutr. 2020;60(20):3475–91. https://doi.org/10.1080/10408398.2019.1693958.

35. Garay-Sevilla ME, Beeri MS, de La Maza MP, Rojas A, Salazar-Villanea S, Uribarri J. The potential role of dietary advanced glycation endproducts in the development of chronic non-infectious diseases: a narrative review. Nutr Res Rev. 2020;33:298–311.

36. Zhao D, Sheng B, Wu Y, Li H, Xu D, Nian Y, Mao S, Li C, Xu X, Zhou G. Comparison of free and bound advanced glycation end products in food: a review on the possible influence on human health. J Agric Food Chem. 2019;67:14007–18.

37. Chen Y, Guo TL. Dietary advanced glycation end-products elicit toxicological effects by disrupting gut microbiome and immune homeostasis. J Immunotoxicol. 2021;18:93–104.

38. Koschinsky T, He CJ, Mitsuhashi T, Bucala R, Liu C, Buenting C, Heitmann K, Vlassara H. Orally absorbed reactive glycation products (glycotoxins): an environmental risk factor in diabetic nephropathy. Proc Natl Acad Sci U S A. 1997;94:6474–9.

39. Grimm S, Ernst L, Grötzinger N, Höhn A, Breusing N, Reinheckel T, Grune T. Cathepsin D is one of the major enzymes involved in intracellular degradation of AGE-modified proteins. Free Radic Res. 2010;44:1013–26.

40. Bansode SB, Chougale AD, Joshi RS, Giri AP, Bodhankar SL, Harsulkar AM, Kulkarni MJ. Proteomic analysis of protease resistant proteins in the diabetic rat kidney. Mol Cell Proteomics. 2013;12:228.

41. He C, Sabol J, Mitsuhashi T, Vlassara H. Dietary glycotoxins: inhibition of reactive products by aminoguanidine facilitates renal clearance and reduces tissue sequestration. Diabetes. 1999;48:1308–15.

42. Delgado-Andrade C, Tessier FÉJ, Niquet-Leridon C, Seiquer I, Navarro MP. Study of the urinary and faecal excretion of Nε-carboxymethyllysine in young human volunteers. Amino Acids. 2012;43:595–602.

43. Kumar Pasupulati A, Chitra PS, Reddy GB. Advanced glycation end products mediated cellular and molecular events in the pathology of diabetic nephropathy. Biomol Concepts. 2016;7:293–9.

44. Politz O, Gratchev A, McCourt PAG, et al. Stabilin-1 and -2 constitute a novel family of fasciclin-like hyaluronan receptor homologues. Biochem J. 2002;362:155–64.

45. Chen M, Nagase M, Fujita T, Narumiya S, Masaki T, Sawamura T. Diabetes enhances lectin-like oxidized LDL receptor-1 (LOX-1) expression in the vascular endothelium: possible role of LOX-1 ligand and AGE. Biochem Biophys Res Commun. 2001;287:962–8.

46. Zhuang A, Forbes JM. Diabetic kidney disease: a role for advanced glycation end-product receptor 1 (AGE-R1)? Glycoconj J. 2016;33:645–52.

47. Fukushi JI, Makagiansar IT, Stallcup WB. NG2 proteoglycan promotes endothelial cell motility and angiogenesis via engagement of galectin-3 and alpha3beta1 integrin. Mol Biol Cell. 2004;15:3580–90.

48. Vlassara H. The AGE-receptor in the pathogenesis of diabetic complications. Diabetes Metab Res Rev. 2001;17:436–43.

49. Cai W, Torreggiani M, Zhu L, Chen X, He JC, Striker GE, Vlassara H. AGER1 regulates endothelial cell NADPH oxidase-dependent oxidant stress via PKC-delta: implications for vascular disease. Am J Physiol Cell Physiol. 2010;298(3):C624–34. https://doi.org/10.1152/AJPCELL.00463.2009.

50. Vlassara H, Cai W, Goodman S, et al. Protection against loss of innate defenses in adulthood by low advanced glycation end products (AGE) intake: role of the antiinflammatory AGE receptor-1. J Clin Endocrinol Metab. 2009;94:4483–91.

51. Cai W, He JC, Zhu L, Chen X, Striker GE, Vlassara H. AGE-receptor-1 counteracts cellular oxidant stress induced by AGEs via negative regulation of p66shc-dependent FKHRL1 phosphorylation. Am J Physiol Cell Physiol. 2008;294(1):C145–52. https://doi.org/10.1152/AJPCELL.00350.2007.

52. Overexpression of AGE-Receptor-1 in Mice Protects against Diabetic Nephropathy | American Diabetes Association. https://professional.diabetes.org/abstract/overexpression-age-receptor-1-mice-protects-against-diabetic-nephropathy. Accessed 7 Feb 2023.

53. Ott C, Jacobs K, Haucke E, Navarrete Santos A, Grune T, Simm A. Role of advanced glycation end products in cellular signaling. Redox Biol. 2014;2:411–29.

54. Dasu MR, Devaraj S, Park S, Jialal I. Increased toll-like receptor (TLR) activation and TLR ligands in recently diagnosed type 2 diabetic subjects. Diabetes Care. 2010;33:861–8.

55. Jules J, Maiguel D, Hudson BI. Alternative splicing of the RAGE cytoplasmic domain regulates cell signaling and function. PLoS One. 2013;8:1. https://doi.org/10.1371/JOURNAL.PONE.0078267.

56. Brett J, Schmidt AM, Du Yan S, et al. Survey of the distribution of a newly characterized receptor for advanced glycation end products in tissues. Am J Pathol. 1993;143:1699.

57. Niu W, Qi Y, Wu Z, Liu Y, Zhu D, Jin W. A meta-analysis of receptor for advanced glycation end products gene: four well-evaluated polymorphisms with diabetes mellitus. Mol Cell Endocrinol. 2012;358:9–17.

58. Yonekura H, Yamamoto Y, Sakurai S, et al. Novel splice variants of the receptor for advanced glycation end-products expressed in human vascular endothelial cells and pericytes, and their putative roles in diabetes-induced vascular injury. Biochem J. 2003;370:1097–109.
59. Yan SF, Ramasamy R, Naka Y, Schmidt AM. Glycation, inflammation, and RAGE: a scaffold for the macrovascular complications of diabetes and beyond. Circ Res. 2003;93:1159–69.
60. Sergi D, Boulestin H, Campbell FM, Williams LM. The role of dietary advanced glycation end products in metabolic dysfunction. Mol Nutr Food Res. 2021;65(1):e1900934. https://doi.org/10.1002/MNFR.201900934.
61. Leung SS, Forbes JM, Borg DJ. Receptor for advanced glycation end products (RAGE) in type 1 diabetes pathogenesis. Curr Diab Rep. 2016;16(10):100. https://doi.org/10.1007/S11892-016-0782-Y.
62. Indyk D, Bronowicka-Szydełko A, Gamian A, Kuzan A. Advanced glycation end products and their receptors in serum of patients with type 2 diabetes. Sci Rep. 2021;11:13264.
63. Vlassara H, Striker GE. AGE restriction in diabetes mellitus: a paradigm shift. Nat Rev Endocrinol. 2011;7:526.
64. Zhao Z, Zhao C, Xu HZ, Zheng F, Cai W, Vlassara H, Ma ZA. Advanced glycation end products inhibit glucose-stimulated insulin secretion through nitric oxide-dependent inhibition of cytochrome c oxidase and adenosine triphosphate synthesis. Endocrinology. 2009;150:2569–76.
65. Böni-Schnetzler M, Thorne J, Parnaud G, Marselli L, Ehses JA, Kerr-Conte J, Pattou F, Halban PA, Weir GC, Donath MY. Increased interleukin (IL)-1beta messenger ribonucleic acid expression in beta -cells of individuals with type 2 diabetes and regulation of IL-1beta in human islets by glucose and autostimulation. J Clin Endocrinol Metab. 2008;93:4065–74.
66. Vlassara H, Uribarri J. Advanced glycation end products (AGE) and diabetes: cause, effect, or both? Curr Diab Rep. 2014;14(1):453. https://doi.org/10.1007/S11892-013-0453-1.
67. Uribarri J, Cai W, Ramdas M, Goodman S, Pyzik R, Xue C, Li Z, Striker GE, Vlassara H. Restriction of advanced glycation end products improves insulin resistance in human type 2 Diabetes: Potential role of AGER1 and SIRT1. Diabetes Care. 2011;34:1610–6.
68. Šebeková K, Saavedra G, Zumpe C, Somoza V, Klenovicsová K, Birlouez-Aragon I. Plasma concentration and urinary excretion of Nε-(carboxymethyl)lysine in breast milk– and formula-fed infants. Ann N Y Acad Sci. 2008;1126:177–80.
69. Wentworth JM, Fourlanos S, Harrison LC. Reappraising the stereotypes of diabetes in the modern diabetogenic environment. Nat Rev Endocrinol. 2009;5:483–9.
70. Coughlan MT, Yap FYT, Tong DCK, et al. Advanced glycation end products are direct modulators of β-cell function. Diabetes. 2011;60:2523–32.
71. Liang F, Kume S, Koya D. SIRT1 and insulin resistance. Nat Rev Endocrinol. 2009;5:367–73.
72. Shu T, Zhu Y, Wang H, Lin Y, Ma Z, Han X. AGEs decrease insulin synthesis in pancreatic β-cell by repressing Pdx-1 protein expression at the post-translational level. PLoS One. 2011;6(4):e18782. https://doi.org/10.1371/JOURNAL.PONE.0018782.
73. le Bagge S, Fotheringham AK, Leung SS, Forbes JM. Targeting the receptor for advanced glycation end products (RAGE) in type 1 diabetes. Med Res Rev. 2020;40:1200–19.
74. Lim M, Park L, Shin G, Hong H, Kang I, Park Y. Induction of apoptosis of Beta cells of the pancreas by advanced glycation end-products, important mediators of chronic complications of diabetes mellitus. Ann N Y Acad Sci. 2008;1150:311–5.
75. Kong X, Lu AL, Yao XM, Hua Q, Li XY, Qin L, Zhang HM, Meng GX, Su Q. Activation of NLRP3 inflammasome by advanced glycation end products promotes pancreatic islet damage. Oxidative Med Cell Longev. 2017;2017:9692546. https://doi.org/10.1155/2017/9692546.
76. Borg DJ, Yap FYT, Keshvari S, et al. Perinatal exposure to high dietary advanced glycation end products in transgenic NOD8.3 mice leads to pancreatic beta cell dysfunction. Islets. 2018;10:10.
77. Raleigh D, Zhang X, Hastoy B, Clark A. The β-cell assassin: IAPP cytotoxicity. J Mol Endocrinol. 2017;59:R121–40.

78. Abedini A, Cao P, Plesner A, et al. RAGE binds preamyloid IAPP intermediates and mediates pancreatic β cell proteotoxicity. J Clin Invest. 2018;128:682–98.
79. Nandipati KC, Subramanian S, Agrawal DK. Protein kinases: mechanisms and downstream targets in inflammation-mediated obesity and insulin resistance. Mol Cell Biochem. 2017;426:27–45.
80. Nowotny K, Jung T, Höhn A, Weber D, Grune T. Advanced glycation end products and oxidative stress in type 2 diabetes mellitus. Biomol Ther. 2015;5:194.
81. Zhang L, Chen Z, Wang Y, Tweardy DJ, Mitch WE. Stat3 activation induces insulin resistance via a muscle-specific E3 ubiquitin ligase Fbxo40. Am J Physiol Endocrinol Metab. 2020;318:E625–35.
82. Puddu A, Viviani LG. Advanced glycation endproducts and diabetes. Beyond vascular complications. Endocr Metab Immune Disord Drug Targets. 2011;11:132–40.
83. Passarelli M, Machado UF. AGEs-induced and endoplasmic reticulum stress/inflammation-mediated regulation of GLUT4 expression and atherogenesis in diabetes mellitus. Cells. 2021;11(1):104. https://doi.org/10.3390/CELLS11010104.
84. Pinto-Junior DC, Silva KS, Michalani ML, et al. Advanced glycation end products-induced insulin resistance involves repression of skeletal muscle GLUT4 expression. Sci Rep. 2018;8:8109. https://doi.org/10.1038/S41598-018-26482-6.
85. Olefsky JM, Glass CK. Macrophages, inflammation, and insulin resistance. Annu Rev Physiol. 2010;72:219–46.
86. Goldin A, Beckman JA, Schmidt AM, Creager MA. Advanced glycation end products: sparking the development of diabetic vascular injury. Circulation. 2006;114:597–605.
87. Hunter SJ, Boyd AC, O'Harte FPM, et al. Demonstration of glycated insulin in human diabetic plasma and decreased biological activity assessed by euglycemic-hyperinsulinemic clamp technique in humans. Diabetes. 2003;52:492–8.
88. Guo Q, Mori T, Jiang Y, et al. Methylglyoxal contributes to the development of insulin resistance and salt sensitivity in Sprague-Dawley rats. J Hypertens. 2009;27:1664–71.
89. Unoki-Kubota H, Yamagishi S, Takeuchi M, Bujo H, Saito Y. Pyridoxamine, an inhibitor of advanced glycation end product (AGE) formation ameliorates insulin resistance in obese, type 2 diabetic mice. Protein Pept Lett. 2010;17:1177–81.
90. Herman WH, Zimmet P. Type 2 diabetes: An epidemic requiring global attention and urgent action. Diabetes Care. 2012;35:943.
91. Groener JB, Oikonomou D, Cheko R, et al. Methylglyoxal and advanced glycation end products in patients with diabetes - what we know so far and the missing links. Exp Clin Endocrinol Diabetes. 2019;127:497–504.
92. Adams JN, Martelle SE, Raffield LM, et al. Analysis of advanced glycation end products in the DHS mind study. J Diabetes Complicat. 2016;30:262–8.
93. Ceriello A. The emerging challenge in diabetes: the "metabolic memory". Vasc Pharmacol. 2012;57:133–8.
94. Ceriello A, Ihnat MA, Thorpe JE. Clinical review 2: the "metabolic memory": is more than just tight glucose control necessary to prevent diabetic complications? J Clin Endocrinol Metab. 2009;94:410–5.
95. Zhang L, Chen B, Tang L. Metabolic memory: mechanisms and implications for diabetic retinopathy. Diabetes Res Clin Pract. 2012;96:286–93.
96. Zhang EL, Wu YJ. Metabolic memory: mechanisms and implications for diabetic vasculopathies. Sci China Life Sci. 2014;57:845–51.
97. Berezin A. Metabolic memory phenomenon in diabetes mellitus: achieving and perspectives. Diabetes Metab Syndr. 2016;10:S176–83.
98. Reddy MA, Zhang E, Natarajan R. Epigenetic mechanisms in diabetic complications and metabolic memory. Diabetologia. 2015;58:443–55.
99. Cai W, Ramdas M, Zhu L, Chen X, Striker GE, Vlassara H. Oral advanced glycation endproducts (AGEs) promote insulin resistance and diabetes by depleting the antioxidant defenses AGE receptor-1 and sirtuin 1. Proc Natl Acad Sci U S A. 2012;109:15888–93.

100. Lotan R, Ganmore I, Livny A, et al. Effect of advanced glycation end products on cognition in older adults with type 2 diabetes: results from a pilot clinical trial. J Alzheimers Dis. 2021;82:1785–95.
101. Papachristou S, Pafili K, Trypsianis G, Papazoglou D, Vadikolias K, Papanas N. Skin advanced glycation end products among subjects with type 2 diabetes mellitus with or without distal sensorimotor polyneuropathy. J Diabetes Res. 2021;2021:6045677. https://doi.org/10.1155/2021/6045677.
102. Yamamoto M, Sugimoto T. Advanced glycation end products, diabetes, and bone strength. Curr Osteoporos Rep. 2016;14:320–6.
103. Karimi J, Goodarzi MT, Tavilani H, Khodadadi I, Amiri I. Relationship between advanced glycation end products and increased lipid peroxidation in semen of diabetic men. Diabetes Res Clin Pract. 2011;91:61–6.
104. Neves D. Advanced glycation end-products: a common pathway in diabetes and age-related erectile dysfunction. Free Radic Res. 2013;47(Suppl 1):49–69.
105. Patel R, Baker SS, Liu W, et al. Effect of dietary advanced glycation end products on mouse liver. PLoS One. 2012;7:e35143.
106. Merhi Z. Advanced glycation end products and their relevance in female reproduction. Hum Reprod. 2014;29:135–45.
107. Gurav A. Advanced glycation end products: a link between periodontitis and diabetes mellitus? Curr Diabetes Rev. 2013;9:355–61.
108. Hu H, Jiang H, Ren H, Hu X, Wang X, Han C. AGEs and chronic subclinical inflammation in diabetes: disorders of immune system. Diabetes Metab Res Rev. 2015;31:127–37.
109. Rojas A, Añazco C, González I, Araya P. Extracellular matrix glycation and receptor for advanced glycation end-products activation: a missing piece in the puzzle of the association between diabetes and cancer. Carcinogenesis. 2018;39:515–21.
110. Ahmad MN, Farah AI, Al-Qirim TM. The cardiovascular complications of diabetes: a striking link through protein glycation. Rom J Intern Med. 2020;58:188–98.
111. Lee J, Yun JS, Ko SH. Advanced glycation end products and their effect on vascular complications in type 2 diabetes mellitus. Nutrients. 2022;14(15):3086. https://doi.org/10.3390/NU14153086.
112. Burke AP, Kolodgie FD, Zieske A, Fowler DR, Weber DK, Varghese PJ, Farb A, Virmani R. Morphologic findings of coronary atherosclerotic plaques in diabetics: a postmortem study. Arterioscler Thromb Vasc Biol. 2004;24:1266–71.
113. Lin L, Park S, Lakatta EG. RAGE signaling in inflammation and arterial aging. Front Biosci. 2009;14:1403.
114. Jansen F, Yang X, Franklin BS, Hoelscher M, Schmitz T, Bedorf J, Nickenig G, Werner N. High glucose condition increases NADPH oxidase activity in endothelial microparticles that promote vascular inflammation. Cardiovasc Res. 2013;98:94–106.
115. Sun L, Ishida T, Yasuda T, Kojima Y, Honjo T, Yamamoto Y, Yamamoto H, Ishibashi S, Hirata KI, Hayashi Y. RAGE mediates oxidized LDL-induced pro-inflammatory effects and atherosclerosis in non-diabetic LDL receptor-deficient mice. Cardiovasc Res. 2009;82:371–81.
116. Rabbani N, Godfrey L, Xue M, Shaheen F, Geoffrion M, Milne R, Thornalley PJ. Glycation of LDL by methylglyoxal increases arterial atherogenicity: a possible contributor to increased risk of cardiovascular disease in diabetes. Diabetes. 2011;60:1973–80.
117. Fukami K, Yamagishi S, Okuda S. Role of AGEs-RAGE system in cardiovascular disease. Curr Pharm Des. 2014;20:2395–402.
118. Vlassara H, Fuh H, Donnelly T, Cybulsky M. Advanced glycation endproducts promote adhesion molecule (VCAM-1, ICAM-1) expression and atheroma formation in normal rabbits. Mol Med. 1995;1:447.
119. Yamagishi S, Fujimori H, Yonekura H, Yamamoto Y, Yamamoto H. Advanced glycation endproducts inhibit prostacyclin production and induce plasminogen activator inhibitor-1 in human microvascular endothelial cells. Diabetologia. 1998;41:1435–41.

120. Quehenberger P, Bierhaus A, Fasching P, et al. Endothelin 1 transcription is controlled by nuclear factor-kappaB in AGE-stimulated cultured endothelial cells. Diabetes. 2000;49:1561–70.
121. Xu B, Chibber R, Ruggiero D, Kohner E, Ritter J, Ferro A. Impairment of vascular endothelial nitric oxide synthase activity by advanced glycation end products. FASEB J. 2003;17:1289–91.
122. Kosmopoulos M, Drekolias D, Zavras PD, Piperi C, Papavassiliou AG. Impact of advanced glycation end products (AGEs) signaling in coronary artery disease. Biochim Biophys Acta Mol basis Dis. 2019;1865:611–9.
123. McNulty M, Mahmud A, Feely J. Advanced glycation end-products and arterial stiffness in hypertension. Am J Hypertens. 2007;20:242–7.
124. Brodeur MR, Bouvet C, Bouchard S, Moreau S, Leblond J, DeBlois D, Moreau P. Reduction of advanced-glycation end products levels and inhibition of RAGE signaling decreases rat vascular calcification induced by diabetes. PLoS One. 2014;9:e85922.
125. Prasad A, Bekker P, Tsimikas S. Advanced glycation end products and diabetic cardiovascular disease. Cardiol Rev. 2012;20:177–83.
126. Hansen LM, Gupta D, Joseph G, Weiss D, Taylor WR. The receptor for advanced glycation end products impairs collateral formation in both diabetic and non-diabetic mice. Lab Investig. 2017;97:34–42.
127. Peppa M, Brem H, Ehrlich P, Zhang JG, Cai W, Li Z, Croitoru A, Thung S, Vlassara H. Adverse effects of dietary glycotoxins on wound healing in genetically diabetic mice. Diabetes. 2003;52:2805–13.
128. Münch G, Westcott B, Menini T, Gugliucci A. Advanced glycation endproducts and their pathogenic roles in neurological disorders. Amino Acids. 2012;42:1221–36.
129. Thornalley PJ. Glycation in diabetic neuropathy: characteristics, consequences, causes, and therapeutic options. Int Rev Neurobiol. 2002;50:37–57.
130. Jack M, Wright D. Role of advanced glycation endproducts and glyoxalase I in diabetic peripheral sensory neuropathy. Transl Res. 2012;159:355–65.
131. Zong H, Ward M, Stitt AW. AGEs, RAGE, and diabetic retinopathy. Curr Diab Rep. 2011;11:244–52.
132. Liu BF, Bhat M, Padival AK, Smith DG, Nagaraj RH. Effect of dicarbonyl modification of fibronectin on retinal capillary pericytes. Invest Ophthalmol Vis Sci. 2004;45:1983–95.
133. Gao X, Zhang H, Schmidt AM, Zhang C. AGE/RAGE produces endothelial dysfunction in coronary arterioles in type 2 diabetic mice. Am J Physiol Heart Circ Physiol. 2008;295(2):H491–8. https://doi.org/10.1152/AJPHEART.00464.2008.
134. Shang L, Ananthakrishnan R, Li Q, et al. RAGE modulates hypoxia/reoxygenation injury in adult murine cardiomyocytes via JNK and GSK-3beta signaling pathways. PLoS One. 2010;5(4):e10092. https://doi.org/10.1371/JOURNAL.PONE.0010092.
135. Ishibashi T, Kawaguchi M, Sugimoto K, Uekita H, Sakamoto N, Yokoyama K, Maruyama Y, Takeishi Y. Advanced glycation end product-mediated matrix metallo-proteinase-9 and apoptosis via renin-angiotensin system in type 2 diabetes. J Atheroscler Thromb. 2010;17:578–89.
136. Ramasamy R, Yan SF, Schmidt AM. The diverse ligand repertoire of the receptor for advanced glycation endproducts and pathways to the complications of diabetes. Vasc Pharmacol. 2012;57:160–7.
137. Kilhovd BK, Juutilainen A, Lehto S, Rönnemaa T, Torjesen PA, Hanssen KF, Laakso M. Increased serum levels of advanced glycation endproducts predict total, cardiovascular and coronary mortality in women with type 2 diabetes: a population-based 18 year follow-up study. Diabetologia. 2007;50:1409–17.
138. Kiuchi K, Nejima J, Takano T, Ohta M, Hashimoto H, Baxter GF. Increased serum concentrations of advanced glycation end products: a marker of coronary artery disease activity in type 2 diabetic patients. Heart. 2001;85:87–91.

139. Bidasee KR, Nallani K, Yu Y, Cocklin RR, Zhang Y, Wang M, Dincer UD, Besch HR. Chronic diabetes increases advanced glycation end products on cardiac ryanodine receptors/calcium-release channels. Diabetes. 2003;52:1825–36.
140. Bidasee KR, Zhang Y, Shao CH, Wang M, Patel KP, Dincer ÜD, Besch HR. Diabetes increases formation of advanced glycation end products on Sarco(endo)plasmic reticulum Ca2+-ATPase. Diabetes. 2004;53:463–73.
141. Candido R, Forbes JM, Thomas MC, et al. A breaker of advanced glycation end products attenuates diabetes-induced myocardial structural changes. Circ Res. 2003;92:785–92.
142. Xie J, Méndez JD, Méndez-Valenzuela V, Aguilar-Hernández MM. Cellular signalling of the receptor for advanced glycation end products (RAGE). Cell Signal. 2013;25:2185–97.
143. Yamazaki KG, Gonzalez E, Zambon AC. Crosstalk between the renin-angiotensin system and the advance glycation end product axis in the heart: role of the cardiac fibroblast. J Cardiovasc Transl Res. 2012;5:805–13.
144. Nielsen JM, Kristiansen SB, Nørregaard R, Andersen CL, Denner L, Nielsen TT, Flyvbjerg A, Bøtker HE. Blockage of receptor for advanced glycation end products prevents development of cardiac dysfunction in db/db type 2 diabetic mice. Eur J Heart Fail. 2009;11:638–47.
145. Persson F. Rossing P (2018) diagnosis of diabetic kidney disease: state of the art and future perspective. Kidney Int Suppl. 2011;8:2–7.
146. Wu XQ, Zhang DD, Wang YN, Tan YQ, Yu XY, Zhao YY. AGE/RAGE in diabetic kidney disease and ageing kidney. Free Radic Biol Med. 2021;171:260–71.
147. Jin Q, Lau ES, Luk AO, et al. Skin autofluorescence is associated with progression of kidney disease in type 2 diabetes: a prospective cohort study from the Hong Kong diabetes biobank. Nutr Metab Cardiovasc Dis. 2022;32:436–46.
148. Koska J, Gerstein HC, Beisswenger PJ, Reaven PD. Advanced glycation end products predict loss of renal function and high-risk chronic kidney disease in type 2 diabetes. Diabetes Care. 2022;45:684–91.
149. Tanji N, Markowitz GS, Fu C, Kislinger T, Taguchi A, Pischetsrieder M, Stern D, Schmidt AM, D'Agati VD. Expression of advanced glycation end products and their cellular receptor RAGE in diabetic nephropathy and nondiabetic renal disease. J Am Soc Nephrol. 2000;11:1656–66.
150. Yamagishi SI, Inagaki Y, Okamoto T, Amano S, Koga K, Takeuchi M. Advanced glycation end products inhibit de novo protein synthesis and induce TGF-beta overexpression in proximal tubular cells. Kidney Int. 2003;63:464–73.
151. Sanajou D, Ghorbani Haghjo A, Argani H, Aslani S. AGE-RAGE axis blockade in diabetic nephropathy: current status and future directions. Eur J Pharmacol. 2018;833:158–64.
152. Bin SS, Ha DS, Min SY, Ha TS. Autophagy precedes apoptosis in angiotensin II-induced podocyte injury. Cell Physiol Biochem. 2019;53:747–59.
153. Yeh WJ, Yang HY, Pai MH, Wu CH, Chen JR. Long-term administration of advanced glycation end-product stimulates the activation of NLRP3 inflammasome and sparking the development of renal injury. J Nutr Biochem. 2017;39:68–76.
154. Tan ALY, Forbes JM, Cooper ME. AGE, RAGE, and ROS in diabetic nephropathy. Semin Nephrol. 2007;27:130–43.
155. Yamagaki SI, Inagaki Y, Okamoto T, Amano S, Koga K, Takeuchi M, Makita Z. Advanced glycation end product-induced apoptosis and overexpression of vascular endothelial growth factor and monocyte chemoattractant protein-1 in human-cultured mesangial cells. J Biol Chem. 2002;277:20309–15.
156. Anil Kumar P, Welsh GI, Saleem MA, Menon RK. Molecular and cellular events mediating glomerular podocyte dysfunction and depletion in diabetes mellitus. Front Endocrinol (Lausanne). 2014;5:151. https://doi.org/10.3389/FENDO.2014.00151.
157. An X, Zhang L, Yao Q, Li L, Wang B, Zhang J, He M, Zhang J. The receptor for advanced glycation endproducts mediates podocyte heparanase expression through NF-κB signaling pathway. Mol Cell Endocrinol. 2018;470:14–25.

158. Rabbani N, Thornalley PJ. Advanced glycation end products in the pathogenesis of chronic kidney disease. Kidney Int. 2018;93:803–13.
159. Vlassara H, Striker LJ, Teichberg S, Fuh H, Li YM, Steffes M. Advanced glycation end products induce glomerular sclerosis and albuminuria in normal rats. Proc Natl Acad Sci. 1994;91:11704–8.
160. Coughlan MT, Patel SK, Jerums G, et al. Advanced glycation urinary protein-bound biomarkers and severity of diabetic nephropathy in man. Am J Nephrol. 2011;34:347–55.
161. Waris S, Winklhofer-Roob BM, Roob JM, Fuchs S, Sourij H, Rabbani N, Thornalley PJ. Increased DNA dicarbonyl glycation and oxidation markers in patients with type 2 diabetes and link to diabetic nephropathy. J Diabetes Res. 2015;2015:915486. https://doi.org/10.1155/2015/915486.
162. Zheng F, He C, Cai W, Hattori M, Steffes M, Vlassara H. Prevention of diabetic nephropathy in mice by a diet low in glycoxidation products. Diabetes Metab Res Rev. 2002;18:224–37.
163. Vlassara H, Cai W, Crandall J, Goldberg T, Oberstein R, Dardaine V, Peppa M, Rayfield EJ. Inflammatory mediators are induced by dietary glycotoxins, a major risk factor for diabetic angiopathy. Proc Natl Acad Sci U S A. 2002;99:15596–601.
164. Cai W, He JC, Zhu L, Chen X, Wallenstein S, Striker GE, Vlassara H. Reduced oxidant stress and extended lifespan in mice exposed to a low glycotoxin diet: association with increased AGER1 expression. Am J Pathol. 2007;170:1893–902.
165. Gutierrez-Mariscal FM, Cardelo MP, de la Cruz S, et al. Reduction in circulating advanced glycation end products by Mediterranean diet is associated with increased likelihood of type 2 diabetes remission in patients with coronary heart disease: from the CORDIOPREV study. Mol Nutr Food Res. 2021;65(1):e1901290. https://doi.org/10.1002/MNFR.201901290.
166. Steenbeke M, de Decker I, Marchand S, Glorieux G, van Biesen W, Lapauw B, Delanghe JR, Speeckaert MM. Dietary advanced glycation end products in an elderly population with diabetic nephropathy: an exploratory investigation. Nutrients. 2022;14:1818. https://doi.org/10.3390/NU14091818.
167. Chilelli NC, Cremasco D, Cosma C, Ragazzi E, Francini Pesenti F, Bonfante L, Lapolla A. Effectiveness of a diet with low advanced glycation end products, in improving glycoxidation and lipid peroxidation: a long-term investigation in patients with chronic renal failure. Endocrine. 2016;54:552–5.
168. Oliveira JS, de Almeida C, de Souza ÂMN, da Cruz LD, Alfenas RCG. Effect of dietary advanced glycation end-products restriction on type 2 diabetes mellitus control: a systematic review. Nutr Rev. 2022;80:294–305.
169. Rowan S, Bejarano E, Taylor A. Mechanistic targeting of advanced glycation end-products in age-related diseases. Biochim Biophys Acta Mol basis Dis. 2018;1864:3631–43.
170. Thornalley PJ. The enzymatic defence against glycation in health, disease and therapeutics: a symposium to examine the concept. Biochem Soc Trans. 2003;31:1341–2.
171. Xue M, Weickert MO, Qureshi S, et al. Improved glycemic control and vascular function in overweight and obese subjects by glyoxalase 1 inducer formulation. Diabetes. 2016;65:2282–94.
172. Maher P, Dargusch R, Ehren JL, Okada S, Sharma K, Schubert D. Fisetin lowers methylglyoxal dependent protein glycation and limits the complications of diabetes. PLoS One. 2011;6(6):e21226. https://doi.org/10.1371/JOURNAL.PONE.0021226.
173. Suantawee T, Thilavech T, Cheng H, Adisakwattana S. Cyanidin attenuates methylglyoxal-induced oxidative stress and apoptosis in INS-1 pancreatic β-cells by increasing glyoxalase-1 activity. Nutrients. 2020;12(5):1319. https://doi.org/10.3390/NU12051319.
174. Sanajou D, Ghorbani Haghjo A, Argani H, Roshangar L, Ahmad SNS, Jigheh ZA, Aslani S, Panah F, Rashedi J, Mesgari Abbasi M. FPS-ZM1 and valsartan combination protects better against glomerular filtration barrier damage in streptozotocin-induced diabetic rats. J Physiol Biochem. 2018;74:467–78.
175. Bucciarelli LG, Wendt T, Qu W, et al. RAGE blockade stabilizes established atherosclerosis in diabetic apolipoprotein E-null mice. Circulation. 2002;106:2827–35.

176. Johnson LL, Johnson J, Ober R, Holland A, Zhang G, Backer M, Backer J, Ali Z, Tekabe Y. Novel receptor for advanced glycation end products-blocking antibody to treat diabetic peripheral artery disease. J Am Heart Assoc. 2021;10:1–12.

177. Puddu A, MacH F, Nencioni A, Viviani GL, Montecucco F. An emerging role of glucagon-like peptide-1 in preventing advanced-glycation-end-product-mediated damages in diabetes. Mediat Inflamm. 2013;2013:591056. https://doi.org/10.1155/2013/591056.

178. Kaida Y, Fukami K, Matsui T, et al. DNA aptamer raised against AGEs blocks the progression of experimental diabetic nephropathy. Diabetes. 2013;62:3241–50.

179. Vlassara H, Uribarri J, Cai W, Goodman S, Pyzik R, Post J, Grosjean F, Woodward M, Striker GE. Effects of sevelamer on HbA1c, inflammation, and advanced glycation end products in diabetic kidney disease. Clin J Am Soc Nephrol. 2012;7:934–42.

180. Urios P, Grigorova-Borsos AM, Sternberg M. Aspirin inhibits the formation of pentosidine, a cross-linking advanced glycation end product, in collagen. Diabetes Res Clin Pract. 2007;77:337–40.

181. Adeshara KA, Bangar NS, Doshi PR, Diwan A, Tupe RS. Action of metformin therapy against advanced glycation, oxidative stress and inflammation in type 2 diabetes patients: 3 months follow-up study. Diabetes Metab Syndr Clin Res Rev. 2020;14:1449–58.

182. Chang KC, Tseng CD, Wu MS, Liang JT, Tsai MS, Cho YL, Tseng YZ. Aminoguanidine prevents arterial stiffening in a new rat model of type 2 diabetes. Eur J Clin Investig. 2006;36:528–35.

183. Tajiri Y, Grill V. Aminoguanidine exerts a beta-cell function-preserving effect in high glucose-cultured beta-cells (INS-1). Int J Exp Diabetes Res. 2000;1:111–9.

184. Fishman SL, Sonmez H, Basman C, Singh V, Poretsky L. The role of advanced glycation end-products in the development of coronary artery disease in patients with and without diabetes mellitus: a review. Mol Med. 2018;24(1):59. https://doi.org/10.1186/S10020-018-0060-3.

185. Alkhalaf A, Klooster A, van Oeveren W, et al. A double-blind, randomized, placebo-controlled clinical trial on benfotiamine treatment in patients with diabetic nephropathy. Diabetes Care. 2010;33:1598–601.

186. Stracke H, Hammes HP, Werkmann D, et al. Efficacy of benfotiamine versus thiamine on function and glycation products of peripheral nerves in diabetic rats. Exp Clin Endocrinol Diabetes. 2001;109:330–6.

187. Lewis EJ, Greene T, Spitalewiz S, et al. Pyridorin in type 2 diabetic nephropathy. J Am Soc Nephrol. 2012;23:131–6.

188. Pereira A, Fernandes R, Crisóstomo J, Seiça RM, Sena CM. The sulforaphane and pyridoxamine supplementation normalize endothelial dysfunction associated with type 2 diabetes. Scientific Rep. 2017;17:1–13.

189. van den Eynde MDG, Houben AJHM, Scheijen JLJM, et al. Pyridoxamine reduces methylglyoxal and markers of glycation and endothelial dysfunction, but does not improve insulin sensitivity or vascular function in abdominally obese individuals: a randomized double-blind placebo-controlled trial. Diabetes Obes Metab. 2023;25(5):1280–91. https://doi.org/10.1111/DOM.14977.

190. Tsunosue M, Mashiko N, Ohta Y, et al. An alpha-glucosidase inhibitor, acarbose treatment decreases serum levels of glyceraldehyde-derived advanced glycation end products (AGEs) in patients with type 2 diabetes. Clin Exp Med. 2010;10:139–41.

191. Beyer-Mears A, Mistry K, Diecke FPJ, Cruz E. Zopolrestat prevention of proteinuria, albuminuria and cataractogenesis in diabetes mellitus. Pharmacology. 1996;52:292–302.

192. Nenna A, Spadaccio C, Lusini M, Ulianich L, Chello M, Nappi F. Basic and clinical research against advanced glycation end products (AGEs): new compounds to tackle cardiovascular disease and diabetic complications. Recent Adv Cardiovasc Drug Discov. 2015;10:10–33.

193. Coughlan MT, Forbes JM, Cooper ME. Role of the AGE crosslink breaker, alagebrium, as a renoprotective agent in diabetes. Kidney Int. 2007;72:S54–60.

194. Toprak C, Yigitaslan S. Alagebrium and complications of diabetes mellitus. Eurasian J Med. 2019;51:285.

195. Abbas G, Al-Harrasi AS, Hussain H, Hussain J, Rashid R, Choudhary MI. Antiglycation therapy: discovery of promising antiglycation agents for the management of diabetic complications. Pharm Biol. 2016;54:198–206.
196. Lee BH, Hsu WH, Hsu YW, Pan TM. Dimerumic acid attenuates receptor for advanced glycation endproducts signal to inhibit inflammation and diabetes mediated by Nrf2 activation and promotes methylglyoxal metabolism into d-lactic acid. Free Radic Biol Med. 2013;60:7–16.
197. Thieme K, da Silva KS, Fabre NT, et al. N-acetyl cysteine attenuated the deleterious effects of advanced glycation end-products on the kidney of non-diabetic rats. Cell Physiol Biochem. 2016;40:608–20.
198. Tao X, Zhang Z, Yang Z, Rao B. The effects of taurine supplementation on diabetes mellitus in humans: a systematic review and meta-analysis. Food Chem. 2022;4:100106.
199. Muellenbach EA, Diehl CJ, Teachey MK, et al. Interactions of the advanced glycation end product inhibitor pyridoxamine and the antioxidant α-lipoic acid on insulin resistance in the obese Zucker rat. Metabolism. 2008;57:1465.
200. Parveen A, Sultana R, Lee SM, Kim TH, Kim SY. Phytochemicals against anti-diabetic complications: targeting the advanced glycation end product signaling pathway. Arch Pharm Res. 2021;44:378–401.
201. Vijaykrishnaraj M, Wang K. Dietary natural products as a potential inhibitor towards advanced glycation end products and hyperglycemic complications: a phytotherapy approaches. Biomed Pharmacother. 2021;144:112336. https://doi.org/10.1016/J.BIOPHA.2021.112336.

Chapter 6
Genetic and Epigenetic Basis of Obesity-Induced Inflammation and Diabetes

Radoslav Stojchevski, Sara Velichkovikj, and Todor Arsov

Abbreviations

ACTH	Adrenocorticotropic hormone
AgRP	Agouti-related protein
ALMS	Alstrom syndrome
ARC	Arcuate nucleus
BBS	Bardet-Biedl syndrome
BDNF	Brain-derived neurotrophic factor
BMI	Body mass index
CCL2	Chemokine (C-C motif) ligand 2 (*s.* MCP-1)
DLK1	Delta-like non-canonical Notch ligand 1 (*s.* Pref-1)
DNMT	DNA methyltransferase

The original version of the chapter has been revised. A correction to this chapter can be found at https://doi.org/10.1007/978-3-031-39721-9_11

R. Stojchevski (✉)
Friedman Diabetes Institute, Lenox Hill Hospital, New York, NY, USA

Donald and Barbara Zucker School of Medicine at Hofstra/Northwell, Hempstead, NY, USA
e-mail: rstojchevski@northwell.edu

S. Velichkovikj
Faculty of Natural Sciences and Mathematics, Institute of Biology, Ss. Cyril and Methodius University, Skopje, Macedonia

Department of Medicine, Lenox Hill Hospital, New York, NY, USA
e-mail: svelichkovik@northwell.edu

T. Arsov
Faculty of Medical Sciences, University Goce Delcev, Shtip, Macedonia
e-mail: todor.arsov@ugd.edu.mk

© The Author(s), under exclusive license to Springer Nature Switzerland AG 2023, corrected publication 2023
D. Avtanski, L. Poretsky (eds.), *Obesity, Diabetes and Inflammation,* Contemporary Endocrinology, https://doi.org/10.1007/978-3-031-39721-9_6

FABP4	Fatty acid-binding protein 4
GWAS	Genome-wide association studies
IL-1β	Interleukin 1 beta
IL-6	Interleukin 6
IR	Insulin receptor
IRS-1	Insulin-receptor substrate 1
JNK	c-Jun N-terminal kinase
LEP-R	Leptin receptor
lncRNA	Long non-coding RNA
MC1R	Melanocortin 1 receptor
MC2R	Melanocortin 2 receptor
MC4R	Melanocortin 4 receptor
miRNA	MicroRNA
ncRNA	Non-coding RNA
NF-κB	Nuclear factor kappa B
NPY	Neuropeptide Y
NTRK2	Neurotrophic receptor tyrosine kinase 2
PC	Proprotein (*s.* prohormone) convertase (*s.* proconvertase)
PCSK1	Proprotein convertase subtilism/kexin type 1
POMC	Proopiomelanocortin
PPARγ	Peroxisome proliferator-activated receptor gamma
pro-GnRH	Progonadotropin-releasing hormone
pro-TRH	Prothyrotropin-releasing hormone
PVN	Paraventricular nucleus
PWS	Prader–Willi syndrome
SIM1	Single-minded homolog 1
T2DM	Type 2 diabetes mellitus
T4	Thyroxine
TNFα	Tumor necrosis factor alpha
TRKB	Tropomyosin receptor kinase B
TSH	Thyroid-stimulating hormone
α-MSH	Alpha melanocyte-stimulating hormone
β-MSH	Beta melanocyte-stimulating hormone
γ-MSH	Gamma melanocyte-stimulating hormone

Introduction

Obesity, defined by the World Health Organization as a body mass index (BMI) >30 kg/m^2, is a complex, chronic disease whose global prevalence has considerably increased in the past several decades. Obesity-induced inflammation may play a role in the pathophysiology of diabetes. As obesity develops, adipose tissue undergoes significant modifications that result in infiltration and activation of pro-inflammatory macrophages (M1) in the metabolic tissues, ultimately leading to chronic low-grade inflammation [1]. There is evidence that in a state of obesity, the excessive pro-inflammatory cytokine production, including tumor necrosis factor α (TNFα), interleukin 6 (IL-6), interleukin 1β (IL-1β), and chemokine (C-C motif) ligand 2 (CCL2) in the adipose tissue, liver, muscle, and pancreas causes inhibition of insulin receptor signaling mainly through activation of c-Jun N-terminal kinase (JNK) and nuclear factor-κB (NF-kB) pathways, thus promoting insulin resistance [2]. Despite the fact that the leading cause of obesity is the imbalance between energy uptake and energy expenditure (high energy-dense foods and sedentary life-style), other factors such as genetics and epigenetics can cause or contribute to excess adiposity. This chapter provides an overview of the known monogenic and some of the syndromic forms of obesity, as well as the epigenetic modifications associated with obesity.

Genetic Cause of Obesity and Leptin-Melanocortin Pathway

The players in the neuroendocrine appetite-regulating pathway in the hypothalamus, also known as the leptin-melanocortin pathway, are at the center of monogenic obesity (Fig. 6.1). Energy homeostasis is regulated by hypothalamic neurons located in the arcuate nucleus (ARC) that respond to various peripheral energy-related signals such as hunger and satiety. These neurons, stimulated by metabolic hormones including leptin, insulin, and ghrelin, synthesize two neuropeptides with antagonistic effects: the anorexigenic proopiomelanocortin (POMC) and the orexigenic agouti-related protein and neuropeptide Y (AgRP/NPY). The binding of leptin or insulin to their receptors on the surface of the POMC neuron activates the conversion of POMC neuropeptide into α-melanocyte-stimulating hormone (α-MSH), a reaction catalyzed by proprotein convertases (PC) 1 and 2 (PC1 and PC2) [3, 4]. In contrast, ghrelin binding to its receptor on the surface of the AgRP/NPY neuron activates the production of AgRP and NPY neuropeptides [5]. Both α-MSH and AgRP exit the ARC and enter the hypothalamus's paraventricular nucleus (PVN), where they compete to attach to their receptor, melanocortin 4 receptor (MC4R). When α-MSH binds to MC4R, it stimulates an anorexigenic response to decrease food intake. On the contrary, when AgRP binds to MC4R, it produces orexigenic signals to increase the appetite [3]. Simultaneously, NPY boosts orexigenic signals by inhibiting POMC neurons, while both leptin and insulin boost anorexigenic signals by inhibiting AgRP/NPY neurons. The signals from MC4R regulate the energy balance by activating various factors and receptors such as brain-derived neurotrophic factor (BDNF), single-minded homolog 1 (SIM1), and tropomyosin-related kinase B (TRKB) in the higher centers of the brain. The presence of pathogenic variants in any of the genes involved in the leptin-melanocortin pathway leads to monogenic forms of obesity.

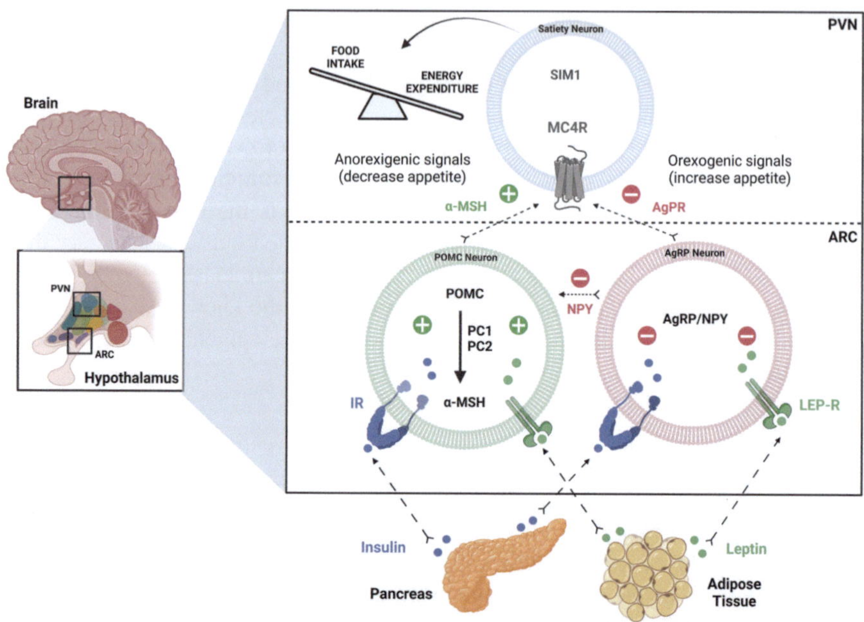

Fig. 6.1 Neuroendocrine appetite-regulating leptin-melanocortin pathway in the hypothalamus: a general scheme. The ARC in the hypothalamus contains neurons that respond to various peripheral signals such as hunger and satiety. When stimulated by LEP, INS, and GHRL, these neurons synthesize two neuropeptides, the anorexigenic POMC and the orexigenic AgRP/NPY. POMC converts to α-MSH when LEP or INS binds to their receptors on the surface of the POMC neuron. This reaction is catalyzed by PC1 and PC2. Moreover, when GHRL binds to its receptor on the surface of the AgRP/NPY neuron, the synthesis of AgRP and NPY neuropeptides begins. Upon exiting the ARC, α-MSH and AgRP enter the PVN in the hypothalamus, where competitive binding to the MC4R takes place. When α-MSH binds to MCR4, anorexigenic signals are generated, triggering appetite decrease. Conversely, when AgRP binds to MC4R, it generates orexigenic signals stimulating increased appetite. Simultaneously, LEP and INS inhibit AgRP/NPY neurons, thus boosting anorexic signaling through MC4R. MC4R's signals activate various receptors and factors in the higher centers of the brain, such as the BDNF, SIM1, and TRKB, which regulate the energy balance. Mutations in genes involved in the leptin-melanocortin pathway lead to monogenic obesity. *ARC* arcuate nucleus, *PVN* paraventricular nucleus, *IR* insulin receptor, *LEP-R* leptin receptor, *POMC* proopiomelanocortin, *PC1* proprotein convertase 1, *PC2* proprotein convertase 2, *α-MSH* α-melanocyte-stimulating hormone, *AgRP* agouti-related protein, *NPY* neuropeptide Y, *MC4R* melanocortin 4 receptor, *SIM1* single-minded homolog 1. (Created with BioRender.com)

Monogenic Obesity

Pathogenic variants in a single gene involved in the leptin-melanocortin pathway cause a rare form of early-onset monogenic obesity associated with extreme polyphagia and various endocrine and reproductive anomalies [6, 7].

Congenital Leptin Deficiency (*LEP*-Related Monogenic Obesity)

Biallelic pathogenic variants disrupting the function of the genes encoding leptin (*LEP*) or leptin receptor (*LEPR*) lead to obesity, hyperphagia, and reduced energy expenditure in rodents, accompanied by increased cortisol secretion, disrupted glucose homeostasis, elevated blood lipid levels, and infertility due to secondary (hypogonadotropic) hypogonadism [8]. The *ob/ob* mouse model of spontaneously occurring monogenic obesity originated from a mouse colony in the Jackson laboratories [8, 9]. The complex "*obese*" phenotype inherited in an autosomal recessive way included hyperphagia, reduced energy expenditure, insulin resistance with hyperglycemia, hyperinsulinemia, hypothyroidism, and infertility [10–12]. The underlying genetic cause was identified through positional cloning of the *ob* gene on mouse chromosome 6 in 1994 [8, 9, 11]. A few years later, it was shown that treating leptin-deficient mice with leptin rescued the obese phenotype by reducing food intake and increasing energy expenditure [10].

The first evidence of the genetic contribution of leptin in human obesity came in 1997 with the identification of two severely obese homozygous cousins for a pathogenic *LEP* frameshift variant (deletion of a single G in codon 133, causing a frameshift with 14 aberrant amino acids after Gly 132 and a premature stop codon), leading to undetectable serum levels of leptin [13, 14]. The treatment of one of the family members with recombinant leptin at age 9 led to a remarkable reversal of the phenotype, with a sustained reduction in body weight, primarily due to the reduction of the body fat content as a result of suppressed hyperphagia [15]. To date, only a few cases of congenital leptin deficiency have been described worldwide, with the prevalence of homozygosity for pathogenic *LEP* variants estimated to be 1 in 15 million [16]. Obese patients with congenital leptin deficiency have an average birth weight, and the exponential weight gain starts during the first 3 months of life [17]. By 1 year of age, patients with congenital leptin deficiency usually weigh more than 20 kg, and by 5 years of age, more than 50 kg. Children with congenital leptin deficiency have increased body fat by up to 50%, compared to 15–25% in unaffected children [18]. In addition, leptin is involved in pubertal development, and many individuals with congenital leptin deficiency have reproductive problems (as do *ob/ob* mice) [19–21]. Persons with congenital leptin deficiency may also have other changes in endocrine parameters, such as low free thyroxine (T4) and high serum inactive thyroid-stimulating hormone (TSH), hypothalamic hypothyroidism, and reduced height in adults (with normal levels of insulin-like growth factors) [22, 23].

Leptin Resistance (*LEPR*-Related Monogenic Obesity)

The leptin receptor is a single-transmembrane domain receptor, a member of the cytokine-receptor family [23, 24]. The diabetic mouse model *db/db* develops remarkable hyperphagic obesity and hyperglycemia due to a spontaneous pathogenic variant in the mouse *db* gene on chromosome 4 that codes for the leptin receptor [11, 25]. The disruption of the signaling through the leptin receptor leads to leptin resistance and obesity, despite elevated levels of leptin [26]. The *db/db* mice share similar phenotype features as the *ob/ob* mouse models, except for insulin resistance which leads to the development of type 2 diabetes mellitus (T2DM) in these mice. The obese Zucker rat, also known as "*fatty*" (*fa/fa*), is another animal model of leptin receptor deficiency [27]. Humans with leptin resistance due to pathogenic variants in the *LEPR* gene are morbidly obese and hyperphagic. Their serum leptin levels are within the range predicted by the percent body fat, suggesting a lack of feedback from leptin receptor signaling on the secretion of leptin from adipocytes. In addition to obesity and hyperglycemia, several other issues have been reported in leptin receptor deficiency, such as delayed pubertal development due to secondary hypogonadism and reduced secretion of growth hormone and thyrotropin [23, 28]. Although early cohort data suggested that leptin receptor deficiency may cause up to 3% of cases with early-onset hyperphagic obesity [28], to date, there are less than 100 known patients with leptin receptor deficiency worldwide, and the estimated prevalence is about 1.3 in one million people [29].

POMC Deficiency (*POMC*-Related Obesity)

POMC is the precursor of multiple peptides, including adrenocorticotropic hormone (ACTH), α melanocyte-stimulating hormone (α-MSH), β melanocyte-stimulating hormone (β-MSH), β-endorphin, and γ melanocyte-stimulating hormone (γ-MSH), involved in regulating energy homeostasis, food intake, adrenal steroidogenesis, melanocyte stimulation, and immune modulation [30]. ACTH acts by binding to the melanocortin 2 receptor (MC2R) in the adrenal cortex and is essential for maintaining normal adrenal cortical function. Pathogenic variants in the *POMC* gene lead to ACTH deficiency and hypocortisolism [31]. Individuals with genetic POMC deficiency are obese and have increased appetite, despite having profound secondary adrenal insufficiency [32]. Transgenic mice with targeted deletion of the *POMC* gene coding region also suffer from obesity [33]. Thus, the regulation of energy homeostasis in genetic POMC deficiency differs from that in typical POMC-deficient hypopituitary patients. The proteolytic cleavage of POMC is catalyzed by PC1/3 and PC2. These enzymes cleave POMC into active peptides, such as the α-MSH that activates melanocortin 1 receptor (MC1R) in the skin, increasing pigment production, and MC4R in the hypothalamus, signaling satiety and suppressing appetite [31].

POMC deficiency is an autosomal recessive disorder with a clinical phenotype that includes a triad of severe hyperphagic obesity, adrenal insufficiency with low cortisol levels, and varying degrees of red hair pigmentation [18, 22, 34]. Patients with this complex phenotype were first described in 1998. To date, less than 50 patients with genetic POMC deficiency have been reported, with an estimated prevalence of 1 in a million [31, 35].

MC4R Mutations

MC4R is a G-protein coupled transmembrane receptor that binds α-MSH, encoded by a single exon *MC4R* gene on chromosome 18q. It is highly expressed in the hypothalamus, the brain region involved in the regulation of feeding behavior and appetite [36, 37]. The role of MC4R in obesity was first reported in MC4R-deficient mice with maturity-onset obesity, hyperphagia, hyperinsulinemia, and hyperglycemia [38].

The first human cases of dominantly inherited MC4R deficiency were described in 1998, recapitulating the mouse phenotype [39, 40]. The clinical spectrum of MC4R deficiency in humans includes hyperphagic obesity, severe hyperinsulinemia, normal puberty development, and no further growth or endocrine problems [18]. Genetic epidemiology studies have shown that MC4R deficiency is the most frequent type of monogenic obesity, and its prevalence is reported to be 1.7–5.8% in obese people [41, 42], the differences in the prevalence likely reflecting the cohort characteristics. Both monoallelic and biallelic forms of MC4R deficiency have been described, and homozygotes usually present with more severe phenotypes. Although recessive forms of MC4R deficiency have been described, for the most part, MC4R deficiency has an autosomal dominant inheritance pattern, with only one pathogenic *MC4R* allele sufficient to cause obesity [39–41]. Although heterozygous loss-of-function pathogenic variants in *MC4R* can cause familial forms of obesity, these variants can also be found in non-penetrant individuals who are not obese [42].

PC1/3 and PC2 Deficiency (*PCSK1*-Related Obesity)

PC1/3 and PC2 are serine endopeptidases that cleave inactive hormone precursors like prothyrotropin-releasing hormone (pro-TRH), proinsulin, proglucagon, progonadotropin-releasing hormone (pro-GnRH), and POMC [43–45]. The peptides derived from the cleavage of these prohormones are involved in regulating energy homeostasis through their effects on energy expenditure and food intake. Pathogenic genetic variants disrupting the function of the genes coding for these enzymes lead to severe obesity [18, 46]. To date, there are only about 35 described cases of proprotein convertase subtilisin/kexin type 1 (*PCSK1*)-related obesity, all carrying biallelic pathogenic variants (either homozygotes or compound heterozygotes), suggesting an autosomal recessive mode of inheritance. The clinical phenotype includes severe early malabsorptive diarrhea in the first 3 months of age, severe early-onset hyperphagic obesity, growth hormone deficiency, impaired glucose homeostasis, secondary hypogonadism, low cortisol levels, and increased proinsulin with low insulin levels [47–49].

SIM1 Deficiency

SIM1 is a key player in neuronal differentiation in the hypothalamic region. *Sim1* haploinsufficient mice are hyperphagic, obese, and prone to diet-induced obesity with regular energy expenditure [50, 51]. A study conducted in 2000 [52] identified a severely obese young girl with hyperphagia, exponential weight gain that started at the age of 3 months, and regular energy expenditure while having no developmental problems, syndromic features, or endocrine dysfunction. Her obesity was associated with the presence of a de novo translocation that included 1p22.1 and 6q12.2, which contain the *SIM1* gene. Other studies show that interstitial chromosome 6q deletions involving *SIM1* are linked to severe obesity in humans [53–55]. Pathogenic *SIM1* variants due to sequence changes have also been shown to cause monogenic obesity in humans with overlapping features of Prader-Willi [50].

BDNF and *NTRK2* Mutations

Processes that occur during the development and plasticity of neurons in the hypothalamus, such as proliferation, survival, and differentiation, are regulated by the brain-derived neurotrophic factor (BDNF) and its receptor TRKB, which are essential for memory, behavior, and cognitive development [56–58]. Partial deficiency of BDNF and TRKB was detected in obese mouse models with hyperphagia [59–61].

The first human case of severe obesity due to mutations in the *BDNF* gene was described recently [62]. The patient was an obese 8-year-old girl with impaired cognition, memory, nociception, and hyperactivity, with a body weight of 20 kg at age 2. Her obesity was linked to a disruption in the *BDNF* locus on chromosome 11 due to a de novo paracentric inversion. To date, only one human case of obesity due to heterozygous de novo missense mutation in neurotrophic receptor tyrosine kinase 2 (*NTRK2*—the gene that encodes TRKB) has been reported. The patient was an 8-year-old boy who presented with early-onset obesity, hyperphagia, developmental delays, impaired memory and learning, and nociception [63]. Only a handful of cases of obesity and developmental delays linked to NTRK2 have been identified, and this remains a rare form of monogenic obesity.

Syndromic Obesity

Syndromic obesity can be described as a condition where, apart from excessive adiposity as a predominant feature, other characteristics such as endocrine dysfunction, limb and facial dysmorphisms, congenital disabilities, and delay in intellectual development may be present [64]. More than 79 obesity syndromes have been reported in the literature [64, 65], of which Bardet–Biedl syndrome, Prader–Willi syndrome, and Alstrom syndrome have been repeatedly mentioned. These three syndromes have a complex genetic basis and are linked to the dysfunction of the primary cilia, also known as primary ciliopathies [66–68].

Bardet–Biedl syndrome (BBS) is a rare autosomal recessive genetic disorder with severe multiorgan impairment and complex genetic etiology [69]. The BBS phenotype is very composite and variable and includes early-onset obesity occurring in the first year of life due to hyperphagia, ranging from mild to severe. In addition, BBS patients may develop other conditions later in life, such as genital abnormalities, renal defects, polydactyly, intellectual disability, hepatic fibrosis, male hypogonadism, female urogenital tract abnormalities, T2DM, hypertension, and congenital heart disease [70, 71]. At least 20 genes have been associated with the development and pathophysiology of BBS so far [72], with most of them affecting the primary cilia's function in signal transduction [73, 74].

Alstrom syndrome (ALMS) is an autosomal recessive disorder caused by pathogenic variants in the gene coding for ALMS1 protein (*ALMS1*) that plays a significant role in maintaining the morphology and function of the primary cilia [75]. Many characteristics associated with BBS are also linked to ALMS, such as early-onset obesity, T2DM, liver and kidney dysfunction, retinal degeneration, cardiomyopathy, and delayed puberty [76].

Prader–Willi syndrome (PWS) is a genetic disorder linked to imprinting, with 65–75% of cases resulting from deletions affecting paternally active genes on chromosome 15q11-q13 region, 20–30% resulting from uniparental maternal disomy, and 1–3% of cases are due to imprinting defects [77, 78]. This disorder has multiple phenotypic similarities with other obesity syndromes, such as developmental delay, hypogonadism, small hands and feet. Patients with PWS are born with neonatal hypotonia and failure to thrive, followed by the development of severe hyperphagic obesity [77, 79].

Role of Epigenetics in Obesity

The set of genes an organism carries in its genome determines its phenotype. If a person has a mutation in a gene, it may develop an altered phenotype, i.e., a single gene mutation in the appetite-regulating pathway can cause an obesity phenotype. Genome-wide association studies (GWAS), which identify associations of genotypes with phenotypes, showed that around 500 genetic loci are associated with BMI [80]. However, genetic predispositions cannot completely elucidate the exponential growth of obesity's global prevalence in the past decades. The concept of epigenetics was first described in 1942 by Conrad Waddington as a "complex of developmental processes that lie between genotype and phenotype" [81]. This idea suggests that epigenetic changes can regulate gene expression by switching the genes on and off without changing the DNA sequence. Humans have a homogenous genome throughout the body; however, the epigenome varies in different cell types. Thus targeted cell gene expression can be allowed or silenced by epigenetic post-transcriptional modifications without changes in the genetic code [82, 83]. Environmental influences and lifestyle factors are known to be the main reasons for causing epigenetic changes and therefore have the ability to alter the expression of genes related to obesity, diabetes, or other pathophysiological conditions (Fig. 6.2). Current known epigenetic factors are DNA methylation, histone tail modifications,

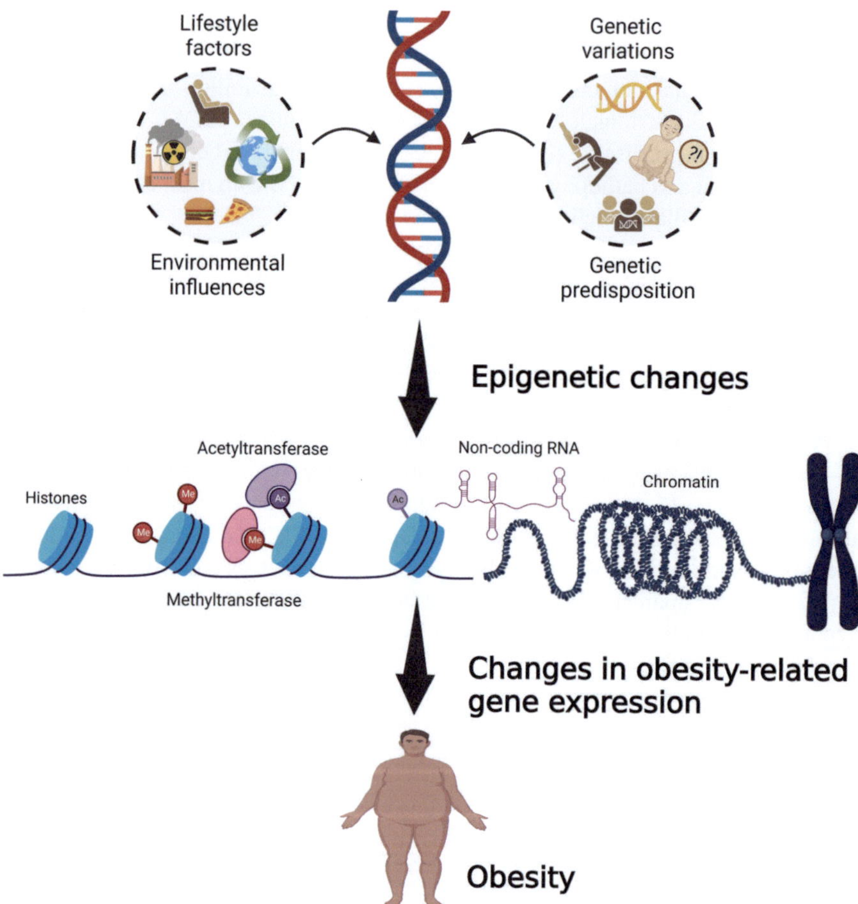

Fig. 6.2 Epigenetic post-transcriptional factors in obesity-related gene expression (DNA methylation, histone modifications, and ncRNAs). Epigenetic changes occur due to environmental and lifestyle factors, which can alter the expression of genes related to obesity, diabetes, or other pathophysiological conditions. Types of epigenetic changes include DNA methylation, histone modifications, and non-coding RNAs (ncRNAs). DNA methylation is catalyzed by DNMTs and works by adding methyl groups to CpG islands in the DNA, which modifies the gene transcriptions and can turn the genes "on" and "off." Histones are spheroproteins that protect and pack DNA molecules forming chromatin. Histone tails are easily modified with acetylation, methylation, or phosphorylation, affecting the histone's interaction with its surrounding DNA. These interactions make DNA more or less accessible to the transcriptional factors, ultimately leading to gene activation or silencing. Lastly, non-coding RNAs work as post-transcriptional gene regulators by binding to transcription factors, histone-modifying enzymes, and RNA polymerase II. (Created with BioRender.com)

and non-coding RNAs (ncRNAs) [84]. They may be passed on to new somatic cells through mitotic cell division or to the fetus by alterations in the parental gametes [85].

DNA Methylation

DNA methylation is a process of covalent binding of methyl groups to CpG islands (a dinucleotide consisting of cytosine and guanine) [86], catalyzed by DNA methyltransferases (DNMTs). These enzymes modify gene expression by methylation in the gene promoter region responsible for transcription initiation. In most instances, this hypermethylation leads to repression of the gene transcription hence causing gene silencing, while hypomethylation or loss of methylation, in general, leads to gene activation [87, 88].

In obesity, DNA methylation alters the expression of the leptin gene (*LEP*) and adiponectin gene (*ADIPOQ*), which regulate energy homeostasis. There are consistent reports of a negative correlation between DNA methylation of the *LEP* promoter in the blood and BMI in obese patients [89, 90]. Hypomethylation of the *LEP* promoter causes upregulation of *LEP* and increased levels of circulating leptin that cannot utilize its anorexigenic effect in leptin-resistant obese patients [91]. Opposite to *LEP*, a positive correlation has been found between DNA methylation of *ADIPOQ* promoter in the adipose tissue and BMI in obese subjects [90]. DNMT-induced hypermethylation of *ADIPOQ* promoter causes downregulation of *ADIPOQ* and decreased adiponectin levels in the adipose tissue, thus decreasing insulin sensitivity and glucose uptake [92, 93]. Obesity-induced promoter hypermethylation also downregulates the expression of insulin-signaling genes, such as insulin (*INS*) and insulin receptor substrate 1 (*IRS1*) [94, 95], impairing glucose metabolism regulation and increasing the risk of developing T2DM. Moreover, anorexigenic *POMC* and the orexigenic *NPY* genes involved in the appetite-regulating pathway have altered methylation in obesity [96]. Lastly, altered methylation in the inflammation and hypoxia-related genes, such as *HIF*, *TNF*, and *IL6*, is also shown to be associated with BMI and obesity [88, 97–99].

Histone Modifications

Histones are spheroproteins abundant in arginine and lysine residues found in the nucleus of eukaryotic cells where DNA is enfolded around them, forming the chromatin. They protect and pack DNA molecules into structural units called nucleosomes. Histone structure consists of a globular domain composed of two copies of four subunits, each having an exposed N-terminal tail, also called a histone tail [100]. Histone tails are known to be easily modified after translation by reactions of acetylation, methylation, or phosphorylation [101]. Acetyltransferases, deacetylases, methyltransferases, and demethylases are enzymes that reversibly catalyze these reactions in the histone tails affecting their close interaction with the DNA surrounding them. Depending on the type of reaction, these interactions between the histone and DNA can be either disrupted or strengthened, resulting in DNA being more or less accessible to the transcriptional factors, ultimately leading to gene activation or silencing.

While histone modifications are part of normal adipogenesis, some histone modifications are directly associated with human obesity and diabetes [102, 103]. Some of the key genes in mice involved in adipogenesis whose expression is altered as a result of histone modifications are those encoding delta-like non-canonical Notch ligand 1 (DLK1) (*Dlk1*), fatty acid-binding protein 4 (FABP4) (*Fabp4*), and peroxisome proliferator-activated receptor γ (PPARγ) (*Pparg*) [102]. Similar to DNA methylation, histone acetylation modulates the expression of *POMC* and *NPY* genes, affecting appetite regulation [88]. Ultimately, obesity-induced inflammation was shown to be mediated via increased histone acetylation at *Tnf* and *Ccl2* genes in high-fat diet (HFD)-fed and *ob/ob* mice [104].

Non-coding RNAs

Post-transcriptional gene expression is regulated by ncRNA molecules. Based on sequence length, ncRNAs are classified into short non-coding RNAs (sncRNAs) (less than 200 nucleotides), which include the microRNAs (miRNAs), and long non-coding RNAs (lncRNAs) (more than 200 nucleotides). miRNAs work mainly as post-translational gene modulators that form base pairs with specific sites in the target mRNA, in most cases either blocking its translation or stimulating its degradation.

Post-transcriptional regulation done by the miRNAs has been observed in practically every biological process, including cell differentiation, development, apoptosis, metabolism, immune responses, and many diseases such as obesity, cancer, cardiovascular disease, neurodegenerative diseases, and viral infections [105]. In the adipose tissue, many miRNAs were found to stimulate or inhibit adipocyte differentiation and proliferation [106–108]. To date, at least 65 miRNAs are reported to be linked to obesity [109]. Some of the reported dysregulated miRNAs associated with obesity were miR-99a, -125b, -130b, -139-5p, -185, -199a-5p, -221, -484, -1229 in adipose tissue [110], miR-15a, -130b, -140-5p, -142-3p, -221, -222, -423-5p, -520c-3p in plasma [111], etc. One meta-analysis reported 40 circulating miRNAs to be dysregulated in T2DM [112], suggesting that their circulating levels may serve as potential early biomarkers for the disease. Long non-coding RNAs exert their gene regulatory function by binding to transcription factors, histone-modifying enzymes, and RNA polymerase II. Many lncRNAs are reported to be associated with obesity and related inflammatory comorbidities; however, their function is still poorly understood [113].

Conclusion and Prospects for the Future

Although lifestyle is the main cause of obesity, there are clear genetic and epigenetic causes and associations. While a lot has been done to understand the obesity-associated gene network using sophisticated genome scanning methods, the fields of epigenomics and epigenetics remain wide open for research. The exact mechanism of how environmental and lifestyle factors affect obesity-related gene expression causing epigenetic changes, like DNA methylation and histone modifications, is yet to be elucidated. The fact that the epigenome is variable, unlike the genome, makes it a potential therapeutic target for obesity. It offers an advantage in detecting early risk factors that can help medical professionals manage obesity by developing prevention plans and treatment.

References

1. Rohm TV, Meier DT, Olefsky JM, Donath MY. Inflammation in obesity, diabetes, and related disorders. Immunity. 2022;55(1):31–55.
2. Esser N, Legrand-Poels S, Piette J, Scheen AJ, Paquot N. Inflammation as a link between obesity, metabolic syndrome and type 2 diabetes. Diabetes Res Clin Pract. 2014;105(2):141–50.
3. Cowley MA, Smart JL, Rubinstein M, Cerdán MG, Diano S, Horvath TL, et al. Leptin activates anorexigenic POMC neurons through a neural network in the arcuate nucleus. Nature. 2001;411(6836):480–4.
4. Qiu J, Zhang C, Borgquist A, Nestor CC, Smith AW, Bosch MA, et al. Insulin excites anorexigenic proopiomelanocortin neurons via activation of canonical transient receptor potential channels. Cell Metab. 2014;19(4):682–93.
5. Chen HY, Trumbauer ME, Chen AS, Weingarth DT, Adams JR, Frazier EG, et al. Orexigenic action of peripheral ghrelin is mediated by neuropeptide Y and agouti-related protein. Endocrinology. 2004;145(6):2607–12.
6. Niazi RK, Gjesing AP, Hollensted M, Have CT, Borisevich D, Grarup N, et al. Screening of 31 genes involved in monogenic forms of obesity in 23 Pakistani probands with early-onset childhood obesity: a case report. BMC Med Genet. 2019;20(1):152.
7. Gale SM, Castracane VD, Mantzoros CS. Energy homeostasis, obesity and eating disorders: recent advances in endocrinology. J Nutr. 2004;134(2):295–8.
8. Zhang Y, Proenca R, Maffei M, Barone M, Leopold L, Friedman JM. Positional cloning of the mouse obese gene and its human homologue. Nature. 1994;372(6505):425–32.
9. Ingalls AM, Dickie MM, Snell GD. Obese, a new mutation in the house mouse. Obes Res. 1996;4(1):101.
10. Pelleymounter MA, Cullen MJ, Baker MB, Hecht R, Winters D, Boone T, et al. Effects of the obese gene product on body weight regulation in ob/ob mice. Science. 1995;269(5223):540–3.
11. Coleman DL. Obese and diabetes: two mutant genes causing diabetes-obesity syndromes in mice. Diabetologia. 1978;14(3):141–8.
12. Mayer J, Bates MW, Dickie MM. Hereditary diabetes in genetically obese mice. Science. 1951;113(2948):746–7.
13. Montague CT, Farooqi IS, Whitehead JP, Soos MA, Rau H, Wareham NJ, et al. Congenital leptin deficiency is associated with severe early-onset obesity in humans. Nature. 1997;387(6636):903–8.

14. Farooqi IS, Keogh JM, Kamath S, Jones S, Gibson WT, Trussell R, et al. Partial leptin deficiency and human adiposity. Nature. 2001;414(6859):34–5.
15. Farooqi IS, Jebb SA, Langmack G, Lawrence E, Cheetham CH, Prentice AM, et al. Effects of recombinant leptin therapy in a child with congenital leptin deficiency. N Engl J Med. 1999;341(12):879–84.
16. Nunziata A, Borck G, Funcke J-B, Kohlsdorf K, Brandt S, Hinney A, et al. Estimated prevalence of potentially damaging variants in the leptin gene. Mol Cell Pediatr. 2017;4(1):10.
17. Farooqi IS, Matarese G, Lord GM, Keogh JM, Lawrence E, Agwu C, et al. Beneficial effects of leptin on obesity, T cell hyporesponsiveness, and neuroendocrine/metabolic dysfunction of human congenital leptin deficiency. J Clin Invest. 2002;110(8):1093–103.
18. Ranadive SA, Vaisse C. Lessons from extreme human obesity: monogenic disorders. Endocrinol Metab Clin N Am. 2008;37(3):733–51. x
19. Gueorguiev M, Góth ML, Korbonits M. Leptin and puberty: a review. Pituitary. 2001;4(1–2):79–86.
20. Strobel A, Issad T, Camoin L, Ozata M, Strosberg AD. A leptin missense mutation associated with hypogonadism and morbid obesity. Nat Genet. 1998;18(3):213–5.
21. Ozata M, Ozdemir IC, Licinio J. Human leptin deficiency caused by a missense mutation: multiple endocrine defects, decreased sympathetic tone, and immune system dysfunction indicate new targets for leptin action, greater central than peripheral resistance to the effects of leptin, and spontaneous correction of leptin-mediated defects. J Clin Endocrinol Metab. 1999;84(10):3686–95.
22. Mantzoros CS, Ozata M, Negrao AB, Suchard MA, Ziotopoulou M, Caglayan S, et al. Synchronicity of frequently sampled thyrotropin (TSH) and leptin concentrations in healthy adults and leptin-deficient subjects: evidence for possible partial TSH regulation by leptin in humans. J Clin Endocrinol Metab. 2001;86(7):3284–91.
23. Clément K, Vaisse C, Lahlou N, Cabrol S, Pelloux V, Cassuto D, et al. A mutation in the human leptin receptor gene causes obesity and pituitary dysfunction. Nature. 1998;392(6674):398–401.
24. Vaisse C, Halaas JL, Horvath CM, Darnell JE, Stoffel M, Friedman JM. Leptin activation of Stat3 in the hypothalamus of wild-type and Ob/Ob mice but not db/db mice. Nat Genet. 1996;14(1):95–7.
25. Chua SC, Chung WK, Wu-Peng XS, Zhang Y, Liu SM, Tartaglia L, et al. Phenotypes of mouse diabetes and rat fatty due to mutations in the OB (leptin) receptor. Science. 1996;271(5251):994–6.
26. Sharma K, McCue P, Dunn SR. Diabetic kidney disease in the db/db mouse. Am J Physiol Renal Physiol. 2003;284(6):F1138–44.
27. Clark JB, Palmer CJ, Shaw WN. The diabetic Zucker fatty rat. Proc Soc Exp Biol Med. 1983;173(1):68–75.
28. Farooqi IS, Wangensteen T, Collins S, Kimber W, Matarese G, Keogh JM, et al. Clinical and molecular genetic spectrum of congenital deficiency of the leptin receptor. N Engl J Med. 2007;356(3):237–47.
29. Kleinendorst L, Abawi O, van der Kamp HJ, Alders M, Meijers-Heijboer HEJ, van Rossum EFC, et al. Leptin receptor deficiency: a systematic literature review and prevalence estimation based on population genetics. Eur J Endocrinol. 2020;182(1):47–56.
30. Raue S, Wedekind D, Wiltfang J, Schmidt U. The role of proopiomelanocortin and α-melanocyte-stimulating hormone in the metabolic syndrome in psychiatric disorders: a narrative mini-review. Front Psych. 2019;10:834.
31. Krude H, Biebermann H, Luck W, Horn R, Brabant G, Grüters A. Severe early-onset obesity, adrenal insufficiency and red hair pigmentation caused by POMC mutations in humans. Nat Genet. 1998;19(2):155–7.
32. Coll AP. Effects of pro-opiomelanocortin (POMC) on food intake and body weight: mechanisms and therapeutic potential? Clin Sci (Lond). 2007;113(4):171–82.

33. Mankowska M, Krzeminska P, Graczyk M, Switonski M. Confirmation that a deletion in the POMC gene is associated with body weight of Labrador Retriever dogs. Res Vet Sci. 2017;112:116–8.
34. Hilado MA, Randhawa RS. A novel mutation in the proopiomelanocortin (POMC) gene of a Hispanic child: metformin treatment shows a beneficial impact on the body mass index. J Pediatr Endocrinol Metab. 2018;31(7):815–9.
35. Krude H, Biebermann H, Gruters A. Mutations in the human proopiomelanocortin gene. Ann N Y Acad Sci. 2003;994:233–9.
36. Yeo GS, Farooqi IS, Challis BG, Jackson RS, O'Rahilly S. The role of melanocortin signalling in the control of body weight: evidence from human and murine genetic models. QJM. 2000;93(1):7–14.
37. Cole SA, Butte NF, Voruganti VS, Cai G, Haack K, Kent JW, et al. Evidence that multiple genetic variants of MC4R play a functional role in the regulation of energy expenditure and appetite in Hispanic children. Am J Clin Nutr. 2010;91(1):191–9.
38. Huszar D, Lynch CA, Fairchild-Huntress V, Dunmore JH, Fang Q, Berkemeier LR, et al. Targeted disruption of the melanocortin-4 receptor results in obesity in mice. Cell. 1997;88(1):131–41.
39. Yeo GS, Farooqi IS, Aminian S, Halsall DJ, Stanhope RG, O'Rahilly S. A frameshift mutation in MC4R associated with dominantly inherited human obesity. Nat Genet. 1998;20(2):111–2.
40. Vaisse C, Clement K, Guy-Grand B, Froguel P. A frameshift mutation in human MC4R is associated with a dominant form of obesity. Nat Genet. 1998;20(2):113–4.
41. Farooqi IS, Keogh JM, Yeo GSH, Lank EJ, Cheetham T, O'Rahilly S. Clinical spectrum of obesity and mutations in the melanocortin 4 receptor gene. N Engl J Med. 2003;348(12):1085–95.
42. Stutzmann F, Tan K, Vatin V, Dina C, Jouret B, Tichet J, et al. Prevalence of melanocortin-4 receptor deficiency in Europeans and their age-dependent penetrance in multigenerational pedigrees. Diabetes. 2008;57(9):2511–8.
43. Seidah NG, Chrétien M. Proprotein and prohormone convertases: a family of subtilases generating diverse bioactive polypeptides. Brain Res. 1999;848(1–2):45–62.
44. O'Rahilly S, Gray H, Humphreys PJ, Krook A, Polonsky KS, White A, et al. Brief report: impaired processing of prohormones associated with abnormalities of glucose homeostasis and adrenal function. N Engl J Med. 1995;333(21):1386–90.
45. Jackson RS, Creemers JWM, Farooqi IS, Raffin-Sanson M-L, Varro A, Dockray GJ, et al. Small-intestinal dysfunction accompanies the complex endocrinopathy of human proprotein convertase 1 deficiency. J Clin Invest. 2003;112(10):1550–60.
46. Chiurazzi M, Cozzolino M, Orsini RC, Di Maro M, Di Minno MND, Colantuoni A. Impact of genetic variations and epigenetic mechanisms on the risk of obesity. Int J Mol Sci. 2020;21(23):9035.
47. Pépin L, Colin E, Tessarech M, Rouleau S, Bouhours-Nouet N, Bonneau D, et al. A new case of PCSK1 pathogenic variant with congenital proprotein convertase 1/3 deficiency and literature review. J Clin Endocrinol Metab. 2019;104(4):985–93.
48. Van Dijck E, Beckers S, Diels S, Huybrechts T, Verrijken A, Van Hoorenbeeck K, et al. Rare heterozygous PCSK1 variants in human obesity: the contribution of the p.Y181H variant and a literature review. Genes (Basel). 2022;13(10):1746.
49. Farooqi IS, Volders K, Stanhope R, Heuschkel R, White A, Lank E, et al. Hyperphagia and early-onset obesity due to a novel homozygous missense mutation in prohormone convertase 1/3. J Clin Endocrinol Metab. 2007;92(9):3369–73.
50. Bonnefond A, Raimondo A, Stutzmann F, Ghoussaini M, Ramachandrappa S, Bersten DC, et al. Loss-of-function mutations in SIM1 contribute to obesity and Prader-Willi-like features. J Clin Invest. 2013;123(7):3037–41.
51. Michaud JL, Boucher F, Melnyk A, Gauthier F, Goshu E, Lévy E, et al. Sim1 haploinsufficiency causes hyperphagia, obesity and reduction of the paraventricular nucleus of the hypothalamus. Hum Mol Genet. 2001;10(14):1465–73.

52. Holder JL, Butte NF, Zinn AR. Profound obesity associated with a balanced translocation that disrupts the SIM1 gene. Hum Mol Genet. 2000;9(1):101–8.
53. Villa A, Urioste M, Bofarull JM, Martínez-Frías ML. De novo interstitial deletion q16.2q21 on chromosome 6. Am J Med Genet. 1995;55(3):379–83.
54. Gilhuis HJ, van Ravenswaaij CM, Hamel BJ, Gabreëls FJ. Interstitial 6q deletion with a Prader-Willi-like phenotype: a new case and review of the literature. Eur J Paediatr Neurol. 2000;4(1):39–43.
55. Faivre L, Cormier-Daire V, Lapierre JM, Colleaux L, Jacquemont S, Geneviéve D, et al. Deletion of the SIM1 gene (6q16.2) in a patient with a Prader-Willi-like phenotype. J Med Genet. 2002;39(8):594–6.
56. Tapia-Arancibia L, Rage F, Givalois L, Arancibia S. Physiology of BDNF: focus on hypotha-lamic function. Front Neuroendocrinol. 2004;25(2):77–107.
57. Huang EJ, Reichardt LF. Neurotrophins: roles in neuronal development and function. Annu Rev Neurosci. 2001;24:677–736.
58. Huang EJ, Reichardt LF. Trk receptors: roles in neuronal signal transduction. Annu Rev Biochem. 2003;72:609–42.
59. Xu B, Goulding EH, Zang K, Cepoi D, Cone RD, Jones KR, et al. Brain-derived neurotrophic factor regulates energy balance downstream of melanocortin-4 receptor. Nat Neurosci. 2003;6(7):736–42.
60. Kernie SG, Liebl DJ, Parada LF. BDNF regulates eating behavior and locomotor activity in mice. EMBO J. 2000;19(6):1290–300.
61. Lyons WE, Mamounas LA, Ricaurte GA, Coppola V, Reid SW, Bora SH, et al. Brain-derived neurotrophic factor-deficient mice develop aggressiveness and hyperphagia in conjunction with brain serotonergic abnormalities. Proc Natl Acad Sci U S A. 1999;96(26):15239–44.
62. Gray J, Yeo GSH, Cox JJ, Morton J, Adlam A-LR, Keogh JM, et al. Hyperphagia, severe obesity, impaired cognitive function, and hyperactivity associated with functional loss of one copy of the brain-derived neurotrophic factor (BDNF) gene. Diabetes. 2006;55(12):3366–71.
63. Yeo GSH, Connie Hung C-C, Rochford J, Keogh J, Gray J, Sivaramakrishnan S, et al. A de novo mutation affecting human TrkB associated with severe obesity and developmental delay. Nat Neurosci. 2004;7(11):1187–9.
64. Kaur Y, de Souza RJ, Gibson WT, Meyre D. A systematic review of genetic syndromes with obesity. Obes Rev. 2017;18(6):603–34.
65. Vos N, Oussaada SM, Cooiman MI, Kleinendorst L, Ter Horst KW, Hazebroek EJ, et al. Bariatric surgery for monogenic non-syndromic and syndromic obesity disorders. Curr Diab Rep. 2020;20(9):44.
66. Valente EM, Rosti RO, Gibbs E, Gleeson JG. Primary cilia in neurodevelopmental disorders. Nat Rev Neurol. 2014;10(1):27–36.
67. Huvenne H, Dubern B, Clément K, Poitou C. Rare genetic forms of obesity: clinical approach and current treatments in 2016. Obes Facts. 2016;9(3):158–73.
68. Stagi S, Bianconi M, Sammarco MA, Artuso R, Giglio S, de Martino M. New thoughts on pediatric genetic obesity: pathogenesis, clinical characteristics and treatment approach. In: Adiposity - omics and molecular understanding. London: IntechOpen; 2017.
69. Suspitsin EN, Imyanitov EN. Bardet-Biedl syndrome. Mol Syndromol. 2016;7(2):62–71.
70. Kulaga HM, Leitch CC, Eichers ER, Badano JL, Lesemann A, Hoskins BE, et al. Loss of BBS proteins causes anosmia in humans and defects in olfactory cilia structure and function in the mouse. Nat Genet. 2004;36(9):994–8.
71. Tobin JL, Beales PL. Bardet-Biedl syndrome: beyond the cilium. Pediatr Nephrol. 2007;22(7):926–36.
72. Manara E, Paolacci S, D'Esposito F, Abeshi A, Ziccardi L, Falsini B, et al. Mutation pro-file of BBS genes in patients with Bardet-Biedl syndrome: an Italian study. Ital J Pediatr. 2019;45(1):72.

73. Nachury MV, Loktev AV, Zhang Q, Westlake CJ, Peränen J, Merdes A, et al. A core complex of BBS proteins cooperates with the GTPase Rab8 to promote ciliary membrane biogenesis. Cell. 2007;129(6):1201–13.
74. Ansley SJ, Badano JL, Blacque OE, Hill J, Hoskins BE, Leitch CC, et al. Basal body dysfunction is a likely cause of pleiotropic Bardet-Biedl syndrome. Nature. 2003;425(6958):628–33.
75. Álvarez-Satta M, Castro-Sánchez S, Valverde D. Alström syndrome: current perspectives. Appl Clin Genet. 2015;8:171–9.
76. Marshall JD, Maffei P, Collin GB, Naggert JK. Alström syndrome: genetics and clinical overview. Curr Genomics. 2011;12(3):225–35.
77. Angulo MA, Butler MG, Cataletto ME. Prader-Willi syndrome: a review of clinical, genetic, and endocrine findings. J Endocrinol Investig. 2015;38(12):1249–63.
78. Kim YJ, Cheon CK. Prader-Willi syndrome: a single center's experience in Korea. Korean J Pediatr. 2014;57(7):310–6.
79. Butler MG, Manzardo AM, Forster JL. Prader-Willi syndrome: clinical genetics and diagnostic aspects with treatment approaches. Curr Pediatr Rev. 2016;12(2):136–66.
80. Yengo L, Sidorenko J, Kemper KE, Zheng Z, Wood AR, Weedon MN, et al. Meta-analysis of genome-wide association studies for height and body mass index in ~700000 individuals of European ancestry. Hum Mol Genet. 2018;27(20):3641–9.
81. Waddington CH. The epigenotype. 1942. Int J Epidemiol. 2012;41(1):10–3.
82. Bird A. Perceptions of epigenetics. Nature. 2007;447(7143):396–8.
83. Al Aboud NM, Tupper C, Jialal I. Genetics, epigenetic mechanism. Treasure Island, FL: StatPearls Publishing; 2022.
84. Qureshi IA, Mehler MF. Epigenetic mechanisms underlying nervous system diseases. Handb Clin Neurol. 2018;147:43–58.
85. Peaston AE, Whitelaw E. Epigenetics and phenotypic variation in mammals. Mamm Genome. 2006;17(5):365–74.
86. Sayols-Baixeras S, Subirana I, Fernández-Sanlés A, Sentí M, Lluís-Ganella C, Marrugat J, et al. DNA methylation and obesity traits: an epigenome-wide association study. The REGICOR study. Epigenetics. 2017;12(10):909–16.
87. Irvine RA, Lin IG, Hsieh C-L. DNA methylation has a local effect on transcription and histone acetylation. Mol Cell Biol. 2002;22(19):6689–96.
88. Mahmoud AM. An overview of epigenetics in obesity: the role of lifestyle and therapeutic interventions. Int J Mol Sci. 2022;23(3):1341.
89. Sadashiv MA, Khokhar M, Sharma P, Joshi R, Mishra SS, et al. Leptin DNA methylation and its association with metabolic risk factors in a northwest Indian obese population. J Obes Metab Syndr. 2021;30(3):304–11.
90. Houde A-A, Légaré C, Biron S, Lescelleur O, Biertho L, Marceau S, et al. Leptin and adiponectin DNA methylation levels in adipose tissues and blood cells are associated with BMI, waist girth and LDL-cholesterol levels in severely obese men and women. BMC Med Genet. 2015;16:29.
91. Izquierdo AG, Crujeiras AB, Casanueva FF, Carreira MC. Leptin, obesity, and leptin resistance: where are we 25 years later? Nutrients. 2019;11(11):2704.
92. Kim AY, Park YJ, Pan X, Shin KC, Kwak S-H, Bassas AF, et al. Obesity-induced DNA hypermethylation of the adiponectin gene mediates insulin resistance. Nat Commun. 2015;6:7585.
93. Houshmand-Oeregaard A, Hansen NS, Hjort L, Kelstrup L, Broholm C, Mathiesen ER, et al. Differential adipokine DNA methylation and gene expression in subcutaneous adipose tissue from adult offspring of women with diabetes in pregnancy. Clin Epigenetics. 2017;9:37.
94. Kuroda A, Rauch TA, Todorov I, Ku HT, Al-Abdullah IH, Kandeel F, et al. Insulin gene expression is regulated by DNA methylation. PLoS One. 2009;4(9):e6953.
95. Rohde K, Klös M, Hopp L, Liu X, Keller M, Stumvoll M, et al. IRS1 DNA promoter methylation and expression in human adipose tissue are related to fat distribution and metabolic traits. Sci Rep. 2017;7(1):12369.

96. Crujeiras AB, Campion J, Díaz-Lagares A, Milagro FI, Goyenechea E, Abete I, et al. Association of weight regain with specific methylation levels in the NPY and POMC promoters in leukocytes of obese men: a translational study. Regul Pept. 2013;186:1–6.

97. Dick KJ, Nelson CP, Tsaprouni L, Sandling JK, Aïssi D, Wahl S, et al. DNA methylation and body-mass index: a genome-wide analysis. Lancet. 2014;383(9933):1990–8.

98. Ali MM, Naquiallah D, Qureshi M, Mirza MI, Hassan C, Masrur M, et al. DNA methylation profile of genes involved in inflammation and autoimmunity correlates with vascular function in morbidly obese adults. Epigenetics. 2022;17(1):93–109.

99. Na YK, Hong HS, Lee WK, Kim YH, Kim DS. Increased methylation of interleukin 6 gene is associated with obesity in Korean women. Mol Cells. 2015;38(5):452–6.

100. Thaker VV. Genetic and epigenetic causes of obesity. Adolesc Med State Art Rev. 2017;28(2):379–405.

101. Zentner GE, Henikoff S. Regulation of nucleosome dynamics by histone modifications. Nat Struct Mol Biol. 2013;20(3):259–66.

102. Zhang Q, Ramlee MK, Brunmeir R, Villanueva CJ, Halperin D, Xu F. Dynamic and distinct histone modifications modulate the expression of key adipogenesis regulatory genes. Cell Cycle. 2012;11(23):4310–22.

103. Okamura M, Inagaki T, Tanaka T, Sakai J. Role of histone methylation and demethylation in adipogenesis and obesity. Organogenesis. 2010;6(1):24–32.

104. Mikula M, Majewska A, Ledwon JK, Dzwonek A, Ostrowski J. Obesity increases histone H3 lysine 9 and 18 acetylation at Tnfa and Ccl2 genes in mouse liver. Int J Mol Med. 2014;34(6):1647–54.

105. Pasquinelli AE. MicroRNAs and their targets: recognition, regulation and an emerging reciprocal relationship. Nat Rev Genet. 2012;13(4):271–82.

106. Cruz KJC, de Oliveira ARS, Morais JBS, Severo JS, Marreiro PDD, do N. Role of microRNAs on adipogenesis, chronic low-grade inflammation, and insulin resistance in obesity. Nutrition. 2017;35:28–35.

107. Xie H, Sun L, Lodish HF. Targeting microRNAs in obesity. Expert Opin Ther Targets. 2009;13(10):1227–38.

108. Arner P, Kulyté A. MicroRNA regulatory networks in human adipose tissue and obesity. Nat Rev Endocrinol. 2015;11(5):276–88.

109. Flórez CAR, García-Perdomo HA, Escudero MM. MicroRNAs associated with overweight and obesity in childhood: a systematic review. MicroRNA. 2020;9(4):255–65.

110. Ortega FJ, Moreno-Navarrete JM, Pardo G, Sabater M, Hummel M, Ferrer A, et al. MiRNA expression profile of human subcutaneous adipose and during adipocyte differentiation. PLoS One. 2010;5(2):e9022.

111. Ortega FJ, Mercader JM, Catalán V, Moreno-Navarrete JM, Pueyo N, Sabater M, et al. Targeting the circulating microRNA signature of obesity. Clin Chem. 2013;59(5):781–92.

112. Zhu H, Leung SW. Identification of microRNA biomarkers in type 2 diabetes: a meta-analysis of controlled profiling studies. Diabetologia. 2015;58(5):900–11.

113. Rey F, Urrata V, Gilardini L, Bertoli S, Calcaterra V, Zuccotti GV, et al. Role of long noncoding RNAs in adipogenesis: state of the art and implications in obesity and obesity-associated diseases. Obes Rev. 2021;22(7):e13203.

Chapter 7
Inflammation and Vascular Pathologies

Angelina Zhyvotovska and Caroline Ong

Abbreviations

ANCHOR	Epanova compared to Lovaza in patients with high triglycerides and mixed dyslipidemia study
ASCVD	Atherosclerotic cardiovascular disease
BMI	Body mass index
CAC	Coronary artery calcification
CANTOS	Canakinumab Anti-inflammatory Thrombosis Outcome Study
CIRT	Cardiovascular Inflammation Reduction Trial
CM	Chylomicrons
COLCOT	Colchicine Cardiovascular Outcomes Trial
CRP	C-reactive protein
CVD	Cardiovascular disease
EPA	Eicosapentaenoic acid
FOURIER	Further cardiovascular outcomes research with PCSK9 inhibition in subjects with elevated risk
FPP	Farnesyl pyrophosphate
GGPP	Geranylgeranyl pyrophosphate
HIF 1α	Hypoxia-inducible factor 1 alpha
HMG-CoA	β-hydroxy-β-methylglutaryl-CoA reductase
hsCRP	High-sensitivity C-reactive protein

A. Zhyvotovska · C. Ong (✉)
Department of Cardiology, Lenox Hill Hospital, New York, NY, USA
e-mail: azhyvotovska@northwell.edu; cong1@northwell.edu

© The Author(s), under exclusive license to Springer Nature Switzerland AG 2023
D. Avtanski, L. Poretsky (eds.), *Obesity, Diabetes and Inflammation*, Contemporary Endocrinology, https://doi.org/10.1007/978-3-031-39721-9_7

ICAM-1	Intercellular adhesion molecule 1
IDL	Intermediate-density lipoprotein
IFN-γ	Interferon-gamma
IL	Interleukins
IMPROVE-IT	Improved Reduction of Outcomes: Vytorin Efficacy International Trial
JELIS	Japan EPA Lipid Intervention Study
JUPITER	Justification for the use of statins in prevention: an intervention Trial Evaluating Rosuvastatin trial
LDL	Low-density lipoprotein
LDL-C	LDL cholesterol
LPL	Lipoprotein lipase
MA	Myocardial infarction
M-CSF	Macrophage colony-stimulating factor
MESA	Multi-Ethnic Study of Atherosclerosis
MMP	Matrix metalloproteinase
NF-κB	Nuclear factor κB
NLRP	NOD-like receptor protein
PAI-1	Plasminogen activator inhibitor 1
PRINCE	Pravastatin Inflammation CRP Evaluation Trial
PROVE-IT	Pravastatin or Atorvastatin Evaluation and Infection Therapy trial
RA	Rheumatoid arthritis
REDUCE-IT	Reduction of Cardiovascular Events with Icosapent Ethyl-Intervention trial
RESPECT-EPA	Randomized trial for evaluation in secondary prevention efficacy of combination therapy-statin and eicosapentaenoic acid trial
ROS	Reactive oxygen species
SPIRE	Reduction of vascular events study
TG	Triglycerides
TGRLP	Triglyceride-rich lipoprotein
Th1 cells	T helper 1 cells
TLR2	Toll-like receptor 2
TNFα	Tumor necrosis factor-alpha
tPA	Tissue plasminogen activator
TRL	Triglyceride-rich lipoprotein
VCAM-1	Vascular cell adhesion molecule 1
VLDL	Very low-density lipoprotein

Introduction

Vascular pathologies such as ischemic heart disease, cerebrovascular disease, and peripheral vascular disease are leading causes of death and disability worldwide [1, 2]. Chronic inflammation is known to play a central role in the development and progression of cardiovascular diseases, including atherosclerosis, acute myocardial infarctions, stroke, heart failure, and atrial fibrillation [3]. The body's response to chronic inflammation leads to the development of vascular plaques. Plaque development is, in turn, mediated by a number of risk factors, such as hypertension, tobacco smoking, diabetes, and obesity [4].

Obesity, in part through chronic low-grade inflammation, promotes the development of clinically significant atherosclerotic cardiovascular disease (ASCVD) [5]. Despite advances in our understanding of the development, progression, and treatment of obesity and ASCVD, obesity rates continue to rise to epidemic levels [6, 7], and ASCVD remains a leading cause of mortality in people with obesity [5, 8].

In this chapter, we will first review the inflammatory pathways and key inflammatory markers implicated in the progression of ASCVD. We will also discuss significant clinical trials on the use of anti-inflammatory agents in the treatment of these conditions. Finally, we will assess the role obesity plays in the development of inflammatory pathways promoting ASCVD.

Pathogenesis of Inflammation in the Development of Atherosclerosis

The development of atherosclerosis is a chronic progressive process that develops over decades; our inflammatory system plays an important role, from the first stages of fatty streak formation to the eventual expansion of complex necrotic plaques [4]. Cells of both the innate and adaptive immune systems regulate the progression of the disease [9].

The first insult in the progression of plaque formation comes from intimal wall disruptions due to shear stress. These disruptions activate endothelial cells, resulting in increased permeability to lipoproteins and upregulation of adhesion receptors. Platelets are the first cells to arrive at the site of endothelial injury, and platelets' glycoproteins Ib and IIb/IIIa engage surface molecules on the endothelial cells. Macrophage colony-stimulating factor (M-CSF), a cytokine produced in the inflamed intima, induces monocytes to differentiate into macrophages [9, 10]. These monocyte-derived macrophages take up modified lipoproteins to become lipid-enriched foam cells. Additionally, activated endothelial cells recruit circulating monocytes and promote transmigration. The natural course of monocytes is to differentiate into macrophages or directly influence the phenotype of other macrophages. As lipids accumulate within the macrophages, they transform into macrophage-derived foam cells; eventually, the rate at which these foam cells develop outpaces the rate of clearance. With time, the fatty streaks of foam cells amalgamate to form a lipid-rich necrotic core [4, 9–11].

Various inflammatory cytokines are also implicated in the development of atherosclerosis [11]. Firstly, monocyte adhesion depends on the upregulation of adhesion molecules such as intercellular adhesion molecule 1 (ICAM-1), P-selectin, and vascular cell adhesion molecule 1 (VCAM-1). Monocytes, macrophages, and dendritic cells express major chemokines which facilitate the transmigration process: CCR2, CCR5, and CX3CR1. Furthermore, T lymphocytes of the adaptive immune system may be stimulated to secrete pro-inflammatory T helper 1 (Th1) cytokines such as interleukins (IL) 1 and 6 (IL-1, IL-6), interferon-gamma (IFN-γ), and tumor necrosis factor-alpha (TNFα). TNFα secretion through various mechanisms causes the restructuring of intracellular junctions, which facilitate leukocyte transmigration. IFN-γ also induces foam cell formation through the upregulation of scavenger receptors on macrophages which have been involved in oxidized low-density lipoprotein (LDL) uptake [5, 9, 12].

At the molecular level, the formation of the NOD-like receptor protein 3 (NLRP3) inflammasome in macrophages propagates inflammation [5, 11, 12]. The result of this inflammasome formation is the production of IL-1β and IL-18. These cytokines activate inflammatory cells, which produce IL-6, which in turn stimulates the production of C-reactive protein (CRP) from the liver. CRP further amplifies the inflammatory cascade. This inflammasome may be one of the significant links between the local inflammation caused by monocytes, macrophages, and T cells, at the sub-endothelial level and systemic inflammation, which further promotes the development of cardiovascular disease (CVD) [5, 9, 11, 12].

At more advanced stages of atherogenesis, cytokines destabilize plaques by promoting apoptosis and matrix degradation [11]. In particular, pro-inflammatory cytokines such as IL-1, TNFα, and IFN-γ have been implicated in macrophage and smooth muscle apoptosis [12]. Macrophage apoptosis generates cell debris which recruits other inflammatory cells and contributes to the enlargement of the lipid core. Smooth muscle cell apoptosis leads to thinning of the fibrous cap, which is further facilitated by IFN-γ via its role in inhibiting collagen synthesis [5, 11]. IL-1 and TNFα further contribute to adverse vascular remodeling by increasing the expression of matrix metalloproteinases (MMPs) which act synergistically with oxidized lipids and other cytokines to promote inflammation [11].

Furthermore, IL-1 and TNFα modify the fibrinolytic properties of endothelial cells: production of tissue plasminogen activator (tPA) is decreased, and plasminogen activator inhibitor 1 (PAI-1) is increased [9]. The plaque itself has important physical properties that play a role in the advancement of atherosclerosis. As the plaque grows, it creates a hypoxic environment for the surrounding endothelium, which prompts angiogenesis via hypoxia-inducible factor 1 alpha (HIF 1α) [11]. Neovascularization plays an important role in the development of arterial stenosis and symptoms, for example, in stable coronary artery disease, as well as in in intra-plaque hemorrhage, which accelerates further plaque expansion, inflammation, and plaque rupture [11].

Inflammation and Lipid Profile

Elevated LDL cholesterol (LDL-C) levels are well-established as an independent risk factor for atherosclerosis. However, there is also an association between hyper-triglyceridemia and atherosclerosis. Some residual risk of atherosclerosis after LDL-C lowering therapy is attributable to triglyceride-rich lipoproteins (TRLs) [5]. Triglycerides (TG) are major components of TRLs, which include chylomicrons (CM), very low-density lipoproteins (VLDLs), and their remnants. Once in circulation, CMs and VLDLs are hydrolyzed by lipoprotein lipase (LPL), generating free fatty acids, CM remnants, smaller VLDLs, and intermediate-density lipoproteins (IDLs). These TRL remnants carry more cholesterol per particle than LDL; each remnant particle contains approximately 40 times more cholesterol compared to LDL [5, 9, 13, 14].

The high atherogenicity of TRLs is thought to be due, in part, to the ease with which they are deposited along arterial walls, subsequently damaging the endothelium and triggering the inflammatory cascade [5, 13]. Additionally, TRLs may enter the arterial lumen via defects in the endothelium at the site of atherosclerotic plaques and, once there, may enhance the recruitment and attachment of monocytes—all of which help to contribute to the development of foam cells [5, 11].

The accumulation of TRLs leads to the retention of remnant particles in the arterial walls and stimulates inflammation and oxidative stress. TRLs participate in inflammation in direct and indirect ways. Oxidized free fatty acids increase the expression of inflammatory interleukins and cytokines [13]. Free fatty acids may cause inflammation by activating toll-like receptor 2 (TLR2) and NOD-like receptors on cells leading to the activation of the nuclear factor κB (NF-κB) signaling pathway. TRL remnants can upregulate the endothelial expression of ICAM-1 and VCAM-1, facilitating further transendothelial migration of remnant particles [11, 13]. TG and VLDL also contribute to plaque rupture via the nucleotide-binding domain-like receptor family pyrin domain-containing protein 1 (NLRP1) inflammasome pathway. NLRP1 inflammasome activation may be a significant source of inflammation in endothelial cells [8, 11, 13].

Additionally, it has been suggested that TRL remnants promote endothelial dysfunction by increasing reactive oxygen species (ROS) and reducing nitrous oxide. These remnant particles are notable because very large TRLs in the plasma may not be atherogenic as they may be too large to enter the arterial wall. ROS enhances vascular endothelial permeability and, at high concentrations, can cause cellular injury and death. The pro-inflammatory imbalance between ROS and nitric oxide may promote endothelial dysfunction and lead to cardiovascular complications [5, 9, 11].

Inflammation in the Development of Acute Myocardial Infarction

Atheromatous disease progress to infarction when the thin fibrous caps of atheromas rupture, leading to occlusion of coronary arteries. The rupture of a plaque exposes the prothrombotic material of the core to the systemic circulation. The cytokines released from foam cells and T cells stimulate the migration of the vascular smooth muscle cells into the intima and the production of interstitial collagens to form an extracellular matrix surrounding the necrotic core [9]. IL-1β plays an important role in the production of MMPs which degrade the collagen in the fibrous cap. Together with lipid core growth, thinning of the fibrous cap leads to plaque instability and increased risk of rupture and acute myocardial infarction or other acute coronary syndromes [9]. Activated macrophages, T cells, and mast cells at sites of plaque rupture secrete various inflammatory cytokines, proteases (such as MMPs and cysteine proteases), ROS, and vasoactive molecules, which can destabilize the thin-capped plaque [4, 11]. These reactions partially inhibit the formation of more stable fibrous caps, weaken collagen stability, and propagate thrombus formation [9].

Myocardial infarction results in the activation of a large-scale immune response, both locally and systemically. Acutely and chronically elevated plasma levels of inflammatory markers, such as high-sensitivity CRP and IL-6, have been associated with worse outcomes [9, 15]. Ischemia leads to cardiomyocyte injury and death, culminating in the release of intracellular contents and recruited platelets, which in turn activate leukocytes, endothelial cells, and neutrophils. Endothelial expression of leukocyte and platelet adhesion molecules compromises the tight junctions, facilitating transmigration. ROS are also released by injured cardiac myocytes, which induce chemokine upregulation, complement activation, and an increased capacity of ICAM-1 ligand to bind neutrophils.

Eventually, blood-derived macrophages, in conjunction with resident macrophages, function to scavenge necrotic debris. This is followed by macrophage-driven repair processes, such as angiogenesis and extracellular matrix deposition. The macrophages communicate with other cell types, such as B cells, neutrophils, and mast cells, for tissue injury and repair functions. It takes approximately 2 weeks before leukocyte numbers return to a baseline in the heart and the blood. Adaptive immunity also plays a role; patients who suffer from complications of acute myocardial infarction, such as cardiogenic shock, are more likely to have amplified levels of Th1 cell cytokines TNFα, IL-1, and IL-6 [11].

Obesity and Inflammation

Chronic inflammation is a common driving factor leading to the adverse metabolic and physiologic sequelae seen in obesity and atherosclerosis. Adipose tissues release adipokines that promote systemic inflammation and induce insulin resistance and hypercoagulability, thereby contributing to the progression of ASCVD [5, 11, 16]. Over the past decades, while there have been improvements in our management of several modifiable risk factors, such as hypertension and cigarette smoking, some of these gains have been undermined by the growing obesity epidemic [17].

As discussed above, just as atherosclerosis activates the innate and adaptive immune systems leading to a chronic, self-propagating, inflammatory condition—so too does obesity. The long-term imbalance in nutrient excess and energy expenditure that results in obesity leads to fatty acid accumulation in the liver, muscle, and adipose tissue. This is partially responsible for worsening insulin resistance [16]. Excess fatty acids are stored as TGs, and high levels of TG which exceed the body's oxidative and storage capabilities also contribute to the accumulation of fatty acid intermediates diacylglycerol and ceramide which are linked to insulin resistance [16]. Free fatty acids bind TLR4, which are present in adipocytes and macrophages, activating innate immune pathways (Fig. 7.1). Activation of TLR4 leads to potent downstream inflammatory responses, in part through mitogen activated protein kinase activator protein 1 and NF-κB signaling pathways [16].

Obesity and insulin resistance cause a number of derangements in lipid metabolism, resulting in elevated TG levels and triglyceride-rich lipoproteins (TGRLPs), increased low-density lipoproteins, and lower levels of high-density lipoprotein [18]. Additionally, apolipoprotein CIII, a constituent of some TGRLPs that accumulate in obesity, is associated with increased cardiovascular disease risk [16]. During obesity, adipose tissue undergoes hyperplasia and hypertrophy, leading to increased adipocyte hypoxia, increased chemokine secretion, and recruitment of inflammatory cells. This "obese" adipose tissue has also been linked to increased expression of TNFα compared with "lean" adipose tissue. Additionally, adipose tissue macrophages in insulin-resistant states express a more inflammatory phenotype [5, 19]. TNFα, in turn, has been shown to worsen glucose intolerance.

Levels of high-sensitivity C-reactive protein (hsCRP) have also been shown to be linearly correlated with both body mass index (BMI) and to waist-to-hip ratio, which are associated with increased cardiovascular disease risk [20, 21]. An interesting link between obesity and cardiovascular disease is that of adiponectin [16]. Adiponectin, an adipocytokine secreted by adipose tissue, helps with insulin sensitivity and inflammation. It has anti-inflammatory, anti-atherogenic, and anti-diabetic properties. Adiponectin levels have been shown to decrease with obesity. Adiponectin is currently being studied as a possible treatment pathway for managing diabetes, obesity, and vascular disease.

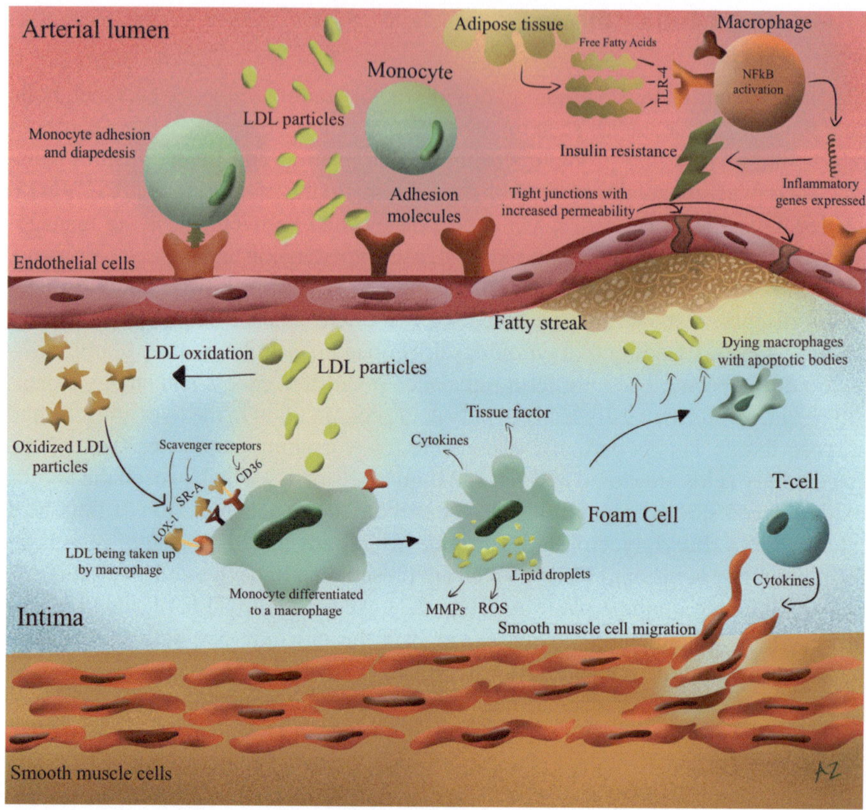

Fig. 7.1 Inflammation in obesity leads to atherogenesis. Increased adipose tissue and free fatty acids in individuals with obesity lead to increased free fatty acids binding to TLR4 and activation of NF-κB. This results in the upregulation of multiple inflammatory genes, which impair insulin signaling and lead to insulin resistance. Circulating LDL particles in the arterial lumen enters the vascular intima, where they undergo LDL oxidation. Oxidized LDL particles are then taken up by macrophages through scavenger receptors (LOX-1, SR-A, CD36). Macrophages are then transformed into "foam cells," lipid-laden macrophages. Foam cells secrete pro-inflammatory cytokines, tissue factors, MMPs, and ROS. Foam cells then undergo apoptosis, and lipids and free cholesterol accumulated in the intima contribute to the formation of the fatty streak. Enhanced inflammation causes the endothelial cell lining to become more permeable to lipids and leukocytes due to the loosening of cellular tight junctions. Once T cells enter the atheroma through interaction with adhesion molecules, they can assume multiple roles contributing to plaque formation. T cells release cytokines to activate macrophages and induce smooth cell proliferation and migration. Eventually, the proliferation of smooth muscles in the intima results in plaque expansion and luminal stenosis

Cigarette Smoking and Inflammation

Tobacco smoking and secondary smoke exposure are major modifiable risk factors for cardiovascular disease. Exposure to smoke induces the release and activation of proatherogenic agents. Active smokers have higher levels of LDL and lower HDL than non-smokers [22]. The mechanisms for this imbalance are not completely understood but are postulated to be at least partly caused by chronic inflammation. By increasing the number of free radicals, smoking upregulates the pro-inflammatory cascade. Nicotine increases the production of TNFα and IL-6. The release of catecholamines caused by smoking leads to an increase in free fatty acids, which can, in turn, increase LDL and VLDL concentrations [23, 24]. Smoking stimulates the peroxidation of lipids resulting in the creation of oxidized LDL, which has been shown to accelerate atherosclerosis in animal models [23]. Smoking may also cause immunosuppression by disrupting key regulatory processes in innate and acquired immunity [25].

The effects of smoking on inflammation and its link to CVD were studied in the Multi-Ethnic Study of Atherosclerosis (MESA) by McEvoy et al. [26]. In a cohort of 6814 participants, the study evaluated the association between smoking and inflammatory biomarkers such as hsCRP, IL-6, and fibrinogen, vascular studies (brachial flow-mediated dilation and carotid distensibility), as well as markers of atherosclerotic disease measured by coronary artery calcification (CAC) (carotid intima-media thickness and ankle-brachial index). The study showed a strong association between active smokers, markers of inflammation, and subclinical atherosclerosis compared to never smokers. Conversely, quitting smoking was associated with lower inflammation and atherosclerosis [26, 27]. A study from the National Health and Nutrition Examination Survey found an improvement in hsCRP levels 5 years after smoking cessation. In the MESA study, it was also found that every 5 years of abstinence from smoking, the odds of developing incident CAC were reduced by 6% [26].

Therapies for Inflammation in Cardiovascular Disease

As we have seen, inflammation plays a critical role in the genesis, propagation, and manifestation of cardiovascular disease. Despite intensive lipid management, persons with heightened systemic inflammation are at greater risk of developing CVD. In two clinical trials (Pravastatin or Atorvastatin Evaluation and Infection Therapy (PROVE-IT) and Improved Reduction of Outcomes: Vytorin Efficacy International Trial (IMPROVE-IT)), residual hsCRP elevation was associated with increased risks of cardiovascular events, even when LDL-C was <70 mg/dL [11]. Data from these and other studies have broadened our understanding of atherosclerotic disease from a disease of chronic passive cholesterol accumulation to a model of disease driven by chronic inflammation.

While the role of systemic inflammatory conditions and the resultant benefits of its treatment for CVD risk reduction is not entirely understood, trials have shown that identifying patients with low=grade inflammation and initiating treatment is beneficial. For example, in the JUPITER (Justification for the Use of Statins in Prevention: An Intervention Trial Evaluating Rosuvastatin) trial, patients with no prior CVD or diabetes with an LDL-C <130 mg/dL but with an hsCRP of >2 mg/L benefited from 20 mg/day of rosuvastatin with a 44% relative risk reduction in a composite endpoint of myocardial infarction, stroke, arterial revascularization, hospitalization for unstable angina or death from cardiovascular causes [28]. While the benefits of statin in the JUPITER trial were confounded by its effects on LDL-C, the more recent CANTOS (Canakinumab Anti-inflammatory Thrombosis Outcome Study) trial showed that using canakinumab, a targeted therapy against IL-1, significantly reduced ASCVD with no effect on LDL-C [29]. This hypothesis was further strengthened by the Colchicine Cardiovascular Outcomes Trial (COLCOT), which showed that non-selective inhibition of inflammation using colchicine significantly reduced ASCVD-related events in patients with high ASCVD risk [30].

Diet, Exercise, and Weight Loss

Certain diets may have anti-inflammatory effects through both weight loss dependent and -independent means. Lifestyle modifications aimed at reducing weight have been shown to decrease inflammatory markers [11]. Insulin=resistant adipose tissue is active and is known to release inflammatory cytokines, such as IL-1, IL-6, and TNFα. Diets high in saturated and trans fats have been linked with low-grade inflammation. For example, high-saturated fat diets are associated with increased CRP and E-selectin. Diabetic patients with high=saturated fat diets have increased IL-6, TNFα, ICAM-1, and VCAM-1 levels. Diets high in trans fats are also associated with increased vascular inflammation by NF-κB, IL-6, hsCRP, and fibrinogen levels, leading to an increased risk of ischemic heart disease. Additionally, higher sugar intake has been directly correlated with elevated plasma CRP, IL-6, ICAM-1, and VCAM-1 levels [11].

Conversely, predominantly fish and plant-based diets high in polyunsaturated fatty acids, such as alpha-linolenic acid, are associated with reduced CRP, VCAM-1, and E-selectin levels. For example, a Mediterranean diet, particularly when supplemented with olive oil and nuts, is rich in monounsaturated and unsaturated omega-3 fats. Such plant-centric diets have been shown to help attenuate the inflammatory milieu caused by adipose tissue independent of weight loss. Mediterranean dietary patterns have also been shown to decrease inflammation by suppressing the levels of CRP, IL-6, and ICAM-1 and increasing beneficial adiponectin. As such, the 2019 ACC/AHA Guideline on the Primary Prevention of Cardiovascular Disease recommends emphasizing dietary vegetables, fruits, legumes, nuts, whole grains, and fish to reduce cardiovascular disease risk [11].

Physical activity is inversely correlated with inflammatory markers expression. The Greek ATTICA study showed that people with reported high levels of physical activity had lower levels of inflammatory mediators, including TNFα and IL-6, as well as lower CRP. These findings were independent of sex, age, smoking status, BMI, or lipid parameters [11, 31]. At a molecular level, exercise initially causes an increase in IL-6 levels and other pro=inflammatory cytokines. However, during exercise, there is also an increase in anti-inflammatory mediators, and exhaustive exercise promotes angiogenesis through various cytokines, including IL-8 [31]. Furthermore, regular exercise leads to increased adiponectin which has both anti-inflammatory and insulin=sensitizing effects, as well as decreases in overall hsCRP levels. Exercise provides additional benefits to cardiovascular health by improving blood pressure and lipid profile [31].

Statin Therapy

Statins lower cholesterol by inhibiting β-hydroxy-β-methylglutaryl-CoA (HMG-CoA) reductase, thus limiting hepatic cholesterol synthesis. The CARE, LIPID, and HPS trials have shown that statin therapy confers a higher-than-anticipated cardio-vascular benefit beyond the magnitude expected by cholesterol=lowering alone. This may be due to the salutary anti-inflammatory effects of statin therapy. Statins have been found to lower CRP levels in a manner that is largely independent of LDL-C levels [32, 33]. Statins exert their anti-inflammatory effects by reducing intracellular isoprenoid intermediates such as farnesyl pyrophosphate (FPP), gera-nylgeranyl pyrophosphate (GGPP), and other post-translational modifications of proteins that are involved in the pro-inflammatory response, which results in down-regulation of IL-1 β, TNF-α, and IL-6 [11]. Statins also have multiple favorable effects on smooth muscle via the upregulation of endothelial nitric oxide synthase and inhibition of NF-κB activation and LDL oxidation [11]. Vascular wall inflam-mation is also reduced through the downregulation of the adhesion molecules ICAM-1 and VCAM-1.

The Pravastatin Inflammation CRP Evaluation (PRINCE) trial was the first to show an independent association between statin therapy and lower levels of hsCRP independent of LDL-C achieved [34]. In the JUPITER trial, persons randomized to low=dose rosuvastatin achieved a 37% reduction in hsCRP and a 50% reduction in LDL-C with a significant 44% relative risk reduction in ischemic events compared with placebo. It was noted that the greatest benefits to CVD risk reduction were achieved when both LDL-C was <70 mg/dL and hsCRP was <1 mg/L [35]. The PROVE-IT trial subsequently demonstrated differences in individual statins on inflammation outside their class effect and cholesterol=lowering efficacy. Patients randomized to atorvastatin who achieved LDL-C <70 mg/dL had lower hsCRP <2 mg/L compared to patients treated with pravastatin who similarly attained LDL-C levels <70 mg/dL [36].

The importance of statin on inflammation is further illustrated by studies on ezetimibe, a non-statin lipid=lowering therapy, which, when given as a monother-apy, reduces LDL levels significantly but has no independent effect on hsCRP. Ezetimibe has been shown to work synergistically with statins to further lower hsCRP compared with statin monotherapy, partly due to the inhibitory effects of ezetimibe on the expression of adhesion molecules and the NF-κB pathway [37].

PCSK9 Inhibitors

The role of PCSK9 inhibitors in attenuating the inflammatory pathway of atherosclerosis remains inconclusive. While PCSK9 inhibitors dramatically lower LDL-C, they do not alter hsCRP levels, a major inflammatory marker that is strongly associated with CVD risk. PCSK9 inhibitors, however, have been found to have anti-inflammatory properties through IL-6-mediated pathways [38–40]. PCSK9 stimulates macrophage production and the release of pro=inflammatory cytokines such as IL-1β and TNFα. Inhibition of PCSK9 may thus attenuate arterial wall inflammation and reverse endothelial dysfunction [11, 38].

While PCSK9 inhibitors do not reduce hsCRP levels, they appear to have greater apparent benefits in individuals with higher levels of inflammatory markers [11, 41]. Even patients with very low levels of LDL-C experience a step-wise risk reduction when stratified by hsCRP values [11]. The seminal Further Cardiovascular Outcomes Research With PCSK9 Inhibition in Subjects With Elevated Risk (FOURIER) study showed that evolocumab resulted in greater absolute risk reductions in patients with higher baseline CRP [42]. Additionally, even patients who achieve substantial LDL-C lowering with PCSK9 inhibitors continue to have a significant residual risk for CVD if they demonstrate high levels of inflammation. Post hoc analysis of Studies of PCSK9 Inhibition and the Reduction of vascular Events studies (SPIRE-1 and SPIRE-2) found that incidence rates for cardiovascular events were 60% higher in patients with hsCRP >3 mg/L, compared with patients in the lowest tertile of hsCRP <1 mg/L, even after achieving similar LDL-C reductions with Bococizumab and statin therapy [43].

Eicosapentaenoic Acid

Diets high in omega-3 fatty acids have been shown to protect against major events associated with CVD. Eicosapentaenoic acid (EPA) is a long-chain n-3 polyunsaturated fatty acid that decreases TG levels by reducing the hepatic production of VLDLs. The Japan EPA Lipid Intervention Study (JELIS) was the first to demonstrate that highly purified EPA could decrease the incidence of cardiovascular events, potentially through its anti-inflammatory effects on plaque stabilization [44]. Subsequently, the Epanova Compared to Lovaza in Patients with High Triglycerides and Mixed Dyslipidemia (ANCHOR) study, which assessed 246 patients with baseline hsCRP ≥2.0 mg/L randomized to 4 g/day of EPA or placebo, supported the anti-inflammatory properties of EPA [45]. While the study found no effect on LDL, hsCRP was reduced by 17.9% [46].

In the Reduction of Cardiovascular Events with Icosapent Ethyl-Intervention (REDUCE-IT) trial, EPA at 4 g/day in patients with elevated triglycerides reduced hsCRP levels by 12.6% (−0.2 mg/L) in the EPA arm, compared to a rise of 29.9% (0.4 mg/L) in the placebo arm. This anti-inflammatory effect could have contributed to the difference between the two groups. The more recent RESPECT-EPA (Randomized trial for Evaluation in Secondary Prevention Efficacy of Combination Therapy-Statin and Eicosapentaenoic Acid) trial further explored the role of inflammation in mediating CVD by targeting a subset of patients with a low ratio of EPA to arachidonic acid (a polyunsaturated fatty acid released following cellular injury that leads to the formation of eicosanoids, a potent group of inflammatory mediators) [47]. Early results from the study suggest that EPA may have additional CVD benefits in patients with a low EPA to arachidonic acid ratio [47, 48].

Colchicine

Colchicine is a potent anti-inflammatory oral medication that inhibits tubulin polymerization, which subsequently leads to cytoskeletal and intracellular transport disruptions [49]. It also accumulates in neutrophils leading to inhibition of neutrophil migration to the site of inflammation and neutrophil adhesion to the endothelium through inhibition of L-selectin adhesion molecule expression. Colchicine has also been shown to suppress tyrosine phosphorylation in neutrophils, thus preventing the release of neutrophil elastase, matrix metalloproteinases, and α-defensins [49].

By reducing the expression of E-selectin adhesion molecules on inflamed endothelium, colchicine similarly inhibits the adhesion of leukocytes to the endothelium. Colchicine also downregulates TNF receptors in macrophages. Additionally, colchicine reduces activation of the NLRP3 inflammasome, thus decreasing the production of IL-1β and IL-18 [50].

IL-1β Inhibition

Canakinumab is a high-affinity human monoclonal antibody against IL-1β that activates the release of IL-6, thus stimulating the liver production of CRP. Canakinumab lowers the incidence of myocardial infarction (MA), as first demonstrated in the CANTOS trial [29, 51]. It was noted that the risk reduction of major adverse cardiovascular events occurred only when the hsCRP levels were <2 mg/L. As Canakinumab was associated with a significant increase in fatal infection or sepsis, it has not been approved by the FDA treating ASCVD [29, 51].

Low-Dose Methotrexate

Methotrexate inhibits the synthesis of DNA, RNA, and proteins by binding and suppressing dihydrofolate reductase activity. It is the most used medication for treating rheumatoid arthritis (RA) to reduce joint damage and pain and improve functional symptoms. In RA, synovial injury is the primary cause of inflammation characterized by increased cytokine (such as IL-6 and TNF) and hsCRP release. TNFα secretion through various mechanisms causes the restructuring of intracellular junctions, ultimately facilitating leukocyte transmigration. IL-6 induces the production and release of CRP. In a systematic literature review performed by Westlake et al. [52], methotrexate was associated with a reduced risk of cardiovascular events in patients with RA.

However, results from the more recent Cardiovascular Inflammation Reduction Trial (CIRT) question this finding. The CIRT study, a randomized, double-blinded, placebo-controlled trial on low-dose methotrexate for the prevention of atherosclerotic events, including MI, nonfatal stroke, and cardiovascular death, failed to demonstrate any reduction in cardiovascular events or CRP, IL-6, and IL-1β levels in the study group compared to placebo. Moreover, the methotrexate group had elevated liver enzyme levels, lower leukocyte counts, and hematocrit levels. It also resulted in a higher incidence of non-basal cell skin cancer than the placebo group [53]. It is to date unclear if and how methotrexate reduces CVD, whether by a direct effect on atherosclerosis or through anti-inflammatory action.

Conclusion

Atherosclerosis, far from merely a disease of lipid metabolism, is strongly mediated by chronic pro-inflammatory conditions such as obesity and diabetes. The response of the innate and adaptive immune system to these conditions results in the activation of a wide array of inflammatory pathways and can lead to the acceleration of vascular disease. Inflammatory markers have been shown to be useful for risk stratification and prognostication of ASCVD. Lifestyle modifications such as diet and exercise along with targeted therapies to lessen our lifetime exposure to inflammation are beneficial in reducing cardiovascular events. As such, therapies that not only target our lipid profile but also reduce inflammation, such as statins, have proven to be some of the most effective treatments in reducing cardiovascular mortality and morbidity.

References

1. Arnett DK, Blumenthal RS, Albert MA, Buroker AB, Goldberger ZD, Hahn EJ, et al. 2019 ACC/AHA guideline on the primary prevention of cardiovascular disease: a report of the American College of Cardiology/American Heart Association Task Force on clinical practice guidelines. Circulation. 2019;140(11):e596–646.
2. United States DoHaHS, Centers for Disease Control and Prevention. National Center for Health Statistics FastStats. 2020 [updated 05/2020]. https://www.cdc.gov/nchs/fastats/default.htm.
3. Meng L-B, Zhang Y-M, Luo Y, Gong T, Liu D-P. Chronic stress a potential suspect zero of atherosclerosis: a systematic review. Front Cardiovasc Med. 2021;8:8.

4. Insull W Jr. The pathology of atherosclerosis: plaque development and plaque responses to medical treatment. Am J Med. 2009;122(1 Suppl):S3–14.
5. Khafagy R, Dash S. Obesity and cardiovascular disease: the emerging role of inflammation. Front Cardiovasc Med. 2021;8:8.
6. Organization WH. Obesity and overweight. 2021. https://www.who.int/news-room/fact-sheets/detail/obesity-and-overweight.
7. Collaborators GBDO, Afshin A, Forouzanfar MH, Reitsma MB, Sur P, Estep K, et al. Health effects of overweight and obesity in 195 countries over 25 years. N Engl J Med. 2017;377(1):13–27.
8. Blüher M. Obesity: global epidemiology and pathogenesis. Nat Rev Endocrinol. 2019;15(5):288–98.
9. Ruparelia N, Chai JT, Fisher EA, Choudhury RP. Inflammatory processes in cardiovascular disease: a route to targeted therapies. Nat Rev Cardiol. 2017;14(3):133–44.
10. Smith JD, Trogan E, Ginsberg M, Grigaux C, Tian J, Miyata M. Decreased atherosclerosis in mice deficient in both macrophage colony-stimulating factor (op) and apolipoprotein E. Proc Natl Acad Sci U S A. 1995;92(18):8264–8.
11. Alfaddagh A, Martin SS, Leucker TM, Michos ED, Blaha MJ, Lowenstein CJ, et al. Inflammation and cardiovascular disease: from mechanisms to therapeutics. Am J Prev Cardiol. 2020;4:100130.
12. Ait-Oufella H, Libby P, Tedgui A. Anticytokine immune therapy and atherothrombotic cardiovascular risk. Arterioscler Thromb Vasc Biol. 2019;39(8):1510–9.
13. Peng J, Luo F, Ruan G, Peng R, Li X. Hypertriglyceridemia and atherosclerosis. Lipids Health Dis. 2017;16(1):233.
14. Basu D, Bornfeldt KE. Hypertriglyceridemia and atherosclerosis: using human research to guide mechanistic studies in animal models. Front Endocrinol (Lausanne). 2020;11:504.
15. Polyakova EA, Mikhaylov EN. The prognostic role of high-sensitivity C-reactive protein in patients with acute myocardial infarction. J Geriatr Cardiol. 2020;17(7):379–83.
16. Rocha VZ, Libby P. Obesity, inflammation, and atherosclerosis. Nat Rev Cardiol. 2009;6(6):399–409.
17. Finucane MM, Stevens GA, Cowan MJ, Danaei G, Lin JK, Paciorek CJ, et al. National, regional, and global trends in body-mass index since 1980: systematic analysis of health examination surveys and epidemiological studies with 960 country-years and 9.1 million participants. Lancet. 2011;377(9765):557–67.
18. Semple RK, Sleigh A, Murgatroyd PR, Adams CA, Bluck L, Jackson S, et al. Postreceptor insulin resistance contributes to human dyslipidemia and hepatic steatosis. J Clin Invest. 2009;119(2):315–22.
19. Khan S, Chan YT, Revelo XS, Winer DA. The immune landscape of visceral adipose tissue during obesity and aging. Front Endocrinol (Lausanne). 2020;11:267.
20. Khan SS, Ning H, Wilkins JT, Allen N, Carnethon M, Berry JD, et al. Association of body mass index with lifetime risk of cardiovascular disease and compression of morbidity. JAMA Cardiol. 2018;3(4):280–7.
21. Cameron AJ, Romaniuk H, Orellana L, Dallongeville J, Dobson AJ, Drygas W, et al. Combined influence of waist and hip circumference on risk of death in a large cohort of European and Australian adults. J Am Heart Assoc. 2020;9(13):e015189.
22. Ambrose JA, Barua RS. The pathophysiology of cigarette smoking and cardiovascular disease: an update. J Am Coll Cardiol. 2004;43(10):1731–7.
23. Michael Pittilo R. Cigarette smoking, endothelial injury and cardiovascular disease. Int J Exp Pathol. 2000;81(4):219–30.
24. Jain RB, Ducatman A. Associations between smoking and lipid/lipoprotein concentrations among US adults aged ≥20 years. J Circ Biomark. 2018;7:1849454418779310.
25. Qiu F, Liang CL, Liu H, Zeng YQ, Hou S, Huang S, et al. Impacts of cigarette smoking on immune responsiveness: up and down or upside down? Oncotarget. 2017;8(1):268–84.
26. McEvoy JW, Nasir K, DeFilippis AP, Lima JA, Bluemke DA, Hundley WG, et al. Relationship of cigarette smoking with inflammation and subclinical vascular disease: the Multi-Ethnic Study of Atherosclerosis. Arterioscler Thromb Vasc Biol. 2015;35(4):1002–10.

27. Reichert V, Xue X, Bartscherer D, Jacobsen D, Fardellone C, Folan P, et al. A pilot study to examine the effects of smoking cessation on serum markers of inflammation in women at risk for cardiovascular disease. Chest. 2009;136(1):212–9.
28. Ridker PM, Danielson E, Fonseca FAH, Genest J, Gotto AM, Kastelein JJP, et al. Rosuvastatin to prevent vascular events in men and women with elevated C-reactive protein. N Engl J Med. 2008;359(21):2195–207.
29. Ridker PM, MacFadyen JG, Glynn RJ, Koenig W, Libby P, Everett BM, et al. Inhibition of interleukin-1β by canakinumab and cardiovascular outcomes in patients with chronic kidney disease. J Am Coll Cardiol. 2018;71(21):2405–14.
30. Tardif J-C, Kouz S, Waters DD, Bertrand OF, Diaz R, Maggioni AP, et al. Efficacy and safety of low-dose colchicine after myocardial infarction. N Engl J Med. 2019;381(26):2497–505.
31. Panagiotakos DB, Georgousopoulou EN, Pitsavos C, Chrysohoou C, Metaxa V, Georgiopoulos GA, et al. Ten-year (2002-2012) cardiovascular disease incidence and all-cause mortality, in urban Greek population: the ATTICA Study. Int J Cardiol. 2015;180:178–84.
32. Sacks FM, Pfeffer MA, Moye LA, Rouleau JL, Rutherford JD, Cole TG, et al. The effect of pravastatin on coronary events after myocardial infarction in patients with average cholesterol levels. Cholesterol and Recurrent Events Trial investigators. N Engl J Med. 1996;335(14):1001–9.
33. Keech A, Colquhoun D, Best J, Kirby A, Simes RJ, Hunt D, et al. Secondary prevention of cardiovascular events with long-term pravastatin in patients with diabetes or impaired fasting glucose: results from the LIPID trial. Diabetes Care. 2003;26(10):2713–21.
34. Albert MA, Staggers J, Chew P, Ridker PM. The pravastatin inflammation CRP evaluation (PRINCE): rationale and design. Am Heart J. 2001;141(6):893–8.
35. Ridker PM. The JUPITER trial: results, controversies, and implications for prevention. Circ Cardiovasc Qual Outcomes. 2009;2(3):279–85.
36. Cannon CP, Braunwald E, McCabe CH, Rader DJ, Rouleau JL, Belder R, et al. Intensive versus moderate lipid lowering with statins after acute coronary syndromes. N Engl J Med. 2004;350(15):1495–504.
37. Ballantyne CM, Houri J, Notarbartolo A, Melani L, Lipka LJ, Suresh R, et al. Effect of ezetimibe coadministered with atorvastatin in 628 patients with primary hypercholesterolemia: a prospective, randomized, double-blind trial. Circulation. 2003;107(19):2409–15.
38. Ruscica M, Tokgözoğlu L, Corsini A, Sirtori CR. PCSK9 inhibition and inflammation: a narrative review. Atherosclerosis. 2019;288:146–55.
39. Navarese EP, Kołodziejczak M, Dimitroulis D, Wolff G, Busch HL, Devito F, et al. From proprotein convertase subtilisin/kexin type 9 to its inhibition: state-of-the-art and clinical implications. Eur Heart J Cardiovasc Pharmacother. 2016;2(1):44–53.
40. Walley KR, Thain KR, Russell JA, Reilly MP, Meyer NJ, Ferguson JF, et al. PCSK9 is a critical regulator of the innate immune response and septic shock outcome. Sci Transl Med. 2014;6(258):258ra143.
41. Ding Z, Pothineni NVK, Goel A, Lüscher TF, Mehta JL. PCSK9 and inflammation: role of shear stress, pro-inflammatory cytokines, and LOX-1. Cardiovasc Res. 2020;116(5):908–15.
42. Bohula EA, Giugliano RP, Leiter LA, Verma S, Park JG, Sever PS, et al. Inflammatory and cholesterol risk in the FOURIER Trial. Circulation. 2018;138(2):131–40.
43. Pradhan AD, Aday AW, Rose LM, Ridker PM. Residual inflammatory risk on treatment with PCSK9 inhibition and statin therapy. Circulation. 2018;138(2):141–9.
44. Yokoyama M, Origasa H, Matsuzaki M, Matsuzawa Y, Saito Y, Ishikawa Y, et al. Effects of eicosapentaenoic acid on major coronary events in hypercholesterolaemic patients (JELIS): a randomised open-label, blinded endpoint analysis. Lancet. 2007;369(9567):1090–8.
45. Ballantyne CM, Bays HE, Kastelein JJ, Stein E, Isaacsohn JL, Braeckman RA, et al. Efficacy and safety of eicosapentaenoic acid ethyl ester (AMR101) therapy in statin-treated patients with persistent high triglycerides (from the ANCHOR study). Am J Cardiol. 2012;110(7):984–92.
46. Miller M, Ballantyne CM, Bays HE, Granowitz C, Doyle RT Jr, Juliano RA, et al. Effects of icosapent ethyl (eicosapentaenoic acid ethyl ester) on atherogenic lipid/lipoprotein, apoli-

poprotein, and inflammatory parameters in patients with elevated high-sensitivity C-reactive protein (from the ANCHOR Study). Am J Cardiol. 2019;124(5):696–701.

47. Bhatt DL, Steg PG, Miller M, Brinton EA, Jacobson TA, Ketchum SB, et al. Cardiovascular risk reduction with icosapent ethyl for hypertriglyceridemia. N Engl J Med. 2019;380(1):11–22.

48. Nishizaki Y, Miyauchi K, Iwata H, Inoue T, Hirayama A, Kimura K, et al. Study protocol and baseline characteristics of randomized trial for evaluation in secondary prevention efficacy of combination therapy-statin and eicosapentaenoic acid: RESPECT-EPA, the combination of a randomized control trial and an observational biomarker study. Am Heart J. 2022;257:1–8.

49. Li Z, Davis GS, Mohr C, Nain M, Gemsa D. Inhibition of LPS-induced tumor necrosis factor-alpha production by colchicine and other microtubule disrupting drugs. Immunobiology. 1996;195(4–5):624–39.

50. Martinon F, Pétrilli V, Mayor A, Tardivel A, Tschopp J. Gout-associated uric acid crystals activate the NALP3 inflammasome. Nature. 2006;440(7081):237–41.

51. Ridker PM, Thuren T, Zalewski A, Libby P. Interleukin-1β inhibition and the prevention of recurrent cardiovascular events: rationale and design of the Canakinumab Anti-inflammatory Thrombosis Outcomes Study (CANTOS). Am Heart J. 2011;162(4):597–605.

52. Westlake SL, Colebatch AN, Baird J, Curzen N, Kiely P, Quinn M, et al. Tumour necrosis factor antagonists and the risk of cardiovascular disease in patients with rheumatoid arthritis: a systematic literature review. Rheumatology (Oxford). 2011;50(3):518–31.

53. Ridker PM, Everett BM, Pradhan A, MacFadyen JG, Solomon DH, Zaharris E, et al. Low-dose methotrexate for the prevention of atherosclerotic events. N Engl J Med. 2018;380(8):752–62.

Chapter 8
Environmental and Lifestyle Factors Influencing Inflammation and Type 2 Diabetes

Varun Reddy and Dimiter Avtanski

Abbreviations

8-OHdG	8-hydroxy-2′-deoxyguanosine
AMPK	AMP-activated protein kinase
BMI	Body mass index
CRP	C-reactive protein
DPP	U.S. Diabetes Prevention Program
DPPOS	Diabetes Prevention Program Outcomes Study
FDPS	Finnish Diabetes Prevention Study
Fiaf	Fasting-inducible adipocyte factor (*s.* angiopoietin-like protein 4)
FMD	Flow-mediated dilation
FMT	Fecal microbiota transplantation
FRAP	Ferric reducing antioxidant potential
FXR-α	Farnesoid X receptor-alpha
GF	Germ-free
GI	Gastrointestinal
GLP	Glucagon-like peptide
GLUT4	Glucose transporter 4
GM	Gut microbiome
GRP120	G protein-coupled receptor
HFD	High-fat diet

V. Reddy
New York Institute of Technology College of Osteopathic Medicine, Old Westbury, NY, USA

D. Avtanski (✉)
Friedman Diabetes Institute, Lenox Hill Hospital, Northwell Health, New York, NY, USA

Feinstein Institutes for Medical Research, Manhasset, NY, USA

Donald and Barbara Zucker School of Medicine at Hofstra/Northwell, Hempstead, NY, USA
e-mail: davtanski@northwell.edu

© The Author(s), under exclusive license to Springer Nature Switzerland AG 2023
D. Avtanski, L. Poretsky (eds.), *Obesity, Diabetes and Inflammation*, Contemporary Endocrinology, https://doi.org/10.1007/978-3-031-39721-9_8

HIIT	High-intensity interval training
HPFS	Health Professionals Follow-Up Survey
IFN-γ	Interferon gamma
IGF-I	Insulin-like growth factor 1
IL	Interleukin
IL-1Ra	Interleukin 1 receptor antagonist
IMCL	Intramyocellular lipid
JNK	c-Jun terminal kinase
LPS	Lipopolysaccharides
LPTA	Leisure time physical activity
MICT	Moderate-intensity continuous training
NOS	Nitric oxide synthase
NSH	Nurses' Health Study
OGTT	Oral glucose tolerance test
PI3K	Phosphoinositide 3-kinase (*s.* phosphatidyl inositol 3-kinase)
PPAR	Peroxisome proliferator-activated receptor
PREDIMED	*Prevención con Dieta Mediterránea* (Spanish for "Prevention with Mediterranean Diet") study
PUFA	Polyunsaturated fatty acid
PYY	Peptide tyrosine tyrosine (*s.* peptide YY)
ROS	Reactive oxygen species
SCFA	Short-chain fatty acid
SIT	Sprint interval training
T1DM	Type 1 *diabetes mellitus*
T2DM	Type 2 *diabetes mellitus*
TCE	Thai chi exercise
TGR5 (*s.* GPBAR1)	G protein-coupled bile receptor 1
TLR	Toll-like receptor
TNFα	Tumor necrosis factor-alpha
TRAP	Total radical-trapping antioxidant parameter
Treg	T-regulatory lymphocyte

Introduction

Diabetes is a global health epidemic, the incidence of which is increasing exponentially. As of 2021 worldwide, 537 million adults were living with diabetes; it is estimated that by 2024 this number will increase to 783 million [1]. Currently, 11.3% of the US adult population is affected by diabetes, and 38% have prediabetes. Diabetes is the leading cause of blindness, heart disease, and kidney failure, affecting the quality of life of patients and caregivers. The healthcare dollars spent on treating diabetes complications and drug therapy are increasing accordingly. Thus, there is an urgent need for effective interventions.

The etiology of diabetes is multifactorial and includes genetic and environmental factors. The management of diabetes emphasizes environmentally modifiable risk factors such as diet, physical activity, and weight management. Recently, the gut microbiome (GM) has gained considerable attention as a potential factor in the pathophysiology of diabetes. Chronic low-grade inflammation is involved in impaired insulin secretion and insulin resistance in diabetes and obesity. Modifying GM with diet and lifestyle changes by decreasing inflammation has been beneficial in preventing and treating diabetes and obesity.

Obesity is a significant risk factor for type 2 *diabetes mellitus* (T2DM). Weight loss of 5% or more improves glycemic control and prevents T2DM in at-risk people. A comprehensive approach to diet and lifestyle is essential to achieve these goals. Diets with various nutrient compositions and food groups have been studied. An increase in T2DM risk has been linked to Western dietary patterns consisting of a diet high in calories, fat, and sodium and low in fruits and vegetables. A sedentary lifestyle can lead to the development of T2DM, and physical exercise can reduce the progression of the disease and its complications.

Randomized controlled studies in various groups worldwide have shown consistent results with lifestyle changes for preventing and treating diabetes. The Da Qing IGT and Diabetes Study performed between 1986 and 1992 in the city of Da Qing, China, involving 110,660 men and women stratified into control, a diet, an exercise, and a combined diet and exercise intervention groups, demonstrated 43% reduction in T2DM in the lifestyle intervention group compared to the control group [2]. A 30-year follow-up of a subgroup from the study continued to show benefits in the incidence of T2DM and related complications [3]. Similarly, the U.S. Diabetes Prevention Program (DPP) in 1996 found a 58% reduction in T2DM in the group with lifestyle intervention [4]. Results from the follow-up outcome study, the Diabetes Prevention Program Outcomes Study (DPPOS), showed a 34% decrease in the incidence of T2DM after 10 years in the lifestyle intervention group [5]. The results from the Finnish Diabetes Prevention Study (FDPS) [6] and others demonstrated similar reductions in the lifestyle intervention groups.

Here, we review some environmental factors and lifestyle changes that play a role in obesity, inflammation, and T2DM.

Role of Diet and Nutrition in Diabetes

Dietary interventions have been proven to be effective in the management of T2DM and related metabolic diseases. Various diets are known to improve T2DM and the accompanying complications through mechanisms inhibiting chronic inflammation characteristics for these conditions. Multiple studies, including the DPP [7] and the FDPS [6], have shown the benefits of lifestyle interventions in reducing the incidence of T2DM. Various diets that were studied in preventing T2DM are discussed below (Fig. 8.1).

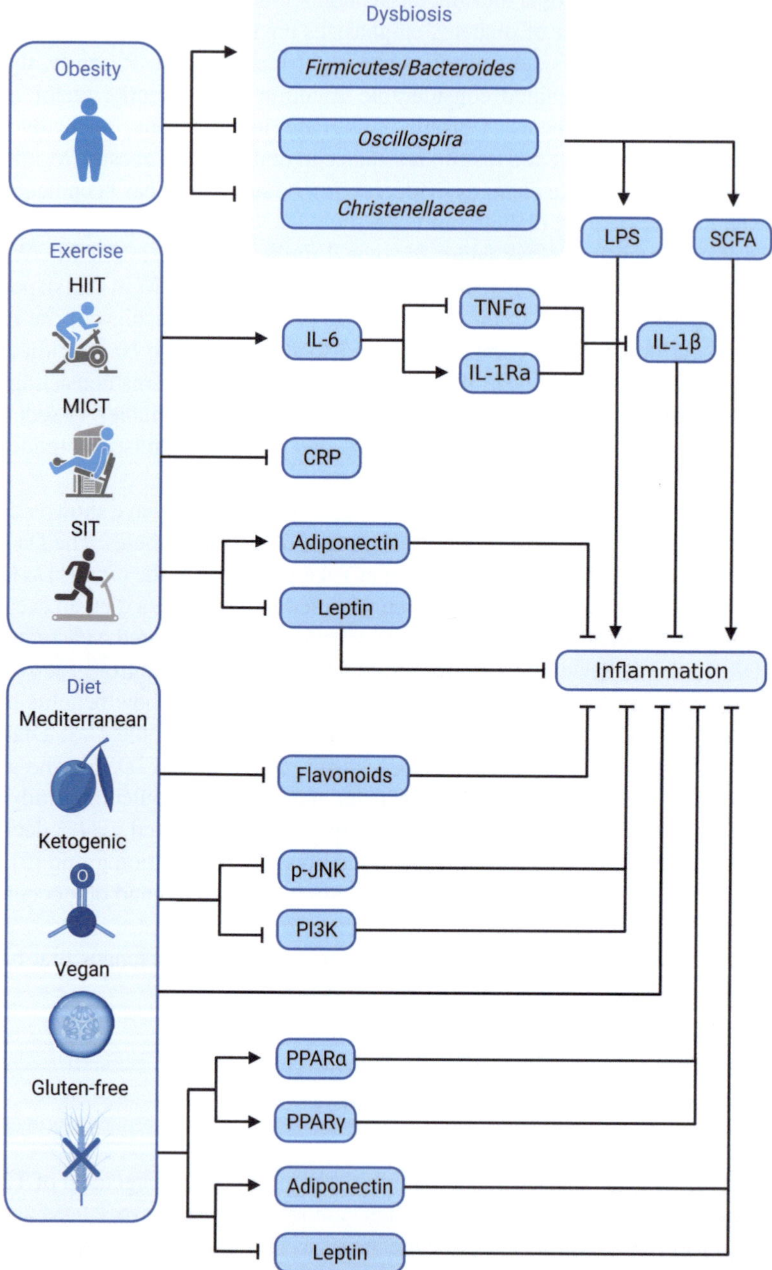

Fig. 8.1 Effects of environmental factors on inflammation. Obesity, exercise, and diet play significant roles in the pathophysiology of obesity-induced inflammation. The figure depicts some of the major molecular players involved in this association. *CRP* C-reactive protein, *HIIT* high-intensity interval training, *IL-1β* interleukin 1 beta, *IL-1Ra* interleukin 1 receptor antagonist, *IL-6* interleukin 6, *LPS* lipopolysaccharides, *MICT* moderate-intensity continuous training, *PI3K* phosphoinositide 3-kinase, *p-JNK* phosphorylated c-Jun terminal kinase, *PPARα* peroxisome proliferator-activated receptor-alpha, *PPARγ* peroxisome proliferator-activated receptor gamma, *SCFA* short-chain fatty acids, *SIT* sprint interval training, *TNFα* tumor necrosis factor-alpha. Created with BioRender.com

Mediterranean Diet

The Mediterranean diet is one of the most studied diets. It consists of whole grains, plenty of fresh vegetables and fruits, nuts, seeds, extra-virgin olive oil as a primary fat source, and low to moderate amounts of dairy products, eggs, fish, and poultry. Mediterranean diet is associated with decreased risk of T2DM because of its anti-inflammatory and antioxidant effects [8], increased plasma ferric reducing antioxidant potential (FRAP), increased total radical-trapping antioxidant parameter (TRAP) as well as lower C-reactive protein (CRP) levels [9]. The Mediterranean diet is rich in phenolic compounds (especially flavonoids, such as quercetin, oleuropein, hydroxytyrosol, and tyrosol), which exert antioxidant and anti-inflammatory effects. The diet is also rich in polyunsaturated fatty acids (PUFAs) and omega-3 fatty acids that improve insulin sensitivity and inhibit NLRP3 inflammasome activity, respectively. PUFA also stimulates glucagon-like peptide (GLP) 1 (GLP-1) secretion from the gut by binding to G protein-coupled receptor 120 (GPR120), thus reducing hyperglycemia.

The study by Al-Aubaidy et al. [10] in T2DM patients consuming citrus fruits as part of the Mediterranean diet showed increased plasma levels of the bioflavonoids naringin, hesperetin, and hesperidin and reduced levels of the proinflammatory cytokine interleukin (IL) 6 (IL-6) and the oxidative stress marker 8-hydroxy-2′-deoxyguanosine (8-OHdG). Meta-analyses by Koloverou et al. [11] and Schwingshackl et al. [12] demonstrated that the Mediterranean diet significantly decreases the onset of T2DM by 19% and 23%, respectively. The PREDIMED (*Prevención con Dieta Mediterránea*, Spanish for "Prevention with Mediterranean Diet") trial [13] showed that consuming a Mediterranean diet with virgin olive oil resulted in a 40% reduction in the onset of T2DM in 4.1 years.

Overall, the present evidence suggests that the Mediterranean diet provides a suitable and sustainable prevention of T2DM.

Ketogenic/Very Low Carbohydrate Diets

A ketogenic diet comprises 55–60% fats, 30–35% proteins, and 5–10% carbohydrates. It replaces glucose with ketone bodies as an energy source. A restricted carbohydrate diet results in lower insulin levels and higher glucagon levels, which increases mitochondrial fatty acid oxidation resulting in the production of acetyl CoA for ketone body formation [14].

Brinkworth et al. [15] demonstrated that in the long term, consumption of a very low-carbohydrate diet results in a significant increase in HDL cholesterol and reduction in triglyceride levels, which benefits patients with prediabetes and obesity. A clinical trial by Myette-Côté et al. [16] that investigated the effects of a short-term low-carbohydrate high-fat diet (HFD) in T2DM has shown an improvement in the inflammatory profile, such as lower levels of peripheral blood mononuclear cells phosphorylated c-Jun N-terminal kinase (p-JNK). JNK is involved in proinflammatory cytokine production, and its phosphorylation is characteristic of dysglycemia and inflammation [17]. Kumar et al. [18] showed that the consumption of a ketogenic diet suppresses the insulin-like growth factor I (IGF-I) and the activation of phosphoinositide 3-kinase (PI3K). However, further studies (more than 2 years long) are needed since the long-term effects of the ketogenic diet are uncertain.

Vegan Diet

A vegan diet is a plant-based diet that includes minimally processed vegetables, fruits, whole grains, legumes, seeds, and nuts and excludes animal and dairy products. It has gained popularity in the Western world in recent years.

Studies have shown that vegan diet decreases the risk of developing T2DM. For example, Adventist Health Study-2 [19] showed a nearly 50% decrease in the risk of T2DM. Similarly, the Rotterdam Study (RS) [20] showed a lower risk of developing insulin resistance, prediabetes, and T2DM. Consuming higher content of vegetables and fruits leads to reduced oxidation and inflammation. The higher fiber content in the vegan diet decreases gastric emptying and slower glucose absorption, and the lower fat content diminishes insulin resistance. Conversely, diets rich in fat increase intramyocellular lipid (IMCL) concentration, thus leading to an increase in reactive oxygen species (ROS) production and cytotoxic effects in mitochondria resulting in insulin resistance [21].

Although the current data are promising, larger randomized studies are needed to prove the effectiveness of the vegan diet in obesity-induced inflammation and T2DM and to point out the potential adverse effects over the long term.

Gluten-Free Diet

A gluten-free diet excludes food containing gluten. Gluten is a protein found in grains, mainly wheat, rye, and barley. Studies demonstrated that gluten peptides increase intestinal permeability and lead to inflammation and T2DM [22]. Animal studies with mice fed a gluten-free diet have shown lower concentrations of the proinflammatory adipokines leptin and resistin and higher levels of the anti-inflammatory adipokine adiponectin concomitant with decreased levels of fasting glucose and insulin [23]. The observed reduction in adiposity, inflammation, and insulin resistance following a gluten-free diet was accompanied by an induction of the expression of the peroxisome proliferator-activated receptors (PPARs) alpha and gamma (PPARα and PPARγ) [23]. The PPARs are crucial in regulating lipid and glucose metabolism, adipocyte differentiation, and inflammatory responses.

It is important to note that the association between gluten intake and the risk of developing T2DM needs to be better defined. For example, the Nurses' Health

Studies I and II (NHS I and NHS II), as well as the Health Professionals Follow-Up Study (HPFS), show that gluten intake is negatively associated with the risk of T2DM [24].

Role of Physical Activity in Diabetes

There is no doubt that regular exercise and high physical activity are beneficial in preventing and managing T2DM, and the lack of physical activity is linked to the development of T2DM. Prediabetes is associated with increased inflammatory markers such as CRP, IL-6, and tumor necrosis factor-alpha (TNFα) [25]. In addition, leptin has been shown to be elevated in individuals at risk for diabetes [26], while adiponectin is inversely associated with prediabetes [27]. In this section, we will discuss the effects of physical activity on inflammatory markers in prediabetes.

Exercise has direct anti-inflammatory effects mediated by acute elevations in IL-6, which inhibits the production of TNFα and stimulates the release of IL-1 receptor antagonist (IL-1Ra), leading to further decreases in the proinflammatory IL-1β signaling [28]. Studies have shown that TNFα mediates insulin resistance and IL-1β causes dysfunction of the pancreatic β-cells [28, 29]. For instance, Larsen et al. [30] achieved an improvement in glucose homeostasis by inhibiting IL-1β. In addition, exercise induces anti-inflammatory effects through indirect mechanisms by decreasing visceral adiposity [31]. Visceral fat is proinflammatory compared to subcutaneous fat [32]. Becic et al. [33] found that exercise increases adiponectin levels and decreases leptin levels in prediabetes. A systematic review and meta-analysis of randomized, controlled trials by Yu et al. [34] demonstrated that exercise (particularly aerobic exercise) decreases leptin and possibly increases adiponectin levels in overweight and obese individuals. Similar results were obtained from a meta-analysis by Jadhav et al. [35], who demonstrated that physical activity in pre-diabetic individuals decreases leptin and IL-6 levels.

Different types of exercise, such as aerobic, resistance training, HIIT (high-intensity interval training), MICT (moderate-intensity continuous training), SIT (sprint interval training), and walking, have been associated with suppressed levels of proinflammatory markers. However, no conclusive evidence indicates which type and intensity of physical activity provides the most significant anti-inflammatory effects. Recent findings revealed that the inflammatory and oxidative stress markers were not different in individuals with T2DM on either HIIT or MICT [36]. A systematic review by Xing et al. [37] showed an improvement in the inflammatory markers IL-6 and TNFα with combined aerobic and resistance exercise. A meta-analysis by Hejazi et al. [38] found an increase in adiponectin and a decrease in the proinflammatory cytokines CRP, TNFα, and CRP levels. A subgroup analysis in this study showed more pronounced effects from aerobic exercises compared to other types of exercise training. A randomized controlled trial by Slentz et al. [39] found that high, moderate-intensity exercises improved oral glucose tolerance in prediabetic individuals. The authors determined moderate-intensity exercise is as effective as other intensive approaches, such as diet and weight loss, in individuals at risk for diabetes. The accumulation of pancreatic fat is believed to result in a dysfunction of the β-cells. Improvement in β-cell function with a decreased pancreatic fat was seen in prediabetic and T2DM individuals on a short-term exercise regimen [40]. Figueiredo et al. [41] highlighted the importance of regular physical exercise as an essential tool in restoring the balance of monocytes and lymphocytes. Regular physical exercise has been shown to increase anti-inflammatory macrophages, CD-16 monocytes, and T-regulatory lymphocytes (Tregs), resulting in improved insulin sensitivity [32]. In T2DM, HIIT led to an increase in CD-16 monocytes, which resulted in a decrease in inflammatory response via TLR2 expression [42]. In addition, TNF-alpha concentrations were reduced, implicating anti-inflammatory effects with HIIT exercises. Balducci et al. [43] found that high-intensity endurance training, together with strength training exhibited enhanced effects on proinflammatory cytokines. In addition, the study of Magalhães et al. [44] found improvements in the circulating levels of IL-6 after 1 year of supervised physical activity of both HIIT and MICT while performing resistance training in type 2 diabetic patients. These findings suggest that long-term exercise ameliorates inflammation in these individuals.

Physical exercise, including aerobic and combined exercises, has been shown to improve endothelial function in T2DM by increasing flow-mediated dilatation (FMD) used as a marker of endothelial function [45]. Parada-Sánchez et al. [46] have shown that irisin, which normally correlates with insulin sensitivity, was positively associated with more intense physical activity. Moreover, an increase in leisure time physical activity (LTPA) was found to diminish diabetes risk in the FDPS [47], and a decrease in the incidence of T2DM with physical activity was seen in a more extended clinical trial—the DPPOS [48].

Other forms of exercise, such as Tai chi, yoga, and pilates, have been studied. Tai chi and yoga include slow, gentle movements and physical postures with controlled breathing during a clear state of mind. Chen et al. [49] showed that Thai chi exercise (TCE) improved BMI and decreased high-sensitive CRP. The goal of pilates is to increase muscle strength as well as to enhance posture and flexibility in a low impact. Pilates has been shown to improve oxidative stress and decrease HbA1c levels [50].

Physical exercise is beneficial in preventing T2DM and should be included as a first-line treatment option for prediabetic individuals. While no long-term randomized controlled studies conclusively indicate the optimal type of physical activity, HIIT is most advantageous for reducing inflammatory markers in prediabetes. However, there are various barriers to implementing physical exercises, such as lack of supervision, access to participation in activities, and long-term compliance. In addition, the aging population, who is at the highest risk and may not be able to perform such training, needs a simplified form of exercise to receive the same benefits. All individuals should decrease sedentary time and engage in regular physical exercise (Fig. 8.1).

Role of the Intestinal Microflora in Obesity-Induced Inflammation and Diabetes

The GM plays an essential role in the host's immune system. It impacts the absorption, breakdown, and storage of nutrients. The human gastrointestinal (GI) tract harbors more than 100 trillion microorganisms, including bacteria, archaea, and eukarya. Bacteria comprise more than half of gut microbes and are dominated by the phyla *Firmicutes* and *Bacteroides* [51]. The archaea are mostly methanogens, predominantly *Methanobrevibacter smithii* and *Methanosphaera stadtmanae*, while the eukarya are mostly yeast.

The development of GM begins in utero and is modulated by various factors that include the mode of neonatal delivery and feeding, age, sex, and body mass index (BMI) [52, 53]. A dysbiosis due to environmental and dietary changes may result in a disruption of intestinal barrier function and cause chronic inflammation, which can further lead to metabolic disorders, such as diabetes (Fig. 8.1).

Intestinal Microflora and Obesity

Relationships between obesity and GM have been studied as potential interventions for treating or preventing obesity. In vivo studies with mice by Bäckhed et al. [54] demonstrated the presence of higher fat mass and insulin resistance in germ-free (GF) C57Bl/6. In the same study, GF mice also displayed higher levels of fasting-inducible adipocyte factor (Fiaf) (also known as angiopoietin-like protein 4) which was reduced after fecal microbiota was transplanted from conventionally raised mice [54]. Conversely, antibiotic use in childhood has been shown to increase the risk of diabetes in adulthood [55]. These observations support the notion that GM can modulate adiposity and thus play a role in energy metabolism.

Genetically obese leptin-deficient (*ob/ob*) mice have a high proportion of *Firmicutes* and a low proportion of *Bacteroidetes* compared to their lean wild-type counterparts [56]. Similarly, findings from Ley et al. [57] and others have shown a higher *Firmicutes/Bacteroidetes* ratio in obese humans. Comparing microbiota from human subjects before and after weight loss over 1 year revealed a decrease in *Firmicutes* and an increase in *Bacteroidetes* regardless of carbohydrate or fat-restrictive diets [58]; however, these findings are not in agreement [59, 60]. Other bacteria, such as *Oscillospira,* were also found to be reduced in obese humans [61]. Goodrich et al. [62] studied the gut microbiota of twins and found that higher levels of *Christensenellaceae* were associated with lower BMI. In the same study, the introduction of *C. minuta* into GF mice resulted in a bodyweight reduction. In addition, Gao et al. [63] found a decreased microbial diversity in obese subjects along with a decrease in the abundance of butyrate-producing bacteria. The same authors also found downregulation of enzymes involved in glucose and insulin signaling pathways in obese subjects.

The methanogenic *Archaea*, including the dominant *Methanobrevibacter smithii*, reduce carbon dioxide into methane during fermentation, which is exhaled in breath [64]. Exhaled methane is an indicator of methanogen colonization and was found to be present in higher amounts in obese individuals [65]. Studies using antibiotics to eradicate breath methane in prediabetic individuals and obese subjects showed an improvement in cholesterol, insulin, and glucose levels during the oral glucose tolerance test (OGTT) [66]. However, animal studies found no differences in the abundance of *M. smithii* in the GI tract of obese and nonobese mice.

Prebiotic supplementation with inulin reduced adiposity in mice with diet-induced obesity [67]. Similarly, inulin-administered streptozotocin-induced diabetes rats had lower glucose levels and elevated serum GLP-1 levels [68]. Studies in obese men found increased short-chain fatty acids (SCFAs) levels with inulin ingestion [69]. Studies with probiotics (live microorganisms) in mice revealed metabolic benefits by reducing inflammation [70] as well as diabetes and obesity. However, human studies are conflicting as it is unclear if consuming live organisms impacts viability in the gut.

Fecal microbiota transplantation (FMT) has been in use for C-difficile colitis (a *Clostridioides difficile* infection). A study by Ridaura et al. [71] examined the effects of microbiota transfer into GF mice from discordant human twins for obesity. The mice receiving microbiota from the lean counterparts remained lean, whereas those receiving microbiota from the obese subjects developed obesity. In a human study, obese diabetic males transplanted with intestinal microflora from lean individuals showed improved microbial diversity with a higher abundance of *Bacteroidetes* and butyrate-producing bacteria after 6 weeks [72]. However, more long-term studies are needed to examine this promising option.

Antibiotic use can alter gut microbiota, thus leading to the progression of T2DM [73]. Studies in type 1 *diabetes mellitus* (T1DM) patients revealed beneficial effects in preventing the viral induction of the disease [74]. However, it should be noted that studies proving this relationship in T1DM are limited.

The emerging evidence suggests that altering gut microbiota may present a promising approach to the prevention and treatment of T2DM. However, future studies are needed to explore and implement this, as well as more personalized treatment options for diabetes.

Intestinal Microflora and Inflammation

The GM is linked to inflammation in numerous studies, both in mice and humans. Intestinal barrier disruption, as seen in dysbiosis, results in increased levels of bacterial endotoxin lipopolysaccharides (LPS). LPS binds to Toll-like receptors (TLR) 4 and 5 (TLR4 and TLR5) and activates proinflammatory cytokines such as TNFα [75]. HFD-fed mice had higher plasma LPS and weight gain, fasting hyperinsulinemia, and hyperglycemia [76]. Similarly, Mehta et al. [77] demonstrated increased insulin resistance in healthy humans after injecting LPS. TLR5 knock-out mice have higher body mass and increased adipose proinflammatory cytokine (interferon-gamma (IFN-γ) and IL-1β) production [78].

Gut bacteria metabolize dietary fibers into SCFA, predominantly butyrate, acetate, and propionate. Butyrate, produced by gut microbiota, has been shown to promote lipolysis, increase energy expenditure, and prevent obesity [79]. Butyrate is also known to inhibit proinflammatory cytokine production [80], and to decrease LPS translocation, thus reducing its inflammatory effects [81]. Butyrate inhibits the expression of nitric oxide synthase (NOS) on intestinal cells via PPARγ signaling, limiting the expansion of pathogenic bacteria such as *Enterobacteriaceae* [82]. In contrast to butyrate, acetate was found to increase insulin resistance and secretion of ghrelin (an appetite-stimulating hormone produced in the gastrointestinal tract), resulting in weight gain [83].

Intestinal Microflora and T2DM

T2DM is associated with changes in gut microbiota. A study by Wu et al. [84] showed a significantly lower abundance of *Bacteroides vulgatus* and *Bifidobacterium* sp. in T2DM patients compared to healthy matched controls. Larsen et al. [85] showed a significant increase in *Firmicutes* bacteria in non-diabetic adults compared to those with T2DM. A study by Qin et al. [86] revealed a decrease in *Clostridium*, *Roseburia*, and *Faecalibacterium* sp. in T2DM subjects as well as all butyrate-producing bacteria of the *Firmicutes* phylum. Other authors [87] have shown a decrease in *Clostridium* species and an increase in *Lactobacillus* and *Bifidobacterium* species in T2DM patients. Diabetic (*db/db* and HFD) mice administered the butyrate-producing bacteria *Clostridium butyricum* improved insulin resistance, glucose, and inflammatory marker levels [88]. Similarly, *Faecalibacterium prausnitzii*, another butyrate producer, was found to be higher in lean non-diabetic individuals compared to obese diabetic patients. In subjects with metabolic syndrome, the transfer of the gut microbiota decreased insulin resistance [72, 89]. Certain dietary fibers alter gut microbiota and increase the abundance of SCFA-producing bacteria, leading to improvements in dysglycemia and decreased HbA1c levels [90].

GM influences glucose homeostasis and insulin resistance. *Bifidobacterium lactis* stimulates the translocation of glucose transporter 4 (GLUT4) to the cell membrane and enhances glucose uptake in addition to decreasing the expression of genes related to hepatic gluconeogenesis and increasing genes involved in glycogen synthesis [91]. Many studies found that bacteria from Lactobacillus phyla improve adiposity, insulin resistance, and hepatic glycogen synthesis by activating PI3K, AMP-activated protein kinase (AMPK), RAC-beta serine/threonine protein kinase (Akt2) signaling, and the expression of GLUT4 and adiponectin [92–94].

As previously discussed, elevated levels of LPS lead to activation of the proinflammatory pathways via adipocyte TLR4 and upregulation of the NF-kB signaling pathway, resulting in insulin resistance [95]. Higher levels of LPS were seen in

T2DM. The highly immune stimulator LPS is predominant in *Enterobacteriaceae*. GF mice exposed to *Enterobacteriaceae* from obese human subjects showed elevation in LPS levels and developed insulin resistance and obesity compared to the GF controls, proving the effects of gut microbes in inflammatory metabolic disorders [96]. In contrast, an animal study demonstrated that *Roseburia intestinalis* promoted increased levels of IL-22 associated with insulin sensitivity in mice. Inhibition of proinflammatory cytokines preventing inflammation was seen with certain microbes. Butyrate-producing bacteria such as *Roseburia* and *Faecalibacterium* inhibit NF-kB activity [97, 98], and various *Lactobacillus* species decrease IL-1β, IL-8, CD36, and CRP levels [99, 100].

Secondary bile acids are formed in the large intestine mainly by *Firmicutes* species. T2DM subjects had lower levels of secondary bile acids compared to their healthy counterparts. They decrease insulin resistance by mediating nuclear receptors such as the nuclear receptor farnesoid X receptor-alpha (FXR-α) and the G protein-coupled receptor TGR5 (also known as G protein-coupled bile receptor 1 or GPBAR1) in various tissues. In the gut, secondary bile acids act on L cells by stimulating GLP-1 and thus activating insulin secretion. Butyrate acts as a ligand for G protein-coupled receptors in the intestine and promotes the release of GLP-1 and -2 and peptide tyrosine tyrosine (PYY) [101–103].

Among the studies in T2DM, *Bifidobacterium* and *Bacteroides* are most frequently reported to be beneficial. Animal studies with *Bifidobacterium* demonstrated improvements in glucose tolerance [104]. Studies with the *Lactobacillus* genus suggested a synergistic role when combined with *Bifidobacterium*. Probiotics containing *Lactobacillus* sp. caused a decrease in endotoxins in mice [105]. Treatment with antibiotics in genetically obese mice fed with HFD resulted in modified gut microbiota and improved weight and insulin resistance. Changes in diet can also alter gut microbiota. The Mediterranean diet was found to modify gut microbiota, including *Bacteroidetes* and *Firmicutes* abundance, and beneficial for preventing T2DM in obese individuals [106].

Conclusions and Further Directions

T2DM is a chronic medical condition that can lead to micro- and macrovascular complications. There is substantial evidence that lifestyle interventions with diet, physical activity, and weight loss can prevent and treat T2DM and reduce the risk of complications. Altering gut microbiota through its anti-inflammatory effects can be a promising treatment for diabetes and obesity.

Individualized dietary interventions would be most beneficial and can be sustained for longer periods. Currently, a Mediterranean diet, which is rich in whole grains, fruits, vegetables, and lean meats, is preferable based on evidence and long-term adherence. Personalized medical nutrition treatment by registered dietitians would be the key to success.

Exercise intervention is clearly beneficial. Structured and guided physical activity would be ideal for decreasing the risk of diabetes. While high-intensity exercise has the most beneficial effects, any degree or intensity of physical activity is helpful. Long-term compliance with physical activity can significantly impact diabetes and its complications.

Targeting gut microbiota is a promising option in treating diabetes. However, the relationship between diabetes, obesity, and microbiota is still unclear. Standardized studies without confounding factors such as health status, race, and geographic location are needed to determine the microbes causative for diabetes. The use of probiotics and the method of their delivery into the gut need to be clarified. Lastly, fecal microbiota transplantation is a promising future therapeutic option for diabetes and obesity.

Structured lifestyle changes are needed to address behavioral changes with diet and physical activity. Providing tools for tracking lifestyle changes and setting goals would help achieve positive changes. Implementing these changes on a large scale is important for the prevention of this massive burden of diabetes and obesity globally.

References

1. International Diabetes Federation. IDF diabetes atlas. 10th ed. Brussels: International Diabetes Federation; 2000.
2. Pan XR, et al. Effects of diet and exercise in preventing NIDDM in people with impaired glucose tolerance. The Da Qing IGT and Diabetes Study. Diabetes Care. 1997;20(4):537–44. https://doi.org/10.2337/diacare.20.4.537.
3. He S, et al. Long-term influence of type 2 diabetes and metabolic syndrome on all-cause and cardiovascular death, and microvascular and macrovascular complications in Chinese adults - a 30-year follow-up of the Da Qing diabetes study. Diabetes Res Clin Pract. 2022;191:110048. https://doi.org/10.1016/j.diabres.2022.110048.
4. Diabetes Prevention Program (DPP) Research Group. The Diabetes Prevention Program (DPP): description of lifestyle intervention. Diabetes Care. 2002;25(12):2165–71. https://doi.org/10.2337/diacare.25.12.2165.
5. Diabetes Prevention Program Research Group et al. 10-year follow-up of diabetes incidence and weight loss in the Diabetes Prevention Program Outcomes Study. Lancet (London, England). 2009;374(9702):1677–86. https://doi.org/10.1016/S0140-6736(09)61457-4.
6. Lindström J, et al. The Finnish Diabetes Prevention Study (DPS): lifestyle intervention and 3-year results on diet and physical activity. Diabetes Care. 2003;26(12):3230–6. https://doi.org/10.2337/diacare.26.12.3230.
7. Knowler WC, et al. Reduction in the incidence of type 2 diabetes with lifestyle intervention or metformin. N Engl J Med. 2002;346(6):393–403. https://doi.org/10.1056/NEJMoa012512.
8. Martín-Peláez S, Fito M, Castaner O. Mediterranean diet effects on type 2 diabetes prevention, disease progression, and related mechanisms. A review. Nutrients. 2020;12(8):2236. https://doi.org/10.3390/nu12082236.
9. Zamora-Ros R, et al. Mediterranean diet and non enzymatic antioxidant capacity in the PREDIMED study: evidence for a mechanism of antioxidant tuning. Nutr Metab Cardiovasc Dis. 2013;23(12):1167–74. https://doi.org/10.1016/j.numecd.2012.12.008.

10. Al-Aubaidy HA, et al. Twelve-week Mediterranean diet intervention increases citrus bioflavonoid levels and reduces inflammation in people with type 2 diabetes mellitus. Nutrients. 2021;13(4):1133. https://doi.org/10.3390/nu13041133.

11. Koloverou E, Esposito K, Giugliano D, Panagiotakos D. The effect of Mediterranean diet on the development of type 2 diabetes mellitus: a meta-analysis of 10 prospective studies and 136,846 participants. Metabolism. 2014;63(7):903–11. https://doi.org/10.1016/j.metabol.2014.04.010.

12. Schwingshackl L, Missbach B, König J, Hoffmann G. Adherence to a Mediterranean diet and risk of diabetes: a systematic review and meta-analysis. Public Health Nutr. 2015;18(7):1292–9. https://doi.org/10.1017/S1368980014001542.

13. Salas-Salvadó J, et al. Prevention of diabetes with Mediterranean diets: a subgroup analysis of a randomized trial. Ann Intern Med. 2014;160(1):1–10. https://doi.org/10.7326/M13-1725.

14. Paoli A. Ketogenic diet for obesity: friend or foe? Int J Environ Res Public Health. 2014;11(2):2092–107. https://doi.org/10.3390/ijerph110202092.

15. Brinkworth GD, Noakes M, Buckley JD, Keogh JB, Clifton PM. Long-term effects of a very-low-carbohydrate weight loss diet compared with an isocaloric low-fat diet after 12 mo. Am J Clin Nutr. 2009;90(1):23–32. https://doi.org/10.3945/ajcn.2008.27326.

16. Myette-Côté É, et al. The effect of a short-term low-carbohydrate, high-fat diet with or without postmeal walks on glycemic control and inflammation in type 2 diabetes: a randomized trial. Am J Physiol Regul Integr Comp Physiol. 2018;315(6):R1210–9. https://doi.org/10.1152/ajpregu.00240.2018.

17. Solinas G, Karin M. JNK1 and IKKbeta: molecular links between obesity and metabolic dysfunction. FASEB J. 2010;24(8):2596–611. https://doi.org/10.1096/fj.09-151340.

18. Kumar S, et al. Implicating the effect of ketogenic diet as a preventive measure to obesity and diabetes mellitus. Life Sci. 2021;264:118661. https://doi.org/10.1016/j.lfs.2020.118661.

19. Tonstad S, Butler T, Yan R, Fraser GE. Type of vegetarian diet, body weight, and prevalence of type 2 diabetes. Diabetes Care. 2009;32(5):791–6. https://doi.org/10.2337/dc08-1886.

20. Chen Z, et al. Plant versus animal based diets and insulin resistance, prediabetes and type 2 diabetes: the Rotterdam study. Eur J Epidemiol. 2018;33(9):883–93. https://doi.org/10.1007/s10654-018-0414-8.

21. Meex RCR, Blaak EE, van Loon LJC. Lipotoxicity plays a key role in the development of both insulin resistance and muscle atrophy in patients with type 2 diabetes. Obes Rev. 2019;20(9):1205–17. https://doi.org/10.1111/obr.12862.

22. Cox AJ, et al. Increased intestinal permeability as a risk factor for type 2 diabetes. Diabetes Metab. 2017;43(2):163–6. https://doi.org/10.1016/j.diabet.2016.09.004.

23. Soares FLP, et al. Gluten-free diet reduces adiposity, inflammation and insulin resistance associated with the induction of PPAR-alpha and PPAR-gamma expression. J Nutr Biochem. 2013;24(6):1105–11. https://doi.org/10.1016/j.jnutbio.2012.08.009.

24. Zong G, et al. Gluten intake and risk of type 2 diabetes in three large prospective cohort studies of US men and women. Diabetologia. 2018;61(10):2164–73. https://doi.org/10.1007/s00125-018-4697-9.

25. Knudsen SH, Pedersen BK. Targeting inflammation through a physical active lifestyle and pharmaceuticals for the treatment of type 2 diabetes. Curr Diab Rep. 2015;15(10):82. https://doi.org/10.1007/s11892-015-0642-1.

26. Kwon H, Pessin JE. Adipokines mediate inflammation and insulin resistance. Front Endocrinol (Lausanne). 2013;4:71. https://doi.org/10.3389/fendo.2013.00071.

27. Jiang Y, Owei I, Wan J, Ebenibo S, Dagogo-Jack S. Adiponectin levels predict prediabetes risk: the Pathobiology of Prediabetes in A Biracial Cohort (POP-ABC) study. BMJ Open Diabetes Res Care. 2016;4(1):e000194. https://doi.org/10.1136/bmjdrc-2016-000194.

28. Donath MY. Targeting inflammation in the treatment of type 2 diabetes: time to start. Nat Rev Drug Discov. 2014;13(6):465–76. https://doi.org/10.1038/nrd4275.

29. Plomgaard P, Bouzakri K, Krogh-Madsen R, Mittendorfer B, Zierath JR, Pedersen BK. Tumor necrosis factor-alpha induces skeletal muscle insulin resistance in healthy human subjects via

inhibition of Akt substrate 160 phosphorylation. Diabetes. 2005;54(10):2939–45. https://doi.org/10.2337/diabetes.54.10.2939.

30. Larsen CM, et al. Interleukin-1-receptor antagonist in type 2 diabetes mellitus. N Engl J Med. 2007;356(15):1517–26. https://doi.org/10.1056/NEJMoa065213.

31. Karstoft K, Pedersen BK. Exercise and type 2 diabetes: focus on metabolism and inflammation. Immunol Cell Biol. 2015;94:146. https://doi.org/10.1038/icb.2015.101.

32. Yudkin JS. Inflammation, obesity, and the metabolic syndrome. Horm Metab Res. 2007;39(10):707–9. https://doi.org/10.1055/s-2007-985898.

33. Becic T, Studenik C, Hoffmann G. Exercise increases adiponectin and reduces leptin levels in prediabetic and diabetic individuals: systematic review and meta-analysis of randomized controlled trials. Med Sci (Basel, Switzerland). 2018;6(4):97. https://doi.org/10.3390/medsci6040097.

34. Yu N, Ruan Y, Gao X, Sun J. Systematic review and meta-analysis of randomized, controlled trials on the effect of exercise on serum leptin and adiponectin in overweight and obese individuals. Horm Metab Res. 2017;49(3):164–73. https://doi.org/10.1055/s-0042-121605.

35. Jadhav RA, Maiya GA, Hombali A, Umakanth S, Shivashankar KN. Effect of physical activity promotion on adiponectin, leptin and other inflammatory markers in prediabetes: a systematic review and meta-analysis of randomized controlled trials. Acta Diabetol. 2021;58(4):419–29. https://doi.org/10.1007/s00592-020-01626-1.

36. Mallard AR, Hollekim-Strand SM, Coombes JS, Ingul CB. Exercise intensity, redox homeostasis and inflammation in type 2 diabetes mellitus. J Sci Med Sport. 2017;20(10):893–8. https://doi.org/10.1016/j.jsams.2017.03.014.

37. Xing H, Lu J, Yoong SQ, Tan YQ, Kusuyama J, Wu XV. Effect of aerobic and resistant exercise intervention on inflammaging of type 2 diabetes mellitus in middle-aged and older adults: a systematic review and meta-analysis. J Am Med Dir Assoc. 2022;23(5):823–830. e13. https://doi.org/10.1016/j.jamda.2022.01.055.

38. Hejazi K, Mohammad Rahimi GR, Rosenkranz SK. Effects of exercise training on inflammatory and cardiometabolic risk biomarkers in patients with type 2 diabetes mellitus: a systematic review and meta-analysis of randomized controlled trials. Biol Res Nurs. 2023;25(2):250–66. https://doi.org/10.1177/10998004221132841.

39. Slentz CA, et al. Effects of exercise training alone vs a combined exercise and nutritional lifestyle intervention on glucose homeostasis in prediabetic individuals: a randomised controlled trial. Diabetologia. 2016;59(10):2088–98. https://doi.org/10.1007/s00125-016-4051-z.

40. Heiskanen MA, et al. Exercise training decreases pancreatic fat content and improves beta cell function regardless of baseline glucose tolerance: a randomised controlled trial. Diabetologia. 2018;61(8):1817–28. https://doi.org/10.1007/s00125-018-4627-x.

41. Figueiredo C, et al. Type and intensity as key variable of exercise in metainflammation diseases: a review. Int J Sports Med. 2022;43(9):743–67. https://doi.org/10.1055/a-1720-0369.

42. Durrer C, Francois M, Neudorf H, Little JP. Acute high-intensity interval exercise reduces human monocyte toll-like receptor 2 expression in type 2 diabetes. Am J Physiol Regul Integr Comp Physiol. 2017;312(4):R529–38. https://doi.org/10.1152/ajpregu.00348.2016.

43. Balducci S, et al. Anti-inflammatory effect of exercise training in subjects with type 2 diabetes and the metabolic syndrome is dependent on exercise modalities and independent of weight loss. Nutr Metab Cardiovasc Dis. 2010;20(8):608–17. https://doi.org/10.1016/j.numecd.2009.04.015.

44. Magalhães JP, et al. Impact of combined training with different exercise intensities on inflammatory and lipid markers in type 2 diabetes: a secondary analysis from a 1-year randomized controlled trial. Cardiovasc Diabetol. 2020;19(1):169. https://doi.org/10.1186/s12933-020-01136-y.

45. Qiu S, et al. Exercise training and endothelial function in patients with type 2 diabetes: a meta-analysis. Cardiovasc Diabetol. 2018;17(1):64. https://doi.org/10.1186/s12933-018-0711-2.

46. Parada-Sánchez SG, Macias-Cervantes MH, Pérez-Vázquez V, Vargas-Ortiz K. The effects of different types of exercise on circulating irisin levels in healthy individuals and in people

with overweight, metabolic syndrome and type 2 diabetes. Physiol Res. 2022;71(4):457–75. https://doi.org/10.33549/physiolres.934896.

47. Laaksonen DE, et al. Physical activity in the prevention of type 2 diabetes: the Finnish diabetes prevention study. Diabetes. 2005;54(1):158–65. https://doi.org/10.2337/diabetes.54.1.158.

48. Kriska AM, et al. The impact of physical activity on the prevention of type 2 diabetes: evidence and lessons learned from the diabetes prevention program, a long-standing clinical trial incorporating subjective and objective activity measures. Diabetes Care. 2021;44(1):43–9. https://doi.org/10.2337/dc20-1129.

49. Chen S-C, Ueng K-C, Lee S-H, Sun K-T, Lee M-C. Effect of t'ai chi exercise on biochemical profiles and oxidative stress indicators in obese patients with type 2 diabetes. J Altern Complement Med. 2010;16(11):1153–9. https://doi.org/10.1089/acm.2009.0560.

50. Vasconcelos Gouveia SS, et al. The effect of pilates on metabolic control and oxidative stress of diabetics type 2 - a randomized controlled clinical trial. J Bodyw Mov Ther. 2021;27:60–6. https://doi.org/10.1016/j.jbmt.2021.01.004.

51. Bäckhed F, Ley RE, Sonnenburg JL, Peterson DA, Gordon JA. Host-bacterial mutualism in the human intestine. Science. 2005;307(5717):1915–20. https://doi.org/10.1126/science.1104816.

52. Al Bander Z, Nitert MD, Mousa A, Naderpoor N. The gut microbiota and inflammation: an overview. Int J Environ Res Public Health. 2020;17(20):7618. https://doi.org/10.3390/ijerph17207618.

53. Aagaard K, Ma J, Antony KM, Ganu R, Petrosino J, Versalovic J. The placenta harbors a unique microbiome. Sci Transl Med. 2014;6(237):237ra65. https://doi.org/10.1126/scitranslmed.3008599.

54. Bäckhed F, et al. The gut microbiota as an environmental factor that regulates fat storage. Proc Natl Acad Sci U S A. 2004;101(44):15718–23. https://doi.org/10.1073/pnas.0407076101.

55. Cox LM, Blaser MJ. Antibiotics in early life and obesity. Nat Rev Endocrinol. 2015;11(3):182–90. https://doi.org/10.1038/nrendo.2014.210.

56. Ley RE, Bäckhed F, Turnbaugh P, Lozupone CA, Knight RD, Gordon JI. Obesity alters gut microbial ecology. Proc Natl Acad Sci U S A. 2005;102(31):11070–5. https://doi.org/10.1073/pnas.0504978102.

57. Ley RE, Turnbaugh PJ, Klein S, Gordon JI. Microbial ecology: human gut microbes associated with obesity. Nature. 2006;444(7122):1022–3. https://doi.org/10.1038/4441022a.

58. Leeming ER, Johnson AJ, Spector TD, Le Roy CI. Effect of diet on the gut microbiota: rethinking intervention duration. Nutrients. 2019;11(12):2862. https://doi.org/10.3390/nu11122862.

59. Turnbaugh PJ, et al. A core gut microbiome in obese and lean twins. Nature. 2009;457(7228):480–4. https://doi.org/10.1038/nature07540.

60. Fernandes J, Su W, Rahat-Rozenbloom S, Wolever TMS, Comelli EM. Adiposity, gut microbiota and faecal short chain fatty acids are linked in adult humans. Nutr Diabetes. 2014;4(6):e121. https://doi.org/10.1038/nutd.2014.23.

61. Konikoff T, Gophna U. Oscillospira: a central, enigmatic component of the human gut microbiota. Trends Microbiol. 2016;24(7):523–4. https://doi.org/10.1016/j.tim.2016.02.015.

62. Goodrich JK, et al. Human genetics shape the gut microbiome. Cell. 2014;159(4):789–99. https://doi.org/10.1016/j.cell.2014.09.053.

63. Gao R, et al. Dysbiosis signatures of gut microbiota along the sequence from healthy, young patients to those with overweight and obesity. Obesity (Silver Spring). 2018;26(2):351–61. https://doi.org/10.1002/oby.22088.

64. Gaci N, Borrel G, Tottey W, O'Toole PW, Brugère J-F. Archaea and the human gut: new beginning of an old story. World J Gastroenterol. 2014;20(43):16062–78. https://doi.org/10.3748/wjg.v20.i43.16062.

65. Mathur R, Amichai M, Chua KS, Mirocha J, Barlow GM, Pimentel M. Methane and hydrogen positivity on breath test is associated with greater body mass index and body fat. J Clin Endocrinol Metab. 2013;98(4):E698–702. https://doi.org/10.1210/jc.2012-3144.

66. Mathur R, et al. Metabolic effects of eradicating breath methane using antibiotics in prediabetic subjects with obesity. Obesity (Silver Spring). 2016;24(3):576–82. https://doi.org/10.1002/oby.21385.

67. Beisner J, Filipe Rosa L, Kaden-Volynets V, Stolzer I, Günther C, Bischoff SC. Prebiotic inulin and sodium butyrate attenuate obesity-induced intestinal barrier dysfunction by induction of antimicrobial peptides. Front Immunol. 2021;12:678360. https://doi.org/10.3389/fimmu.2021.678360.

68. Zhang Q, Yu H, Xiao X, Hu L, Xin F, Yu X. Inulin-type fructan improves diabetic phenotype and gut microbiota profiles in rats. PeerJ. 2018;6:e4446. https://doi.org/10.7717/peerj.4446.

69. van der Beek CM, et al. The prebiotic inulin improves substrate metabolism and promotes short-chain fatty acid production in overweight to obese men. Metabolism. 2018;87:25–35. https://doi.org/10.1016/j.metabol.2018.06.009.

70. Wang J, et al. Modulation of gut microbiota during probiotic-mediated attenuation of metabolic syndrome in high fat diet-fed mice. ISME J. 2015;9(1):1–15. https://doi.org/10.1038/ismej.2014.99.

71. Ridaura VK, et al. Gut microbiota from twins discordant for obesity modulate metabolism in mice. Science. 2013;341(6150):1241214. https://doi.org/10.1126/science.1241214.

72. Vrieze A, et al. Transfer of intestinal microbiota from lean donors increases insulin sensitivity in individuals with metabolic syndrome. Gastroenterology. 2012;143(4):913–6.e7. https://doi.org/10.1053/j.gastro.2012.06.031.

73. Wen L, Duffy A. Factors influencing the gut microbiota, inflammation, and type 2 diabetes. J Nutr. 2017;147(7):1468S–75S. https://doi.org/10.3945/jn.116.240754.

74. Kriegel MA, Sefik E, Hill JA, Wu H-J, Benoist C, Mathis D. Naturally transmitted segmented filamentous bacteria segregate with diabetes protection in nonobese diabetic mice. Proc Natl Acad Sci U S A. 2011;108(28):11548–53. https://doi.org/10.1073/pnas.1108924108.

75. Janssen AWF, Kersten S. Potential mediators linking gut bacteria to metabolic health: a critical view. J Physiol. 2017;595(2):477–87. https://doi.org/10.1113/JP272476.

76. Cani PD, et al. Metabolic endotoxemia initiates obesity and insulin resistance. Diabetes. 2007;56(7):1761–72. https://doi.org/10.2337/db06-1491.

77. Mehta NN, et al. Experimental endotoxemia induces adipose inflammation and insulin resistance in humans. Diabetes. 2010;59(1):172–81. https://doi.org/10.2337/db09-0367.

78. Vijay-Kumar M, et al. Metabolic syndrome and altered gut microbiota in mice lacking toll-like receptor 5. Science. 2010;328(5975):228–31. https://doi.org/10.1126/science.1179721.

79. Jia Y, et al. Butyrate stimulates adipose lipolysis and mitochondrial oxidative phosphorylation through histone hyperacetylation-associated $\beta3$ -adrenergic receptor activation in high-fat diet-induced obese mice. Exp Physiol. 2017;102(2):273–81. https://doi.org/10.1113/EP086114.

80. Lührs H, et al. Cytokine-activated degradation of inhibitory kappaB protein alpha is inhibited by the short-chain fatty acid butyrate. Int J Color Dis. 2001;16(4):195–201. https://doi.org/10.1007/s003840100295.

81. Hartstra AV, Bouter KEC, Bäckhed F, Nieuwdorp M. Insights into the role of the microbiome in obesity and type 2 diabetes. Diabetes Care. 2015;38(1):159–65. https://doi.org/10.2337/dc14-0769.

82. Byndloss MX, et al. Microbiota-activated PPAR-γ signaling inhibits dysbiotic Enterobacteriaceae expansion. Science. 2017;357(6351):570–5. https://doi.org/10.1126/science.aam9949.

83. Perry RJ, et al. Acetate mediates a microbiome-brain-β-cell axis to promote metabolic syndrome. Nature. 2016;534(7606):213–7. https://doi.org/10.1038/nature18309.

84. Wu X, et al. Molecular characterisation of the faecal microbiota in patients with type II diabetes. Curr Microbiol. 2010;61(1):69–78. https://doi.org/10.1007/s00284-010-9582-9.

85. Larsen N, et al. Gut microbiota in human adults with type 2 diabetes differs from non-diabetic adults. PLoS One. 2010;5(2):e9085. https://doi.org/10.1371/journal.pone.0009085.

86. Qin J, et al. A metagenome-wide association study of gut microbiota in type 2 diabetes. Nature. 2012;490(7418):55–60. https://doi.org/10.1038/nature11450.

87. Grigorescu I, Dumitrascu DL. Implication of gut microbiota in diabetes mellitus and obesity. Acta Endocrinol (Bucharest, Rom 2005). 2016;12(2):206–14. https://doi.org/10.4183/aeb.2016.206.

88. Jia L, et al. Anti-diabetic effects of Clostridium butyricum CGMCC0313.1 through promoting the growth of gut butyrate-producing bacteria in type 2 diabetic mice. Sci Rep. 2017;7(1):7046. https://doi.org/10.1038/s41598-017-07335-0.

89. van der Vossen EWJ, et al. Effects of fecal microbiota transplant on DNA methylation in subjects with metabolic syndrome. Gut Microbes. 2021;13(1):1993513. https://doi.org/10.1080/19490976.2021.1993513.

90. Zhao L, et al. Gut bacteria selectively promoted by dietary fibers alleviate type 2 diabetes. Science. 2018;359(6380):1151–6. https://doi.org/10.1126/science.aao5774.

91. Kim S-H, et al. The anti-diabetic activity of Bifidobacterium lactis HY8101 in vitro and in vivo. J Appl Microbiol. 2014;117(3):834–45. https://doi.org/10.1111/jam.12573.

92. Arora T, Singh S, Sharma RK. Probiotics: interaction with gut microbiome and antiobesity potential. Nutrition. 2013;29(4):591–6. https://doi.org/10.1016/j.nut.2012.07.017.

93. Park S, et al. Lactobacillus plantarum HAC01 regulates gut microbiota and adipose tissue accumulation in a diet-induced obesity murine model. Appl Microbiol Biotechnol. 2017;101(4):1605–14. https://doi.org/10.1007/s00253-016-7953-2.

94. Wang G, Li X, Zhao J, Zhang H, Chen W. Lactobacillus casei CCFM419 attenuates type 2 diabetes via a gut microbiota dependent mechanism. Food Funct. 2017;8(9):3155–64. https://doi.org/10.1039/c7fo00593h.

95. Chung S, Lapoint K, Martinez K, Kennedy A, Boysen Sandberg M, McIntosh MK. Preadipocytes mediate lipopolysaccharide-induced inflammation and insulin resistance in primary cultures of newly differentiated human adipocytes. Endocrinology. 2006;147(11):5340–51. https://doi.org/10.1210/en.2006-0536.

96. Fei N, Zhao L. An opportunistic pathogen isolated from the gut of an obese human causes obesity in germfree mice. ISME J. 2013;7(4):880–4. https://doi.org/10.1038/ismej.2012.153.

97. Inan MS, Rasoulpour RJ, Yin L, Hubbard AK, Rosenberg DW, Giardina C. The luminal short-chain fatty acid butyrate modulates NF-kappaB activity in a human colonic epithelial cell line. Gastroenterology. 2000;118(4):724–34. https://doi.org/10.1016/s0016-5085(00)70142-9.

98. Kinoshita M, Suzuki Y, Saito Y. Butyrate reduces colonic paracellular permeability by enhancing PPARgamma activation. Biochem Biophys Res Commun. 2002;293(2):827–31. https://doi.org/10.1016/S0006-291X(02)00294-2.

99. Liu W-C, Yang M-C, Wu Y-Y, Chen P-H, Hsu C-M, Chen L-W. Lactobacillus plantarum reverse diabetes-induced Fmo3 and ICAM expression in mice through enteric dysbiosis-related c-Jun NH2-terminal kinase pathways. PLoS One. 2018;13(5):e0196511. https://doi.org/10.1371/journal.pone.0196511.

100. Tian P, et al. Antidiabetic (type 2) effects of Lactobacillus G15 and Q14 in rats through regulation of intestinal permeability and microbiota. Food Funct. 2016;7(9):3789–97. https://doi.org/10.1039/c6fo00831c.

101. Ipharraguerre IR, et al. Bile acids induce glucagon-like peptide 2 secretion with limited effects on intestinal adaptation in early weaned pigs. J Nutr. 2013;143(12):1899–905. https://doi.org/10.3945/jn.113.177865.

102. Brighton CA, et al. Bile acids trigger GLP-1 release predominantly by accessing basolaterally located G protein-coupled bile acid receptors. Endocrinology. 2015;156(11):3961–70. https://doi.org/10.1210/en.2015-1321.

103. Christiansen CB, et al. Bile acids drive colonic secretion of glucagon-like-peptide 1 and peptide-YY in rodents. Am J Physiol Gastrointest Liver Physiol. 2019;316(5):G574–84. https://doi.org/10.1152/ajpgi.00010.2019.

104. Le TKC, et al. Bifidobacterium species lower serum glucose, increase expressions of insulin signaling proteins, and improve adipokine profile in diabetic mice. Biomed Res. 2015;36(1):63–70. https://doi.org/10.2220/biomedres.36.63.
105. Qi SR, Cui YJ, Liu JX, Luo X, Wang HF. Lactobacillus rhamnosus GG components, SLP, gDNA and CpG, exert protective effects on mouse macrophages upon lipopolysaccharide challenge. Lett Appl Microbiol. 2020;70(2):118–27. https://doi.org/10.1111/lam.13255.
106. Santos-Marcos JA, Perez-Jimenez F, Camargo A. The role of diet and intestinal microbiota in the development of metabolic syndrome. J Nutr Biochem. 2019;70:1–27. https://doi.org/10.1016/j.jnutbio.2019.03.017.

Chapter 9
Inflammation in Pregnant Women with Obesity and Gestational Diabetes Mellitus

Tara S. Kim

Abbreviations

ACOG	American College of Obstetricians and Gynecologists
ADA	American Diabetes Association
AT	Adipose tissue
BMI	Body mass index
BPA	Bisphenol A
DASH	Dietary Approaches to Stop Hypertension
DC	Dendritic cell
DM	Diabetes mellitus
EDC	Endocrine-disrupting chemicals
EPA	Eicosapentaenoic acid
EPOCH	Exploring Perinatal Outcomes among Children
FA	Folic acid
FDA	Food and Drug Administration
FPG	Fasting plasma glucose
FSH	Follicle-stimulating hormone
GD	Grave's disease
GDM	Gestational diabetes mellitus
GWG	Gestational weight gain
HAPO	Hyperglycemia and Adverse Pregnancy Outcome
HbA1c	Hemoglobin A1c
HT	Hashimoto's thyroiditis
IFN	Interferon

T. S. Kim (✉)
Donald and Barbara Zucker School of Medicine at Hofstra/Northwell, Hempstead, NY, USA

Department of Internal Medicine, Division of Endocrinology, Lenox Hill Hospital,
New York, NY, USA
e-mail: TKim1@northwell.edu

© The Author(s), under exclusive license to Springer Nature
Switzerland AG 2023
D. Avtanski, L. Poretsky (eds.), *Obesity, Diabetes and Inflammation*,
Contemporary Endocrinology, https://doi.org/10.1007/978-3-031-39721-9_9

IL	Interleukin
IOM	Institute of Medicine
LGA	Large-for-gestational-age
M	Macrophage
M1	M1 macrophages
M2	M2 macrophages
MG	Myasthenia gravis
MI	Myo-inositol
MMP	Matrix metalloproteinases
MMR	Maternal mortality rate
MO	Maternal obesity
Mono	Monocytes
MP	Macrophage
MS	Multiple sclerosis
NF	Nuclear factor
NIH	National Institutes of Health
NK	Natural killer
NP	Neutrophils
NTD	Neural tube defect
OGTT	Oral glucose tolerance test
PPT	Postpartum thyroiditis
PRIMS	Pregnancy in multiple sclerosis
RA	Rheumatoid arthritis
RCT	Randomized control trial
RPG	Random plasma glucose
SGA	Small-for-gestational-age
SPRING	Study of PRobiotics IN Gestation
T2DM	Type 2 diabetes mellitus
TGFβ	Transforming growth factor-beta
Th	T helper cell type
TNF	Tumor necrosis factor
TNFα	Tumor necrosis factor-alpha
Treg	Regulatory T-cell
TSH	Thyroid stimulating hormone
WAT	White adipose tissue
WHO	World Health Organization

Introduction

Over the past two decades, the science has become increasingly clear that obesity results in a chronic state of inflammation and is associated with serious diseases including, but not limited to, cardiovascular diseases, fatty liver, airway diseases, diabetes mellitus (DM), certain cancers, and mental disorders [1, 2]. However, a particularly unique group of patients—pregnant women with obesity and gestational diabetes mellitus (GDM)—warrants further attention.

Obesity or GDM are both risk factors for perinatal and fetal complications. Women with obesity in pregnancy have an increased risk of preeclampsia, eclampsia, delivery of a macrosomic infant, thromboembolism, cardiovascular diseases, and GDM [3–5]. Women with GDM also have an increased frequency of adverse outcomes, including preeclampsia or gestational hypertension, need for maternal transfusions, infant admission to the neonatal intensive care unit, higher incidence of cesarean section, macrosomia, and progression to type 2 diabetes mellitus (T2DM) [6, 7]. There is considerable overlap between these two entities.

While other chapters in this book have addressed inflammation in obesity and DM in general, this chapter focuses specifically on the role of inflammation in pregnant women with obesity and/or GDM. The author believes the gestation period is a critical window of opportunity for patient education and disease prevention. Understanding the metabolic milieu of a pregnant woman with obesity or GDM is vital to the development of successful prevention and management strategies.

The metabolic changes in obesity, gestational diabetes, and pregnancy are physiologically complex and clinically challenging to address. To organize this chapter, we will review the epidemiologic impact of obesity in pregnancy and GDM, present the general concepts of fetal programming, and describe immune system function in pregnancy. This will be followed by a review of physiology and definitions/diagnostic criteria of obesity in pregnancy and GDM, respectively. The role of inflammation in pregnant women with obesity and women with GDM will be reviewed as well. Finally, we will present management considerations and discuss implications for future research.

Epidemiology of Obesity and Gestational Diabetes

The epidemiologic and clinical significance of obesity and GDM in pregnant women is staggering. The pre-pregnancy obesity rate in the USA was 29% in 2019, which is an increase of 11% from 2016. Increases occurred across all maternal ages, all states except for Vermont, race, and educational levels [8]. The prevalence of GDM is estimated to be 7–10% and continues to increase with higher rates of obesity. Among women with GDM, up to 20% are subsequently diagnosed with diabetes [9]. The maternal complications associated with obesity and GDM in pregnancy are well established.

Maternal obesity (MO) influences morbidity and mortality, with states like Illinois reporting 44% of pregnancy-related maternal deaths [10]. Severe maternal morbidity from 20 weeks gestation and 1 year postpartum in Medicaid beneficiaries in Ohio is reported to be 6.4% in women with obesity (class 3 obesity having the highest rate at 8.1%) compared to 4.6% in healthy weight women. Mortality rates are higher in class 3 obesity (8.8 per 10,000 pregnancies) compared to women with healthy pregnancy weights (7.7 per 10,000 pregnancies) [11]. It is reported that there is up to a threefold to fivefold increase in the risk of composite neonatal injuries in the offsprings of mothers with overweight and obesity, specifically affecting the skeletal and peripheral nervous system [12]. Additional studies report U-shaped associations between gestational weight gain and risk of infant death, with the risk of infant death remaining higher in mothers with underweight, overweight, and obesity than in normal-weight counterparts [13, 14].

Maternal morbidity and mortality data for women with GDM is not very clear. A retrospective analysis based on administrative data by Tavera et al. [15] reported that in contrast to mothers with DM, those with GDM have lower risks of in-hospital death compared to mothers without pre-pregnancy diabetes or GDM, with maternal mortality rate (MMR) dropping by 18.7%. These potential protective effects of GDM may be explained by women with GDM having higher rates of private insurance coverage than women with diabetes (53.7% vs. 42%) [15]. Birth weight greater than 90th percentiles, newborn percent body fat >90th percentile, cord c-peptide >90th percentile have been reported in women with GDM. Long-term risks of offspring born to women with GDM include increased childhood/adult obesity rates and cardiometabolic risks such as insulin resistance and atherogenic lipid profile [16, 17].

While the general population may be intrigued by the impact of maternal health during the pregnancy window on the short- and long-term effects on children, the medical and scientific community are tasked with addressing the ever-growing obesity epidemic and optimizing the health of future generations to come. To effectively address generational health, we need to understand the concept of fetal programming.

Fetal Programming

Population-wide studies dating back to the mid-1930s recognize that the early growth environment has long-term effects on child and subsequent adult health. This is true for atherosclerotic, cardiovascular, and ischemic diseases. The endocrine system is no exception. In addition to epidemiological studies, pathological and immunological explanations show that both the endocrine cell populations and proportion of endocrine tissue in the pancreas change markedly in early life—volume density of total endocrine tissue being 15% in neonates, 6–7% in infants, and 2–3% in adults [18]. Research also shows cytologic changes in the fetal pancreas of offspring born to mothers with and without diabetes with higher proportions of endocrine tissue and abnormalities of islets described in neonates born to mothers with diabetes than in non-diabetes counterparts [19, 20]. Mounting evidence has recognized a relationship between early growth and the subsequent development of glucose intolerance and T2DM as well [21]. This evidence supports what the famed English physician Dr. David Barker postulated and later became known as "the Barker hypothesis." The Barker hypothesis of "fetal origins" or "fetal programming" proposes that organ systems and associated functions undergo programming during early embryonic life, which sets the tone for adult health and susceptibility to developing chronic disease [22]. In 1992, the "thrifty phenotype hypothesis" was coined as a synonym for the Barker hypothesis to elucidate the associations between poor fetal growth and increased risk of developing impaired glucose and metabolic disease. Dr. Barker hypothesized that one major consequence of inadequate nutrition is the impaired development of the endocrine pancreas, which increases the risk of developing T2DM. Further, he purported that those individuals who starved in utero were more likely to become overweight as adults and more likely to experience obesity-related diseases, including diabetes and cardiovascular diseases [21, 23, 24]. Major skepticism that persists surrounding the Barker hypothesis pertains to the mainly correlational associations and the existence of potential confounding factors. Despite these criticisms, the concept of fetal programming provides a significant and radical paradigmatic framework for understanding health and disease. The implications of fetal programming are far-reaching and can deepen our understanding of epigenetics and transgenerational health.

Role of the Immune System in Pregnancy

The natural role of the immune system is to protect the host from pathogens that cause illness. Pregnancy is a unique and medically fascinating puzzle wherein the mother's immune system does not attack the fetus but adapts to support fetal development. There is a traditional belief that the pregnant state is associated with immune suppression and immunologic vulnerability, increasing susceptibility to infectious diseases. This concept is being challenged. While the details of the immunologic response to pregnancy and implantation are far beyond the scope of this chapter, normal pregnancy elicits both pro- and anti-inflammatory responses during specific stages of gestation. Figure 9.1 illustrates the predominant inflammatory state, major (but not exhaustive) immunologic/cytokine profiles, and clinical manifestations from pregestational to postpartum stages.

Proinflammatory risk factors before pregnancy include obesity and GDM. Obesity is characterized by an imbalance between T helper cell type-1 (Th1) which are proinflammatory, and T helper cell type-2 (Th2) cytokines which produce an anti-inflammatory response. In chronic obesity, there is also accumulation of M1 macrophages, increased levels of tumor necrosis factor-alpha (TNFα), and interleukins (IL) 10, 1, and 6 [25, 26]. In GDM, there is an increase in Th1 and Th17 responses, macrophage infiltration, and overactivation of neutrophils (NP) which may suggest immune dysregulation [27]. Clinically, these changes can contribute to insulin resistance.

Mor et al. [28] proposed that depending on the stage of pregnancy, pregnancy is both a pro- and anti-inflammatory condition. At implantation, there are high levels of proinflammatory Th1 cells and cytokines. The first trimester of pregnancy, when implantation occurs, evokes a robust inflammatory response. The embryo interrupts the uterine lining and the mother's vasculature to secure an adequate blood supply.

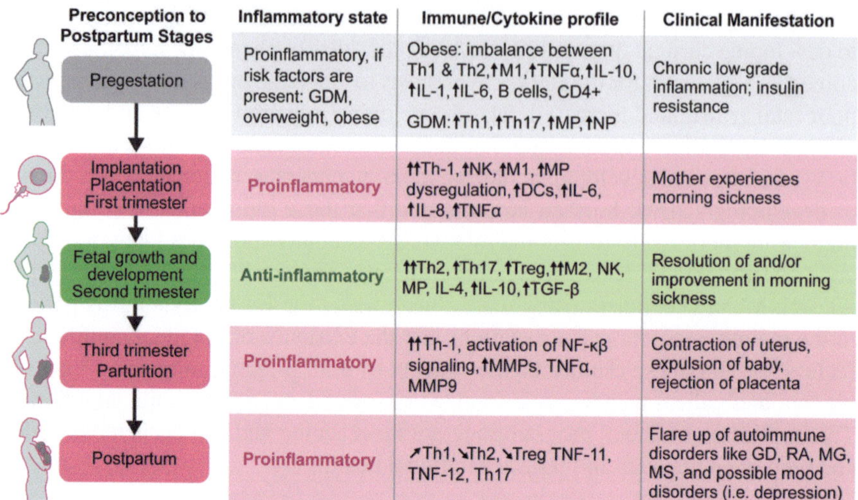

Preconception to Postpartum Stages	Inflammatory state	Immune/Cytokine profile	Clinical Manifestation
Pregestation	Proinflammatory, if risk factors are present: GDM, overweight, obese	Obese: imbalance between Th1 & Th2,↑M1,↑TNFα,↑IL-10, ↑IL-1,↑IL-6, B cells, CD4+ GDM:↑Th1,↑Th17,↑MP,↑NP	Chronic low-grade inflammation; insulin resistance
Implantation Placentation First trimester	Proinflammatory	↑↑Th-1,↑NK,↑M1,↑MP dysregulation,↑DCs,↑IL-6, ↑IL-8,↑TNFα	Mother experiences morning sickness
Fetal growth and development Second trimester	Anti-inflammatory	↑↑Th2,↑Th17,↑Treg,↑↑M2, NK, MP, IL-4,↑IL-10,↑TGF-β	Resolution of and/or improvement in morning sickness
Third trimester Parturition	Proinflammatory	↑↑Th-1, activation of NF-κβ signaling,↑MMPs, TNFα, MMP9	Contraction of uterus, expulsion of baby, rejection of placenta
Postpartum	Proinflammatory	↗Th1,↘Th2,↘Treg TNF-11, TNF-12, Th17	Flare up of autoimmune disorders like GD, RA, MG, MS, and possible mood disorders (i.e. depression)

Fig. 9.1 Inflammation from pregestation to postpartum. Predominant inflammatory states from pregestation through postpartum, associated cytokine profiles and clinical manifestation. *GDM* gestational diabetes, *MP* macrophages, *M1* M1 macrophages, *M2* M2 macrophages, *mono* monocytes, *TNFα* tumor necrosis factor-alpha, *MMP* matrix metalloproteinases, *IL* interleukin, *NK* natural killer, *DC* dendritic cells, *NP* neutrophil, *TGFβ* transforming growth factor-beta, *Th* T helper, *GD* Grave's disease, *RA* rheumatoid arthritis, *MG* myasthenia gravis, *MS* multiple sclerosis

An inflammatory response is needed to repair the uterus and remove dying cells. Systemic inflammation may explain why, during this first trimester of pregnancy, women develop "morning sickness." Morning sickness is proposed to be an adaptive response to fetal presence.

Subsequently, the second trimester has been hypothesized to be an anti-inflammatory state where the mother and fetus have reached a symbiotic stage. A shift from Th1 to Th2 and regulatory T-cell (Treg) production is observed during fetal growth and development [29]. There is also a predominance of alternatively activated macrophages (M2) during the second trimester of pregnancy after placental development is complete [30]. The M2 macrophage microenvironment prevents rejection of the fetus and supports fetal growth through parturition [31]. Evidence to support the achievement of a symbiotic relationship is the resolution of symptoms during this gestational period.

The third trimester of pregnancy prepares women for labor and delivery and requires an inflammatory response. In this stage of pregnancy, there is a shift to proinflammatory Th1 and nuclear factor-κB (NF-κB) signaling pathway which initiates labor and continues through delivery. Cervical ripening, dilatation, myometrial contractions, and fetal membrane rupture/placental detachment are regulated by NF-κB. NF-κB also regulates the expression of matrix metalloproteinases (MMPs) which are regulators of uteroplacental and vascular remodeling [32, 33]. These proinflammatory processes provoke the release of hormones that induce labor, contraction of the uterus, and ultimately delivery of the fetus.

Lastly, in the postpartum stage, several cytokines return to the baseline to facilitate wound healing and lactation [28, 29]. The cytokine profile of Th1 and Th2 postpartum is somewhat controversial. Shimaoka et al. [34] reported elevations in Th1 that peak 2–4 months postpartum and remain elevated until 11 months postpartum. Th2 cytokines peaked 6–7 months postpartum and plateaued until 11 months. Somerset et al. [35] investigated the prevalence of the T-cell subset in human pregnancy and found a decline of Treg cells postpartum. The Th1/Th2 balance and role of proinflammatory cytokines have been implicated in numerous autoimmune disorders in pregnancy. Clinical observations include the remittance of rheumatoid arthritis (RA) and multiple sclerosis (MS) (both Th1-related diseases) during pregnancy, followed by an exacerbation or onset in the postpartum period [36]. After delivery, the shift from Th2 to Th1 and the decline of Treg may explain the presence of autoimmune thyroid diseases such as Grave's disease (GD), Hashimoto's thyroiditis (HT), and postpartum thyroiditis (PPT) [37]. New onset or exacerbation of GD or HT generally occurs 4–12 months or 1–4 months postpartum, respectively. The timing of postpartum thyroid disease may reflect the serial changes in cytokines and postpartum rebound in humoral immunity [34]. The Pregnancy In Multiple Sclerosis (PRIMS) study was a prospective study of 227 pregnant women with a live infant. Study participants were followed for up to 2 years postpartum. Major findings from the study include (1) a significant decrease in the relapse rate during pregnancy and (2) a marked increase in relapse 3 months after delivery. The rates of relapse were not affected by breast-feeding, analgesia, age at MS onset, or previous pregnancies [38]. In a smaller study of 8 pregnant women, Al-Shammri et al. [39] confirmed these findings and investigated the relationship between clinical status and cytokine levels. Six out of eight women observed a shift toward Th1 after delivery, with results indicating that clinical remission during pregnancy was associated with Th2 predominance during pregnancy.

Interest in the potential role of inflammation in postpartum mood disorders is also growing. Some research suggests that proinflammatory changes in the postpartum period may be associated with mood disorders such as perinatal depression and anxiety [40, 41].

Obesity

Physiology

The anabolic state in early pregnancy is necessary for healthy fetal growth and development. While some energy needs can be met by maternal stores, maternal dietary intake is critical. Appropriate gestational weight gain (GWG) is essential to meet the increased demands of pregnancy and lactation, but excessive GWG is associated with weight retention postpartum and long-term obesity [42, 43]. This necessitates an evaluation of what is considered "healthy weight gain" during pregnancy.

Maternal components of GWG consist of total body water accretion, fat-free mass or protein accretion, and fat mass or fat accretion. Although variable, total body water accretion averages about 6–8 L, and plasma volume expansion approaches up to 45% as pregnancy advances. Protein accrual mainly occurs later in pregnancy and accounts for approximately 1% of physiologic GWG. Most fat deposited during pregnancy is subcutaneous and contributes 1–6 kg of GWG [44]. This last detail is important to note because white adipose tissue (WAT) and the placenta are the primary sites of inflammation during pregnancy.

Definition/Diagnosis

The most used measure to define overweight and obesity is the body mass index (BMI). Although BMI is a convenient clinical tool, it is a *surrogate* of percentage fat mass, and its application to clinical settings can be misleading. It must be noted up front that there is controversy surrounding BMI as it relates to its effectiveness for people of all races and ethnicities, it does not take into account the natural physiologic changes in aging, inaccurate utility in people with increased muscle mass such as athletes, fluid status in diseases like heart failure and physiologic changes associated with pregnancy. Despite criticism and shortfalls of the use of BMI in pregnancy, MO is defined as BMI $\geq$ 30 kg/m^2, with maternal overweight defined as having a BMI between 25 and 29.9 kg/m^2. Practically, most clinicians use pregestational BMI and weight gain during pregnancy to monitor health.

Recognizing the importance of both balancing GWG and meeting nutrition requirements in pregnancy, the Institute of Medicine (IOM) published recommendations for desirable weight gain during pregnancy in 1990 [45]. The committee used body mass index (BMI) cutoffs from the Metropolitan Life Insurance Company (1959) with classifications as follows: underweight BMI < 19.8 kg/m^2; normalweight BMI 19.8–26.0 kg/m^2; overweight BMI 26.0–29.0 kg/m^2; and obese BMI > 29.0 kg/m^2. The committee recommended that women with normal prepregnancy weight carrying a single fetus aim for a weight gain of 11.5–16 kg, while women with low pre-pregnancy BMI aim for the weight gain of about 12.5–18 kg. Target ranges for women with BMI > 26 were 7–11.5 kg [45].

Over two decades later, the obesity epidemic continued unabated, and the original guidelines were reexamined in 2009. These updated guidelines were published to recognize the significance of racial/ethnic subgroups, older age at pregnancy, and chronic conditions of women entering pregnancy including hypertension or diabetes. The 2009 guidelines differed from original guidelines in two ways. First, the World Health Organization (WHO) cutoff points for BMI were used rather than utilizing the Metropolitan Life Insurance Company standards for height-weight. The four WHO-defined categories include underweight BMI < 18 kg/m^2, normalweight BMI 18.5–24.9 kg/m^2, overweight BMI 25–29.9 kg/m^2, and obese $\geq$30 kg/ m^2. Second, the updated guidelines include a specific and relatively narrow range of recommended weight gain for women with obesity and provide a range of weight

Table 9.1 Recommendations for weight gain during pregnancy

Year	1990[a]	2009[b]
Pre-pregnancy BMI cutoff values		
Underweight	<19.8	<18.5
Normal weight	19.8–26.0	18.5–24.9
Overweight	>26.0–29.0	25.0–29.9
Obese	>29	>30.0
Recommended total weight gain ranges (lbs)		
Underweight	28–40	28–40
Normal weight	25–35	25–35
Overweight	15–25	15–25
Obese	At least 15	11–20
Rates of weight gain second and third trimester (lbs/wk)		
Underweight		1
Normal weight		1
Overweight		0.6
Obese		0.5

[a]BMI categories based on Metropolitan Life Insurance tables; Institute of Medicine. *Nutrition during pregnancy; part I: weight gain, part II: nutrient supplements.* Washington, DC: National Academy, 1990
[b]BMI categories based on WHO BMI categories; Institute of Medicine. *Weight gain during pregnancy: reexamining the guidelines.* Washington, DC: National Academy Press, 2009

gain per week for each category of pre-pregnancy BMI [46]. Table 9.1 provides a side-by-side comparison of the original IOM recommendations from 1990 and the updated recommendations published in 2009.

Interestingly, the IOM summarized that: (1) variance in GWG is accounted for by an increase in fat mass and (2) an increase in fat mass during gestation is inversely proportional to pregravid obesity [44]. The role of fat mass is of particular importance, as we will discuss its central role in inflammation next.

Inflammation in Pregnant Women with Obesity

Obesity, in general, involves a state of low-grade chronic inflammation. Evolving research has revealed the complex nature of the maternal-fetal immune interaction, as described earlier in this chapter. Specifically, WAT and the placenta are the primary sites of inflammation during pregnancy.

Adipose tissue (AT) is recognized as an active endocrine organ that secretes various adipokines and proinflammatory cytokines involved in inflammatory processes and metabolism. AT secretes adipocytokines (leptin, adiponectin, TNFα, IL-6, etc.). Studies in the 1990s [47, 48] revealed that individuals with obesity express up to 2.5-fold more TNFα relative to lean controls, the presence of a positive correlation of TNFα mRNA expression levels in fat tissue, and hyperinsulinemia (an indirect measure of insulin resistance). It is proposed that TNFα likely inhibits insulin receptor's tyrosine kinase activity, which then interferes with insulin action [47, 48].

Research studies to date have shown that mothers with pre-pregnancy obesity also have elevated levels of proinflammatory cytokines IL-6, C-reactive protein (CRP), TNFα, and IFNγ. Challier et al. [49] examined the inflammatory status in pregnant women with obesity compared to lean women and reported that obesity in pregnancy is associated with peripheral inflammation. While the authors did not find changes in TNFα, there were (1) increased circulating concentrations of IL-6 and CRP, (2) doubling insulin concentrations associated with a fourfold increase in insulin resistance, (3) higher leptin levels, and (4) increased gene expression of inflammatory markers CD14 and CD68 (monocyte maturation and differentiation antigens) [49].

Importantly, inflammation is not limited to maternal sources of AT. The placental production of cytokines is also vital to pregnancy. Compared to lean women, the placenta of women with obesity can have up to a twofold to threefold increase in the number of placental macrophages indicated by markers CD68+ and CD14+. Associations between MO and lipid-rich placental environments have also been described, with Saben et al. [50] reporting up to 50% greater placental lipid droplet accumulation in mothers with obesity than in lean women. This MO is associated with a lipotoxic placental environment characterized by increased placental lipids and increased oxidative stress and inflammation markers [50, 51]. The inflammatory response in pregnancy is a balance between pro- and anti-inflammatory cytokines, and MO may shift this balance toward a more proinflammatory state.

Fetal Programming

MO is linked to metabolic dysregulation in offspring with increased incidence of obesity, hyperglycemia, T2DM, and metabolic syndrome. Percentage body fat is greater in offspring of women with higher antenatal BMI—offspring percentage body fat is independently associated with higher maternal BMI, pregnancy weight gain, and parity. Higher maternal BMI in pregnancy, greater GWG, and being first-born are independent predictors of offspring-estimated fat mass and BMI (independent of lifestyle factors like smoking, social class, and mother's age) [52].

The fetal effects of MO are implicated to have reached far beyond endocrine and cardiac pathology to include adverse neurodevelopmental outcomes such as autism spectrum disorders, cerebral palsy, and attention deficit hyperactivity disorder. Animal models have found hypomethylation in offspring brains, altered gene expressions involved in circadian rhythm and feeding behavior, and changes in skeletal muscle, glucose, and lipid homeostasis. Pregestational MO can have fetal effects as early as implantation. Results from animal studies provide mechanistic insight for humans and have advanced our understanding of the effects of obesity on maternal and infant gut microbiome [53].

Gestational Diabetes Mellitus

Physiology

Normal glucose metabolism is characterized by relative insulin sensitivity early in pregnancy. The increased sensitivity during early gestation promotes glucose uptake into adipose stores to meet the energy demands of pregnancy later on. However, insulin sensitivity decreases sharply beginning in the second trimester due to a surge of hormones, including estrogen, progesterone, leptin, cortisol, placental growth hormone, and placental lactogens. Decreased insulin sensitivity and a state of insulin resistance promote endogenous glucose production breakdown of fat stores with increased transport of glucose and free fatty acid to support fetal growth [54].

In GDM, insulin levels are insufficient to meet demands. Insulin deficiency can be caused by autoimmune β-cell dysfunction, highly penetrant genetic abnormalities that lead to impaired insulin secretion, β-cell dysfunction associated with chronic insulin resistance, and neurohormonal dysfunction [54, 55]. Further, a number of organ systems contribute to and are affected by GDM. GDM is associated with upregulated gluconeogenesis in the liver, reduced number and function within skeletal muscle cells, changes in the gut microbiome, and increased levels of proinflammatory cytokines. The placenta is also affected by GDM, with reports of placental DNA hypermethylation and potential differences in proteome modifications [54].

Diagnosis

Significant effort has been undertaken to develop universal diagnostic criteria for GDM. To date, however, no universally accepted consensus for screening methods, the timing of testing, and diagnostic cutoff values has been established.

In 2012, the American Diabetes Association (ADA) published results from an epidemiologic study of 23,316 pregnancies to compare associations of maternal HbA_{1c} and glucose with pregnancy outcomes. A primary aim of the hyperglycemia and adverse pregnancy outcomes (HAPO) study was to determine the level of glucose intolerance during pregnancy, short of a diagnosis of diabetes, associated with adverse outcomes [56]. All participants underwent a 75-g oral glucose tolerance test (OGTT) between 24 and 32 weeks gestation, fasting plasma glucose (FPG), and random plasma glucose (RPG) collection at 34–37 weeks gestation. Primary outcomes included: (1) birth weight >90th percentile (macrosomia), (2) primary cesarean section, (3) clinical neonatal hypoglycemia, and (4) cord C-peptide >90th percentile (hyperinsulinemia). Secondary outcomes were preeclampsia, preterm delivery, a sum of skinfolds >90th percentile, and percent body fat >90th percentile [57].

The HAPO study found that associations were significantly stronger with glucose measures than hemoglobin A1c (HbA_{1c}) for birth weight, sum of skinfolds, and percent body fat >90th percentile, as well as for fasting and 1-h glucose for C-peptide. After adjusting for glucose measures, HbA_{1c} was associated with some pregnancy outcomes but not others which suggested measurement of HbA_{1c} was not a useful alternative to an OGTT in pregnant women. There was also a stronger association between a single measure of glucose at 28 weeks gestation with pregnancy outcomes than associations of HbA_{1c} with the same outcomes [57]. The study did not identify a clear inflection point associated with various adverse outcomes and did not make specific recommendations for diagnostic criteria [56]. International professional societies have convened multitudes of conferences and workshops over the past decade to formulate universal guidelines to assist clinicians with the diagnosis of GDM. At the time of this writing, no universal guideline exists. Clinically relevant and commonly used diagnostic criteria specified by professional societies are summarized in Table 9.2.

Several risk factors for GDM, including overweight and obesity, advanced maternal age, family history of diabetes, cigarette smoking, having a macrosomic baby, and non-Caucasian race/ethnicity, have been identified [58]. Exposure to endocrine-disrupting chemicals (EDC), such as phenols and bisphenol A (BPA) has also gained attention in recent years as being a potential risk factor for developing GDM [59].

Role of Inflammation in Gestational Diabetes

Both obesity and GDM are associated with increased adipose tissue macrophages that secrete proinflammatory cytokines. These proinflammatory cytokines impair insulin signaling and inhibit the release of insulin from β-cells. Chronic states of inflammation may be important to the pathogenesis of GDM but this hypothesis requires ongoing research [54]. Plasma TNFα is the primary mediator of increases in insulin resistance in normal pregnancy, and increased concentrations of these proinflammatory cytokines have been observed in studies. In a prospective cohort study by Wolf et al. [60], increased maternal leukocyte count at 10–12 weeks gestation was associated with an increased risk of developing GDM. This observation was independent of various factors including obese status, advanced maternal age, non-Caucasian race, and multiple gestations. Authors recognize, however, that leukocyte count is a non-specific marker of inflammation that is influenced by various factors including, but not limited to, gestation [60].

While increased expression of TNFα and inflammatory cytokines have been reported in placenta from GDM patients [61], others report placenta obtained from women with GDM have increased antioxidant gene expression and blunted cytokine release to an oxidative challenge which may be protective or adaptive mechanisms [62]. No conclusive statements can be made about the effect of maternal GDM on placental inflammation.

Table 9.2 Recommendations for screening and diagnosis of GDM by professional society

Society	Test	Time	Plasma glucose (mg/dL)	
ADA[a]	One step 75-g OGTT	Fasting	≥92	
		1-h	≥180	
		2-h	≥153	
	Two step Step one: 50-g OGTT (non-fasting) Step two: 100-g OGT (fasting)	1-h	≥130–140* proceed to 100-g OGTT	
		Fasting	≥95	
		1-h	≥180	
		2-h	≥155	
		3-h	≥140	
ACOG[b]	Two step Step one: 50-g OGTT	1-h	≥135* or ≥140 proceed to 100-g OGTT	
	Step two: 100-g OGTT	Fasting 1-h	Carpenter and Coustan	National Diabetes Data Group
		2-h 3 h	≥95	≥105
			≥180	≥190
			≥155	≥165
			≥140	≥145
Endocrine Society[c]/ IADSPG	Two h 75-g OGTT (fasting)	Fasting	92–125	
		1-h	≥180	
		2-h	153–199	
WHO[d]	Plasma glucose 75-g OGTT	Fasting	92–125	
		1-h	≥180	
		2-h	153–199	

OGTT oral glucose tolerance test

[a]American Diabetes Association Professional Practice Committee; 2. Classification and Diagnosis of Diabetes: *Standards of Medical Care in Diabetes-2022. Diabetes Care*: 45 (Supplement_1) January 2022. Testing at 24–28 weeks gestation in women not previously diagnosed with diabetes. *U.S. Preventive Service Task Force compared cutoffs of 130 mg/dL and 140 mg/dL. Higher cutoff yielded sensitivity of 70–80% and specificity of 69–89%, while lower cutoff was 88–99% sensitive and 66–77% specific. Data on cutoff value of 135 mcg/dL limited

[b]American College of Obstetrics and Gynecology Practice Bulletin No. 190: Gestational Diabetes Mellitus. *Obstetrics & Gynecology* 131 (2); February 2022. *Some experts use a threshold of ≥130 mg/dL

[c]Endocrine Society recommendations based on the International Association of Diabetes and Pregnancy Study Group (IADPSG) criteria. Diabetes and Pregnancy: An Endocrine Society Clinical Practice Guidelines, JCEM, 98 (11), 2013. Two hour 75-g OGTT performed after an overnight fast for at least 8 h (but not more than 14 h)

[b]World Health Organization. Diagnostic Criteria and Classification of Hyperglycemia First Detected in Pregnancy. 2013, Geneva Switzerland

Fetal Programming

Since GDM is considered an early manifestation of diabetes unmasked by pregnancy, it may play a role in fetal programming. A literature review by Kim et al. [63] indicates associations between maternal GDM and offspring with overweight and obesity after adjusting for pre-pregnancy BMI, which could suggest fetal programming. There is some early evidence that fetal exposure to GDM is associated with higher childhood adiposity [63]. Analyses of offspring from the US Exploring

Perinatal Outcomes among Children (EPOCH) study found alterations in a number of gene methylations associated with adiposity-related outcomes in a cohort of patients exposed to GDM [64]. The fetal-placental vasculature has also displayed alterations from GDM pregnancies, such as altered adenosine metabolism, increased oxidative stress, and increased proinflammatory and procoagulant states. These alterations may impair vasoreactivity and nutrient transport [65].

Recommendations

The ideal approach to decreasing pregnancy risks associated with obesity and GDM is, ultimately, preconception optimization of BMI, preventing excess weight gain during pregnancy, and risk reduction strategies for GDM. Unfortunately, strategies to address overweight and obesity have not been successful, as evidenced by the growing global pandemic of population obesity. Mitigating obesity requires a complex and vast network of factors on individual, political, community, health-systems, and business-based levels. Health counseling specific to women with pregestational obesity and GDM has been conducted but with mixed results.

Antenatal and Natal Nutritional and Behavioral Modifications

A multicenter randomized trial in Australia [66] evaluated the effect of antenatal dietary and lifestyle interventions on the health outcomes of pregnant women with overweight and obesity. Over 2000 women with BMI ≥ 25 kg/m^2 were included in the study. Women were randomized to intervention which included comprehensive dietary counseling and exercise recommendations. Dietary advice encouraged maintaining the balance of carbohydrates, fat, and protein while reducing foods high in refined carbohydrates and saturated fats. Additional advice on fiber intake, vegetables, and fruits serving, along with the promotion of increasing walking and physical activity, was also provided. Between the study and control participants, there was no difference in risks of infants born large-for-gestational-age (LGA), preterm birth before 37 weeks, or admission to the neonatal intensive care unit. For women, no significant differences in complications were observed.

Results of a smaller, randomized trial ($n = 118$) in the USA of women within the Kaiser Permanente system [67] found that group-based dietary intervention helped women with obesity to minimize GWG and reduce the prevalence of LGA newborns. The intervention included a combination of diet (Dietary Approaches to Stop Hypertension (DASH) without sodium restriction) and exercise (30 min of moderate physical activity in the absence of complications) recommendations.

Physical activity confers health benefits to the general population. It is widely recognized as an effective strategy for primary and secondary prevention of cardiovascular diseases, diabetes, osteoporosis, depression, and premature death. A meta-analysis of 13 studies was conducted to assess the effects of exercise on maternal and infant outcomes in pregnant women with overweight and obesity. Recommendations varied from study to study, ranging widely from the type of exercise (daily step goals vs. treadmill vs. cycling, etc.), duration (25–100 min), and frequency (one, several times a week vs. monthly) of exercise. The study concluded that while prenatal exercise interventions reduced GWG and risk of GDM for women with overweight and obesity, no evidence was found about infant benefit/harm [68].

Cumulative research evaluating successful intervention strategies for achieving healthy weight in pregnant women is characterized by individual study limitations like limited racial and ethnic diversity, the timing of intervention, degree of counseling (simple advice vs. intensive nutritional plans), and types of behavioral therapy. The mixed outcomes/results from individual studies, health disparities, and social determinants of health remain barriers to overcome if we are to achieve effective solutions and recommendations in this unique patient population.

Optimizing BMI Prior to Pregnancy

Medications

To date, pharmaceutical and medical researchers are reluctant to conduct studies on pregnant women due to potential fetal risks, the threat of legal liability, and ethical concerns. Generally, expectant mothers and unborn fetuses are considered vulnerable populations and are excluded from drug development clinical trials. Although organizations like the National Institutes of Health (NIH) and the U.S. Food and Drug Administration (FDA) are providing research guidance and pursuing a legislative change to encourage the inclusion of pregnant women in medical research, pregnant women remain underrepresented in clinical research. The underrepresentation of women also exists in medication/treatment studies for weight loss medicines and GDM.

Metformin, a commonly used medicine in T2DM and polycystic ovarian syndrome (PCOS), is being used increasingly in clinical practice for managing GDM. It reduces glucose production by the liver, decreases absorption by the intestines and the stomach, and is not associated with weight gain. Studies in women with GDM taking metformin have reported safety, improved neonatal morbidity, and a healthier neonatal period [69, 70].

A Cochrane review published by Australian investigators Dodd et al. [71] evaluated the role of metformin in pregnant women with obesity (but not diabetes) on maternal and infant outcomes. Women who received metformin or a placebo had similar risk for LGA infants, slightly lower gestational weight gain, and no differences in gestational hypertension or preeclampsia. Metformin made little or no difference in the risk of developing gestational diabetes and was associated with adverse side effects, including abdominal pain, diarrhea, and headache. The authors concluded that there is insufficient evidence to support the use of metformin for improving maternal and fetal outcomes in pregnant women with obesity.

Bariatric Surgery

Compared to nutritional and behavioral interventions, bariatric surgery to optimize pre-pregnancy BMI is being considered. Promising studies report that bariatric surgery is associated with reduced risks of GDM and excessive fetal growth, lower maternal complication rates such as postpartum hemorrhage, and LGA infants. Neonatal outcomes of bariatric surgery are more conflicting but may result in small-for-gestational-age (SGA) infants, increased preterm delivery, and possibly increased perinatal mortality [72, 73].

The timing and type of surgery require a serious discussion and shared decision-making as excessive and rapid weight loss can lead to significant malnutrition and vitamin deficiencies. Malabsorptive and restrictive procedures, independently or combined, can lead to vitamin deficiencies, especially fat-soluble vitamins, and affect iron absorption. Current guidelines recommend avoiding pregnancy for 12–24 months after bariatric surgery.

Supplementation

A randomized control trial by Haghiac et al. [74] evaluated the role of long-chain omega-3 fatty acid supplementation in pregnant women with obesity. The study randomized 72 women with overweight/obesity to receive the intervention—1200 mg of eicosapentaenoic acid (EPA) and 800 mg of docosahexaenoic acid (DHA)—from weeks 10 to 16 until term. The study was completed in 24 women and had a high dropout rate secondary to the discomfort of taking 4 capsules/day. The findings supported murine models that omega-3 supplementation decreased inflammation in overweight/obese women. After 25 weeks, there was a lower expression of inflammatory genes in AT and the placenta and decreased CRP levels at the time of delivery [74]. How these findings contribute to clinical outcomes remains under study.

Folic acid (FA) supplementation is a widely and commonly recommended nutritional intervention in pregnancy to decrease neural tube defect (NTD) rates. There has been a suggestion that women with obesity have an absolute folate deficiency due to suboptimal intake. A potential mechanism for folate deficiency in women with obesity has been proposed. It includes chronic low-grade inflammation, which increases metabolic demand for folate, higher intestinal permeability in obesity that leads to suboptimal uptake of micronutrients, relative malnutrition, and lower adherence to supplementation [75]. The relationship between FA supplementation and the prevention of GDM remains unclear [76]. Recommendations for folic acid supplementation vary by organization. In general, folic acid of 400 µg is recommended during the periconceptional period with considerations for higher doses in select patient groups.

Myo-inositol (MI), an inositol produced in humans and present in food sources like fresh fruits and vegetables, has been studied in pregnant women for GDM prevention. It is a six-carbon (C_6) ring structure that is a precursor for derivatives that act as secondary messengers and regulate several hormones like the thyroid-stimulating hormone (TSH), follicle-stimulating hormone (FSH), and insulin. Altered levels of MI and its derivatives have been observed in several pathologies, such as Alzheimer's disease, PCOS, various cancers, insulin resistance, and psychiatric diseases [77–79]. MI supplementation is emerging as a treatment for various diseases with favorable results, particularly in women with PCOS [80]. Early results are promising, with MI-treated groups showing a significantly decreased prevalence of GDM [81, 82]. A metanalysis of four trials with 690 participants [82] showed that MI supplementation was accompanied by a significant reduction in the incidence of GDM (OR 0.32, 95% CI 0.21 to 0.48; $P < 0.001$), reductions fasting, 1- and 2-h OGTT glucose values and gestational hypertension. Three trials were from Italy, one from Iran, and only included studies of pregnant women with overweight and obesity. MI may emerge as a new and preventive strategy for reducing GDM in pregnant women with overweight and obesity. Large, well-designed, and adequately powered trials are needed to assess safety and generalizability.

Studies evaluating the association between vitamin D deficiency and the risk of GDM have been conflicting. A systematic review by Zhang et al. [83], including 87 observational studies and 25 randomized controlled trials, show that pregnant women with low vitamin D levels had an 85% higher risk of GDM compared to women with normal vitamin D levels (OR 1.850, 95% CI 1.471–2.328). Randomized control trials (RCT) studying the role of vitamin D and its effects on inflammation and oxidative stress are limited and difficult to validate. Lastly, vitamin D studies vary based on what researchers use as a cutoff for low vitamin D level.

Finally, the gut microbiome is emerging as a new clinical and scientific frontier that necessitates discussion. Changes in gut microbiota are reported in obesity, diabetes, liver diseases, cancers, and neurodegenerative diseases. Pregnancy is also associated with significant changes in the composition of gut microbiota. Koren et al. [84] describe dramatic changes in the gut microbiota during pregnancy. In the first trimester of pregnancy, the gut microbiota is healthy and diverse, similar to healthy non-pregnant female and male controls. By the third trimester, the structure and composition of the microbiota resemble a disease-associated dysbiosis. No differences between gut microbiotas of GDM+ and GDM- mothers were detected. Interestingly, the women in this study had reduced insulin sensitivity and increased adiposity during gestation. The authors observed increased inflammation markers in the stool from trimester 1 to trimester 3. The dysbiosis in the third trimester was similar to obesity-associated microbiomes, including low taxonomic richness [84]. More research is needed to establish the underlying mechanisms. The Study of PRobitics IN Gestation (SPRING) was conducted to evaluate probiotics for the prevention of GDM in women with overweight and obesity. Volunteers were strati-fied by BMI and randomized to a probiotic capsule (mixture of *Lactobacillus rhamnosus* and *Bifidobacterium animalis lactis*) versus a placebo administered throughout pregnancy. Study results showed no statistical difference in GDM between arms of the study but noted higher fasting glucose in women randomized to the probiotics arm. Lower rates of excessive weight gain in women on probiotics ($P = 0.01$) were observed but with no difference in mean weight gain between the study and control groups [85].

Conclusions and Implications for Future Research

Pregnancy is a fascinating period of metabolic change and physiologic adaptations. This chapter presents a brief review of the role of inflammation in pregnant women with obesity and/or GDM. As the rates of obesity and diabetes continue to rise, it is essential to identify at-risk populations, make proper clinical diagnoses, and imple-ment mitigation strategies. While critical evaluations and evolving research con-tinue, concepts of fetal and epigenetic programming can potentially affect transgenerational health. Therefore, education during the pregnancy window is vital for maternal and fetal health optimization.

Perhaps, the very complex and dynamic nature of pregnancy contributes to the lack of "universal" diagnostic criteria for obesity and GDM and the dearth of suc-cessful management strategies to date. The need for larger-scale studies addressing health disparities, racial inequities, and social determinants of health in overweight and obese populations is well known. However, more research is needed to deter-mine effective ways to educate individual physicians and providers on the proper screening of women at risk for obesity in pregnancy and GDM. This may require critical reviews of medical school and residency curricula. Improving access to pre-conception/conception care for all interested women can include creative and eco-nomic strategies like web-based learning, telehealth visits, and group-based support groups.

Clinical inertia in treating women of childbearing age with medicines and thera-peutics, including supplements, persists. This may be attributed to the underrepre-sentation of women in clinical trials. Improving female participation and diversity in medical research, with appropriate safety and ethical standards, can elucidate issues of drug safety, timing, dose efficacy, side effect profile, and fetal outcomes.

Daily scientific advances and medical breakthroughs in genomics, drug develop-ment, targeted gene therapy, and machine learning are promising. The interconnect-edness of the global medical community, facilitated through technology and social networks, provides a ripe environment for tackling some of the clinical challenges presented in this chapter. It is incumbent on the medical community to invest time and resources to optimize maternal and fetal health while decreasing disease burden.

References

1. Hotamisligil GS. Inflammation and metabolic disorders. Nature. 2006;444:860–7.
2. Rohm TV, Meier DT, Olefsky JM, Donath MY. Inflammation in obesity, diabetes, and related disorders. Immunity. 2022;55:31–55.
3. Baeten JM, Bukusi EA, Lambe M. Pregnancy complications and outcomes among overweight and obese nulliparous women. Am J Public Health. 2001;91:436–40.
4. Sebire NJ, Jolly M, Harris JP, et al. Maternal obesity and pregnancy outcome: a study of 287,213 pregnancies in London. Int J Obes Relat Metab Disord. 2001;25:1175–82.
5. Ehrenberg HM, Mercer BM, Catalano PM. The influence of obesity and diabetes on the prevalence of macrosomia. Am J Obstet Gynecol. 2004;191:964–8.
6. Hartling L, Dryden DM, Guthrie A, Muise M, Vandermeer B, Donovan L. Diagnostic thresholds for gestational diabetes and their impact on pregnancy outcomes: a systematic review. Diabet Med. 2014;31:319–31.
7. Lowe WL Jr, Scholtens DM, Lowe LP, et al. Association of gestational diabetes with Maternal disorders of glucose metabolism and childhood adiposity. JAMA. 2018;320:1005–16.
8. Driscoll AK, Gregory ECW. Increases in prepregnancy obesity: United States, 2016–2019. NCHS Data Brief; 2020.
9. Casagrande SS, Linder B, Cowie CC. Prevalence of gestational diabetes and subsequent type 2 diabetes among U.S. women. Diabetes Res Clin Pract. 2018;141:200–8.
10. Thornton P, Abrams R, Briller J, Geller S. Illinois maternal morbidity and mortality report October 2018. University of Illinois at Chicago; 2020.
11. Frey HA, Ashmead R, Farmer A, et al. Association of Prepregnancy Body Mass Index with Risk of severe maternal morbidity and mortality among medicaid beneficiaries. JAMA Netw Open. 2022;5:e2218986-e.
12. Blomberg M. Maternal obesity, mode of delivery, and neonatal outcome. Obstet Gynecol. 2013;122:50–5.
13. Bodnar LM, Siminerio LL, Himes KP, et al. Maternal obesity and gestational weight gain are risk factors for infant death. Obesity (Silver Spring). 2016;24:490–8.
14. Chen A, Feresu SA, Fernandez C, Rogan WJ. Maternal obesity and the risk of infant death in the United States. Epidemiology. 2009;20:74–81.
15. Tavera G, Dongarwar D, Salemi JL, et al. Diabetes in pregnancy and risk of near-miss, maternal mortality and foetal outcomes in the USA: a retrospective cross-sectional analysis. J Public Health. 2021;44:549–57.
16. Murray SR, Reynolds RM. Short- and long-term outcomes of gestational diabetes and its treatment on fetal development. Prenat Diagn. 2020;40:1085–91.
17. Kaseva N, Vääräsmäki M, Sundvall J, et al. Gestational diabetes but not Prepregnancy overweight predicts for cardiometabolic markers in offspring twenty years later. J Clin Endocrinol Metabol. 2019;104:2785–95.
18. Rahier J, Wallon J, Henquin JC. Cell populations in the endocrine pancreas of human neonates and infants. Diabetologia. 1981;20:540–6.
19. Wellmann KF, Volk BW. The islets of infants of diabetic mothers. In: Volk BW, Wellmann KF, editors. The diabetic pancreas. Boston, MA: Springer; 1977. p. 365–80.
20. Holemans K, Aerts L, Van Assche FA. Lifetime consequences of abnormal fetal pancreatic development. J Physiol. 2003;547:11–20.
21. Ozanne SE, Hales CN. Early programming of glucose–insulin metabolism. Trends Endocrinol Metabol. 2002;13:368–73.
22. Barker DJ, Osmond C, Kajantie E, Eriksson JG. Growth and chronic disease: findings in the Helsinki Birth Cohort. Ann Hum Biol. 2009;36:445–58.
23. Hales CN, Barker DJ. Type 2 (non-insulin-dependent) diabetes mellitus: the thrifty phenotype hypothesis. Diabetologia. 1992;35:595–601.
24. Hales CN, Barker DJP. The thrifty phenotype hypothesis: type 2 diabetes. Br Med Bull. 2001;60:5–20.

25. Ignacio RM, Kim CS, Kim SK. Immunological profiling of obesity. J Lifestyle Med. 2014;4:1–7.
26. Esposito K, Pontillo A, Giugliano F, et al. Association of low Interleukin-10 levels with the metabolic syndrome in obese women. J Clin Endocrinol Metabol. 2003;88:1055–8.
27. McElwain CJ, McCarthy FP, McCarthy CM. Gestational diabetes mellitus and maternal immune dysregulation: what we know so far. Int J Mol Sci. 2021;22:4261.
28. Mor G, Cardenas I, Abrahams V, Guller S. Inflammation and pregnancy: the role of the immune system at the implantation site. Ann N Y Acad Sci. 2011;1221:80–7.
29. Meyyazhagan A, Kuchi Bhotla H, Pappuswamy M, Tsibizova V, Al Qasem M, Di Renzo GC. Cytokine see-saw across pregnancy, its related complexities and consequences. Int J Gynaecol Obstet. 2023;160(2):516–25.
30. Brown MB, von Chamier M, Allam AB, Reyes L. M1/M2 macrophage polarity in normal and complicated pregnancy. Front Immunol. 2014;5:606.
31. Zhang YH, He M, Wang Y, Liao AH. Modulators of the balance between M1 and M2 macrophages during pregnancy. Front Immunol. 2017;8:120.
32. Lindström TM, Bennett PR. The role of nuclear factor kappa B in human labour. Reproduction (Cambridge, England). 2005;130:569–81.
33. Chen J, Khalil RA. Matrix metalloproteinases in normal pregnancy and preeclampsia. Prog Mol Biol Transl Sci. 2017;148:87–165.
34. Shimaoka Y, Hidaka Y, Tada H, et al. Changes in cytokine production during and after normal pregnancy. Am J Reprod Immunol. 2000;44:143–7.
35. Somerset DA, Zheng Y, Kilby MD, Sansom DM, Drayson MT. Normal human pregnancy is associated with an elevation in the immune suppressive CD25+ CD4+ regulatory T-cell subset. Immunology. 2004;112:38–43.
36. Elenkov IJ, Wilder RL, Bakalov VK, et al. IL-12, TNF-α, and hormonal changes during late pregnancy and early postpartum: implications for autoimmune disease activity during these times. J Clin Endocrinol Metabol. 2001;86:4933–8.
37. Gaberšček S, Zaletel K. Thyroid physiology and autoimmunity in pregnancy and after delivery. Expert Rev Clin Immunol. 2011;7:697–707.
38. Vukusic S, Hutchinson M, Hours M, et al. Pregnancy and multiple sclerosis (the PRIMS study): clinical predictors of post-partum relapse. Brain J Neurol. 2004;127:1353–60.
39. Al-Shammri S, Rawoot P, Azizieh F, et al. Th1/Th2 cytokine patterns and clinical profiles during and after pregnancy in women with multiple sclerosis. J Neurol Sci. 2004;222:21–7.
40. Szpunar MJ, Malaktaris A, Baca SA, Hauger RL, Lang AJ. Are alterations in estradiol, cortisol, and inflammatory cytokines associated with depression during pregnancy and postpartum? An exploratory study. Brain, Behav Immun Health. 2021;16:100309.
41. Osborne LM, Yenokyan G, Fei K, et al. Innate immune activation and depressive and anxious symptoms across the peripartum: an exploratory study. Psychoneuroendocrinology. 2019;99:80–6.
42. Vesco KK, Dietz PM, Rizzo J, et al. Excessive gestational weight gain and postpartum weight retention among obese women. Obstet Gynecol. 2009;114:1069.
43. Rooney BL, Schauberger CW. Excess pregnancy weight gain and long-term obesity: one decade later. Obstet Gynecol. 2002;100:245–52.
44. Institute of Medicine, National Research Council Committee to Reexamine IOMPWG. The National Academies Collection: reports funded by National Institutes of Health. In: Rasmussen KM, Yaktine AL, editors. Weight gain during pregnancy: reexamining the guidelines. Washington, DC: National Academies Press (US), National Academy of Sciences; 2009.
45. Institute of Medicine Committee on Nutritional Status During Pregnancy and Lactation. Nutrition during pregnancy: part I weight gain: part II nutrient supplements. Washington, DC: National Academies Press (US) 1990 by the National Academy of Sciences; 1990.
46. Institute of Medicine. Weight gain during pregnancy: reexamining the guidelines. Report Brief; 2009.

47. Hotamisligil GS, Arner P, Caro JF, Atkinson RL, Spiegelman BM. Increased adipose tissue expression of tumor necrosis factor-alpha in human obesity and insulin resistance. J Clin Invest. 1995;95:2409–15.
48. Dandona P, Weinstock R, Thusu K, Abdel-Rahman E, Aljada A, Wadden T. Tumor necrosis factor-α in sera of obese patients: fall with weight loss. J Clin Endocrinol Metabol. 1998;83:2907–10.
49. Challier JC, Basu S, Bintein T, et al. Obesity in pregnancy stimulates macrophage accumulation and inflammation in the placenta. Placenta. 2008;29:274–81.
50. Saben J, Lindsey F, Zhong Y, et al. Maternal obesity is associated with a lipotoxic placental environment. Placenta. 2014;35:171–7.
51. Basu S, Haghiac M, Surace P, et al. Pregravid obesity associates with increased maternal endotoxemia and metabolic inflammation. Obesity (Silver Spring). 2011;19:476–82.
52. Reynolds RM, Osmond C, Phillips DIW, Godfrey KM. Maternal BMI, parity, and pregnancy weight gain: influences on offspring adiposity in young adulthood. J Clin Endocrinol Metabol. 2010;95:5365–9.
53. Neri C, Edlow AG. Effects of maternal obesity on fetal programming: molecular approaches. Cold Spring Harb Perspect Med. 2015;6:a026591.
54. Plows JF, Stanley JL, Baker PN, Reynolds CM, Vickers MH. The pathophysiology of gestational diabetes mellitus. Int J Mol Sci. 2018;19:19.
55. Metzger BE, Buchanan TA, Coustan DR, et al. Summary and recommendations of the fifth international workshop-conference on gestational diabetes mellitus. Diabetes Care. 2007;30:S251–S60.
56. Coustan DR, Lowe LP, Metzger BE, Dyer AR. The Hyperglycemia and Adverse Pregnancy Outcome (HAPO) study: paving the way for new diagnostic criteria for gestational diabetes mellitus. Am J Obstet Gynecol. 2010;202(654):e1–6.
57. Lowe LP, Metzger BE, Dyer AR, et al. Hyperglycemia and Adverse Pregnancy Outcome (HAPO) study: associations of maternal A1C and glucose with pregnancy outcomes. Diabetes Care. 2012;35:574–80.
58. Solomon CG, Willett WC, Carey VJ, et al. A prospective study of Pregravid determinants of gestational diabetes mellitus. JAMA. 1997;278:1078–83.
59. Ehrlich S, Lambers D, Baccarelli A, Khoury J, Macaluso M, Ho S-M. Endocrine disruptors: a potential risk factor for gestational diabetes mellitus. Am J Perinatol. 2016;33:1313–8.
60. Wolf M, Sauk J, Shah A, et al. Inflammation and glucose intolerance: a prospective study of gestational diabetes mellitus. Diabetes Care. 2004;27:21–7.
61. Marseille-Tremblay C, Ethier-Chiasson M, Forest J-C, et al. Impact of maternal circulating cholesterol and gestational diabetes mellitus on lipid metabolism in human term. Placenta. 2008;75:1054–62.
62. Lappas M, Mitton A, Permezel M. In response to oxidative stress, the expression of inflammatory cytokines and antioxidant enzymes are impaired in placenta, but not adipose tissue, of women with gestational diabetes. J Endocrinol. 2010;204:75–84.
63. Kim SY, Sharma AJ, Callaghan WM. Gestational diabetes and childhood obesity: what is the link? Curr Opin Obstet Gynecol. 2012;24:376–81.
64. Yang IV, Zhang W, Davidson EJ, Fingerlin TE, Kechris K, Dabelea D. Epigenetic marks of in utero exposure to gestational diabetes and childhood adiposity outcomes: the EPOCH study. Diabet Med. 2018;35:612–20.
65. Silva L, Plösch T, Toledo F, Faas MM, Sobrevia L. Adenosine kinase and cardiovascular fetal programming in gestational diabetes mellitus. Biochim Biophys Acta (BBA) - Mol Basis Dis. 2020;1866:165397.
66. Dodd JM, Turnbull D, McPhee AJ, et al. Antenatal lifestyle advice for women who are overweight or obese: LIMIT randomised trial. BMJ. 2014;348:g1285.
67. Vesco KK, Karanja N, King JC, et al. Efficacy of a group-based dietary intervention for limiting gestational weight gain among obese women: a randomized trial. Obesity (Silver Spring). 2014;22:1989–96.

68. Du M-C, Ouyang Y-Q, Nie X-F, Huang Y, Redding SR. Effects of physical exercise during pregnancy on maternal and infant outcomes in overweight and obese pregnant women: a meta-analysis. Birth. 2019;46:211–21.
69. Rowan JA, Hague WM, Gao W, Battin MR, Moore MP. Metformin versus insulin for the treatment of gestational diabetes. N Engl J Med. 2008;358:2003–15.
70. Balani J, Hyer SL, Rodin DA, Shehata H. Pregnancy outcomes in women with gestational diabetes treated with metformin or insulin: a case–control study. Diabet Med. 2009;26:798–802.
71. Dodd JM, Grivell RM, Deussen AR, Hague WM. Metformin for women who are overweight or obese during pregnancy for improving maternal and infant outcomes. Cochrane Database Syst Rev. 2018;2018:CD010564.
72. Johansson K, Cnattingius S, Näslund I, et al. Outcomes of pregnancy after bariatric. Surgery. 2015;372:814–24.
73. Lesko J, Peaceman A. Pregnancy outcomes in women after bariatric surgery compared with obese and morbidly obese controls. Obstet Gynecol. 2012;119:547–54.
74. Haghiac M, Yang X-h, Presley L, et al. Dietary Omega-3 fatty acid supplementation reduces inflammation in obese pregnant women: a randomized double-blind controlled clinical trial. PLoS One. 2015;10:e0137309.
75. van der Windt M, Schoenmakers S, van Rijn B, Galjaard S, Steegers-Theunissen R, van Rossem L. Epidemiology and (patho)physiology of folic acid supplement use in obese women before and during pregnancy. Nutrients. 2021;13:331.
76. Keating E, Martel F, Araújo J. Folic acid and gestational diabetes: foundations for further studies. In: Nutrition and diet in maternal diabetes; 2018. p. 465–77.
77. Voevodskaya O, Poulakis K, Sundgren P, et al. Brain myoinositol as a potential marker of amyloid-related pathology. Neurology. 2019;92:e395.
78. Unfer V, Carlomagno G, Papaleo E, Vailati S, Candiani M, Baillargeon J-P. Hyperinsulinemia alters myoinositol to d-chiroinositol ratio in the follicular fluid of patients with PCOS. Reprod Sci. 2014;21:854–8.
79. Chhetri DR. Myo-inositol and its derivatives: their emerging role in the treatment of human diseases. Front Pharmacol. 2019;10:1172.
80. Unfer V, Facchinetti F, Orrù B, Giordani B, Nestler J. Myo-inositol effects in women with PCOS: a meta-analysis of randomized controlled trials. Endocr Connect. 2017;6:647–58.
81. D'Anna R, Santamaria A. Myo-inositol supplementation in gestational diabetes. In: Rajendram R, Preedy VR, Patel VB, editors. Nutrition and diet in maternal diabetes: an evidence-based approach. Cham: Springer; 2018. p. 229–35.
82. Mashayekh-Amiri S, Mohammad-Alizadeh-Charandabi S, Abdolalipour S, Mirghafourvand M. Myo-inositol supplementation for prevention of gestational diabetes mellitus in overweight and obese pregnant women: a systematic review and meta-analysis. Diabetol Metab Syndr. 2022;14:93.
83. Zhang Y, Gong Y, Xue H, Xiong J, Cheng G. Vitamin D and gestational diabetes mellitus: a systematic review based on data free of Hawthorne effect. BJOG. 2018;125:784–93.
84. Koren O, Goodrich Julia K, Cullender Tyler C, et al. Host remodeling of the gut microbiome and metabolic changes during pregnancy. Cell. 2012;150:470–80.
85. Callaway LK, McIntyre HD, Barrett HL, et al. Probiotics for the prevention of gestational diabetes mellitus in overweight and obese women: findings from the SPRING double-blind randomized controlled trial. Diabetes Care. 2019;42:364–71.

Chapter 10
Potential Pharmaceutical and Non-pharmaceutical Approaches to Obesity and Diabetes: Focus on Inflammation

Raihan El-Naas, Sarah R. Barenbaum, Alpana P. Shukla, and Louis J. Aronne

Abbreviations

AHA	American Heart Association
AMPK	Adenosine monophosphate-activated protein kinase
ATM	Adipose tissue macrophages
BMI	Body mass index
CRP	C-reactive protein
CVD	Cardiovascular disease
DASH	Dietary Approaches to Stop Hypertension diet
DII	Dietary inflammatory index
FDA	Food and Drug Administration
GIP	Glucose-dependent insulinotropic polypeptide
GLP-1	Glucagon-like peptide 1
HbA1c	Glycosylated hemoglobin
hsCRP	High-sensitivity C-reactive protein
IL-10	Interleukin 10
IL-1Ra	Interleukin 1 receptor antagonist
IL-1β	Interleukin 1 beta

R. El-Naas
Department of Internal Medicine, New York-Presbyterian Hospital/Weill Cornell Medical Center, New York, NY, USA
e-mail: rae2018@nyp.org

S. R. Barenbaum (✉) · A. P. Shukla · L. J. Aronne
Division of Endocrinology, Diabetes and Metabolism, Comprehensive Weight Control Center, Weill Cornell Medicine, New York, NY, USA
e-mail: srb9023@med.cornell.edu; aps2004@med.cornell.edu; ljaronne@med.cornell.edu

© The Author(s), under exclusive license to Springer Nature Switzerland AG 2023
D. Avtanski, L. Poretsky (eds.), *Obesity, Diabetes and Inflammation*, Contemporary Endocrinology, https://doi.org/10.1007/978-3-031-39721-9_10

IL-6	Interleukin 6
LPS	Lipopolysaccharide
MRCC-I	Mitochondrial respiratory chain complex I
NLRP-3	NOD-like receptor protein 3
PPARγ	Peroxisome proliferator-activated receptor gamma
SGLT2	Sodium-glucose cotransporter 2
T2D	Type 2 diabetes
TNFα	Tumor-necrosis factor alpha
Treg	T regulatory cells

Introduction

Obesity, a complex chronic disease characterized by increased adiposity, has been shown to be strongly correlated with several obesity-related disorders, including impaired glucose tolerance, dyslipidemia, and hypertension, collectively known as metabolic syndrome [1]. These heterogeneous disorders have been studied for decades, but more recently, the relationship between obesity, type 2 diabetes (T2D), and the immune system has come to light. Particularly, the role of inflammation in obesity and diabetes is of growing interest and will be the central topic of discussion in this chapter. Chronic, systemic low-grade inflammation has been shown to be a pathological feature in multiple diseases, including obesity and T2D, and more importantly, is an independent risk factor for diabetes [2, 3]. Moreover, several studies illustrate that a reduction in weight is associated with decreased expression of pro-inflammatory cytokines [4, 5]. This reduction in systemic inflammation also correlates with increased insulin sensitivity [5]. Hence, interventions targeting weight loss are a fundamental part of the clinical management of obesity and its associated disorders. This chapter will discuss both the pharmacologic and non-pharmacologic management of obesity and T2D with a special emphasis on their role in chronic systemic inflammation. To better understand the anti-inflammatory roles of these approaches, some of the most pertinent molecular mechanisms involved in creating the inflammatory milieu in obesity and T2D will be addressed prior to diving into the management approaches.

Molecular Mechanisms

The key sites of inflammation in obesity and in T2D are adipose tissue, the pancreas, the liver, and skeletal muscle [2]. Several studies have illustrated that there is an upregulation and increased gene expression of multiple pro-inflammatory cytokines in obesity such as tumor necrosis factor alpha (TNFα), interleukin-1 beta (IL-1β), interleukin-6 (IL-6), C-reactive protein (CRP), and others [4, 6]. These cytokines are thought to originate either from the adipose tissue itself or from macrophages that infiltrate the adipose tissue, also known as "adipose tissue macrophages" (ATMs) [1, 4]. In addition, there are an abundance of other immune cells (specifically, the cytotoxic or CD8+ T cells) in adipose tissue that stimulate monocyte chemotaxis and differentiation into ATMs [7]. Conversely, the T regulatory cells, or T regs, which inhibit monocyte migration and promote an anti-inflammatory state, appear to be reduced in obesity, thereby further exacerbating the chronic inflammatory state [7]. The following sections will briefly discuss adipose tissue, ATMs, and the major pro- and anti-inflammatory cytokines released by both, with a focus on the molecular mechanisms involved.

Adipose Tissue

Adipose tissue is an endocrine organ that secretes various pro-and anti-inflammatory cytokines, or "adipokines" [4]. These adipokines vary in expression depending on the depot site of the adipose tissue, namely either visceral or subcutaneous adipose tissue [4]. One characteristic feature of the unique adipokine profile of visceral fat, for example, is that it contains a larger number of ATMs and fewer Tregs than subcutaneous fat [8]. This physiologic and functional difference between the two fat depots could potentially explain why visceral fat is more closely associated with metabolic syndrome and obesity-related pathological disorders than subcutaneous fat [1, 2].

ATMs

ATMs are the primary source of pro-inflammatory cytokines as elucidated by gene expression analysis of both macrophage and non-macrophage cells (adipocytes, stromal cells, etc.) within adipose tissue [1]. Moreover, the accumulation of macrophages appears to be directly proportional to the adipocyte size [1]. Once the macrophages are activated, they release a variety of bioactive molecules that result in an increased production of the classic acute phase reactants such as CRP [1].

Pro-inflammatory Cytokines

TNFα

TNFα levels have consistently been shown to be elevated in plasma and the adipose tissue of individuals with obesity [4]. Furthermore, the levels were positively correlated with impaired glucose tolerance and insulin resistance [4]. The mechanism is hypothesized to involve the TNFα inhibition of the peroxisome proliferator-activated receptor gamma (PPARγ) protein, which is a key regulator of insulin sensitivity in the body [7]. However, when translated to clinical practice, the effects of TNFα on insulin resistance are inconsistent. A randomized controlled trial investigating the effects of TNFα inhibitor etanercept on inflammatory markers and insulin sensitivity in patients with obesity and T2D revealed that although etanercept significantly decreased plasma levels of inflammatory markers such as CRP and IL-6, no improvement in insulin sensitivity was observed [9]. Conversely, when TNFα inhibitors were investigated in patients with rheumatoid arthritis and psoriasis, the reduction in TNFα levels was associated with improved insulin sensitivity [10, 11]. This suggests that TNFα inhibitors can improve insulin resistance only in severe or highly inflammatory states.

IL-1β

IL-1β is one of the chief pro-inflammatory cytokines involved in the pathogenesis of T2D [12]. This cytokine is activated when its precursor pro-IL-1β is cleaved by caspase-1. Caspase-1 is stimulated within a large multimeric protein called the NOD-like receptor protein 3 inflammasome or NLRP3 inflammasome [12]. This inflammasome detects certain obesity-associated proteins such as the "lipotoxicity-associated ceramide" and induces caspase-1 followed by pro-IL-1β activation and IL-1β secretion [12]. In the pancreas, IL-1β mediates immune cell recruitment and an inflammatory cascade that subsequently induces pancreatic β-cell apoptosis resulting in decreased insulin production [6]. Thus, the NLRP3 inflammasome-induced inflammation in obesity may contribute to insulin resistance [12]. Therefore, decreased NLRP3 expression in adipose tissue results in reduced inflammation and enhanced insulin sensitivity in patients with obesity and T2D [12]. A trial investigating the effects of IL-1 antagonist anakinra in patients with T2D revealed that blockade of the IL-1β-mediated inflammatory pathway was coupled with reduced inflammatory markers, enhanced pancreatic β-cell insulin secretion, and improved glycemic control [13].

IL-6 and CRP

Other key inflammatory players in obesity and T2D are CRP and its inducer, IL-6. A 2012 systemic review and meta-analysis evaluating the association between CRP and T2D illustrated that increased levels of CRP were significantly correlated with a higher risk of T2D [14]. In addition, the meta-analysis revealed a positive correlation between IL-6 and the risk of developing T2D [14]. However, the pathophysiological mechanisms of IL-6 and CRP in T2D and obesity are not very well understood [14].

Leptin

Leptin is an adipokine that regulates energy intake and storage, feeding behavior, and insulin sensitivity [15]. Animal studies show that mice that lack leptin demonstrate hyperphagic eating patterns, insulin resistance, and obesity with subsequent reversal of these metabolic changes upon the administration of leptin [16]. Nevertheless, leptin plasma levels are directly proportional to adipose mass, and individuals with obesity have elevated leptin levels without the anticipated anorectic responses indicating that leptin resistance develops in obesity [16]. Moreover, these high levels of leptin can stimulate the proliferation of monocytes and promote their production of TNFα and IL-6, suggesting that leptin has pro-inflammatory effects that contribute to the chronic low-grade inflammatory state in obesity and T2D [17].

Anti-inflammatory Cytokines

Adiponectin

Adiponectin is a major anti-inflammatory cytokine whose production in adipose tissue is inhibited by pro-inflammatory cytokines such as TNFα and IL-6 [4]. Animal studies revealed that mice with adiponectin deficiency had higher TNFα mRNA expression in the adipose tissue and higher levels of TNFα in the blood with subsequent normalization of the TNFα levels upon administration of adiponectin [18]. In humans, plasma levels of adiponectin were low in patients with obesity or T2D and were inversely proportional to the amount of visceral fat [19]. Adiponectin is hypothesized to exert its anti-inflammatory effects in a couple of ways. First, it activates adenosine monophosphate-activated protein kinase (AMPK) in the liver and muscle, and hence, inhibits gluconeogenesis in the former and increases fatty acid oxidation and glucose uptake in the latter [20]. Second, adiponectin prevents macrophage transformation into foam cells, facilitates phagocytosis of apoptotic cells, and promotes the secretion of other anti-inflammatory cytokines, such as interleukin-10 (IL-10) [4, 21].

Non-pharmacological Approaches

Diet, exercise, and behavioral modification are the cornerstone of treating obesity and the initial therapy for T2D. Although the weight loss induced by dietary interventions and exercise routines can reduce inflammation, certain diets and types of exercise appear to have intrinsic anti-inflammatory benefits independent of weight loss [4, 5]. The following section will discuss the role that various dietary interventions and exercise play in the systemic inflammation in obesity and T2D.

Nutrition and Dietary Interventions

In addition to the chronic low-grade background inflammation seen in obesity and T2D [3], inflammatory mediators appear to rise acutely post-meals [22]. This acute inflammatory response typically lasts only a few hours but can occur several times a day following each meal [5]. Certain meals or food components contain lipopoly-saccharides (LPS) or can alter the gut's penetrability and absorption of bacterial LPS [3, 5]. LPS, a powerful inflammatory stimulant, triggers systemic inflammation [3, 5]. However, the pathophysiological relationship between post-prandial inflammation and metabolic syndrome or insulin resistance remains unclear and is under investigation [5]. A plethora of studies have explored the relationship between nutrition in metabolic disorders and inflammation, from the various diet types to the different eating patterns to the assorted macro- and micronutrients. The following sections will briefly discuss a few of the common diet types and some of the every-day whole foods as they relate to inflammation and insulin resistance.

One caveat is that while there are general associations of foods that may cause inflammation and evidence of specific diets that may help reduce inflammation, there is no specific "anti-inflammatory" diet. The "anti-inflammatory diet" appears to typically be an elimination diet, and much more research is needed in this area.

Diet Types

The effects of different diet types on inflammatory marker expression are summarized in Table 10.1.

The "Healthy" Diet Numerous studies have investigated the correlation of inflammatory markers with consuming a "healthy" diet [5]. One cohort study [22] compared a "healthy" diet, defined as one rich in whole grains, fruits, vegetables, poultry, fish, and soy products, to a Western diet, defined as one with high consumption of refined grains, red, processed meat, fried food, and sweets. The Western diet

Table 10.1 Types of dietary approaches and their effects on various inflammatory markers

	Inflammatory markers		
Diet type	TNFα	IL-6	CRP
"Healthy"		↓	↓
Hypo-energetic	↓	↓	↓
Mediterranean		↓	↓
DASH			↓
Ketogenic			↓
Low-carb diet			↓
Low-fat diet			↔
Vegetarian			↓
Vegan			↓

was associated with higher plasma concentrations of CRP and IL-6 and a higher BMI and fat mass compared to the "healthy diet" [22, 23]. Supporting the above findings, other studies also revealed that consuming these "healthy" diets was negatively correlated with plasma CRP levels even after correcting for confounding factors such as BMI and waist circumference [24, 25].

Hypo-energetic Diet One particular diet type that shown to decrease long-standing low-grade inflammation is a hypo-energetic diet [5]. The energy restriction, defined in most studies as a deficit of 500 calories from the baseline diet, promotes weight loss and is associated with reduced concentrations of inflammatory mediators, namely TNFα, IL-6, and CRP [5]. Although it is challenging to assess whether the weight loss or the diet type used to induce weight loss is responsible for the reduction in inflammation, it seems that energy or caloric restriction itself may have anti-inflammatory benefits [5]. Moreover, early studies investigating low-energy carbohydrate and low-energy fat diets revealed that both reduced levels of the inflammatory markers including TNFα, CRP, and others [26]. This illustrates that the energy restriction itself may be of greater significance than the type of low-energy food consumed [26].

Mediterranean Diet This popular diet is typically known for its use of extra-virgin olive oil as the primary source of fat [27]. It is also rich in vegetables, fruits, fish, nuts, and low-fat dairy products [27]. The Mediterranean diet has been shown to be inversely correlated with inflammatory markers such as IL-6 and CRP [28]. Furthermore, compared to other nutritional interventions, such as low-fat diets, the Mediterranean diet resulted in the greatest improvement in glycosylated hemoglobin (HbA1c), fasting glucose, and insulin resistance in individuals with obesity and diabetes [27, 29]. Interestingly, these beneficial metabolic changes seem to be independent of the changes in body weight and are sustained over long periods, which does not occur with other types of weight loss nutritional interventions [27, 29].

Dietary Approaches to Stop Hypertension (DASH) Diet The DASH diet emphasizes fruits, vegetables, and low-fat dairy products, includes whole grains, fish, nuts, and poultry, and focuses on a reduction of total fat, saturated fat, cholesterol, sweets, and sugary beverages [30]. It is similar to the Mediterranean diet, though it includes more dairy and does not specifically encourage the use of extra-virgin olive oil or fish. The DASH-Sodium trial specifically randomized participants to either a DASH diet or control, which was designed to reflect a typical diet in the USA and additionally randomized the subjects to 3 different levels of sodium intake. This study found that over 12 weeks, the DASH diet alone reduced high-sensitivity CRP (hsCRP) compared to the typical American diet. In this study, sodium reduction led to an increase in hsCRP; the reasons for this are unclear but are postulated to be related to an increase in aldosterone in the low-sodium state, which has pro-inflammatory effects [31].

Ketogenic or Very Low-Carb Diets Ketogenic or very low-carb diets (defined as less than 50 g of carbohydrates per day) are diets that focus on depleting the body of glucose stores forcing it to rely on ketones for energy. These diets decrease not only visceral obesity but also reduce systemic markers of inflammation and improve insulin sensitivity [32]. Recent trials show that adherence to a ketogenic diet can even lead to the reversal of T2D in more than 50% of individuals [32]. However, ketogenic diets are very restrictive and are, therefore, hard to maintain long-term.

Low-Carb Diet There is a consistent positive correlation between the dietary glycemic index and certain markers of oxidative stress in healthy individuals suggesting that high-glycemic index carbohydrates can lead to chronic oxidative stress and contribute to the chronic low-grade inflammation [33]. Low-carb diets (defined as 50–100 g of carbohydrates per day) are associated with reduced CRP levels supporting their therapeutic anti-inflammatory potential [33].

Low-Fat Diet Although low-fat diets lower the risk of developing metabolic syndrome [34], the LIPGENE randomized controlled trial demonstrated a lack of significant effect of adjusting dietary fat on inflammatory markers or insulin sensitivity [35]. Moreover, a high-fat diet was shown to have no association with plasma CRP levels [25]. Nevertheless, high-fat meals can lead to post-prandial hyperlipidemia and contribute to the acute post-prandial inflammatory response [5]. However, the clinical significance of this acute inflammatory response is still unclear.

Vegetarian Diet Multiple cross-sectional studies have explored the inflammatory effects of the vegetarian diet, which is mainly plant-based with dairy and eggs but without any seafood, meat, or poultry [5]. The vegetarian diet was associated with superior antioxidant status and lower plasma concentrations of CRP compared with the non-vegetarian diet [36]. However, given that these were mostly observational studies and not clinical trials, it is important to note that there may be confounding lifestyle factors when comparing vegetarians with non-vegetarians, such as smoking, physical activity, and socioeconomic status.

Vegan Diet Recently, vegan diets have become more popular due to their reported effects on reducing cholesterol, blood pressure, and weight. They may also reduce inflammation [37]. Vegan diets, which are rich in fresh fruits, vegetables, whole grains, legumes, nuts, and seeds, exclude all animal products and by-products. One residential study [38] enrolled 604 subjects for 3 weeks and placed them on a vegan diet. After three weeks, most participants had a reduction in their CRP levels. Interestingly, the males in this study had a more significant decrease in CRP than females. Another study [39] enrolled 100 participants with a history of known coronary artery disease and randomized them 1:1 to either a vegan diet or the American Heart Association (AHA)-recommended diet for 8 weeks. After 8 weeks, those on a vegan diet had a significantly lower concentration of hsCRP compared to the AHA diet. Of note, this study showed no significant change in BMI or waist circumference, and there were no significant differences in glycemic control.

Specific Foods

Whole Grains Intake of whole grains was associated with increased adiponectin concentration [40] and lower plasma CRP levels, and hence, negatively correlated with markers of insulin resistance, obesity, and T2D [41]. Additionally, one study revealed that replacing a refined-grain meal with a similar whole-grain meal reduced the post-prandial levels of pro-inflammatory cytokines in both healthy individuals without diabetes and those with diabetes [42].

Fruits and Vegetables Intriguingly, the variety of fruits and vegetables consumed rather than the quantity is inversely correlated with plasma CRP levels [43]. This implies that specific micronutrients within the fruits and vegetables, such as flavonoids, rather than the whole fruit or vegetable, may be contributing to the anti-inflammatory benefits [3, 5].

Fish, Nuts, and Coffee The data for fish, nuts, and coffee are mixed with some studies showing an inverse correlation between these individual ingredients and CRP or a positive correlation between them and plasma adiponectin levels, while other studies show no association between either variable [5].

Processed Foods The oxidative stress induced by processed foods can result in advanced glycation and advanced lipo-oxidation end products [44]. However, the role of these end products in inflammation and their potentially harmful effects on humans remain controversial [5] and hence will not be discussed in this chapter.

Finally, one tool that can help summarize the inflammatory potential of an individual's diet is the dietary inflammatory index (DII). The DII was created to gauge an individual diet's inflammatory potential based on its constituents and place it on a scale from maximally anti-inflammatory to maximally pro-inflammatory [23]. The higher the DII score and the more pro-inflammatory the diet was, the greater the risk of obesity, T2D, and other chronic illnesses [23]. This correlation supports the inflammatory role that diet and nutrition play in obesity and its related metabolic disorders. Thus, this tool could be used by clinicians and dieticians as a highly individualized approach to dietary counseling.

Exercise and Physical Activity

Exercise and physical activity have countless health benefits in the general healthy population and chronic illnesses such as obesity, T2D, cardiovascular disease (CVD), and others [45]. It is important to note, however, that although the terms exercise and physical activity may be used interchangeably, they are slightly different. Physical activity is any physical movement our bodies engage in, whereas exercise is an intentional, planned, and structured form of physical activity [45].

Analogous to hormones, the term "exerkines" was first created in 2016 to describe the signaling molecules originating from different tissues, including skeletal muscle, released in response to both acute and chronic exercise [45, 46]. A key exerkine released by contracted skeletal muscle during acute exercise is IL-6, which rises exponentially with exercise and correlates with the intensity and duration of exercise [47]. However, despite the pro-inflammatory nature of IL-6, the physiological levels of muscle-derived IL-6 stimulate the release of pro-inflammatory cytokine inhibitors such as IL-1 receptor antagonist (IL-1Ra) and certain TNFα inhibitors in addition to the secretion of anti-inflammatory cytokines such as IL-10 [47]. Hence, although acute exercise may initially be pro-inflammatory due to IL-6 release, this acute inflammatory response is rapidly counteracted by an anti-inflammatory reaction [45, 47].

Furthermore, with time and regular exercise, the IL-6 plasma concentrations along with plasma CRP tend to decrease through various mechanisms, including enhanced antioxidant capacity and improved glucose tolerance and insulin sensitivity [48]. Therefore, long-term exercise can have both direct and indirect anti-inflammatory benefits through changes in body composition [48]. Moreover, several studies show that physical inactivity is associated with increased inflammation [49], and thus, further support the anti-inflammatory advantages of exercise and physical activity.

With regard to the type of exercise, both aerobic and resistance exercises can be recommended for individuals with metabolic syndrome given the lack of any clinically significant difference between them, as seen in a systematic review and meta-analysis comparing the two [50, 51]. In terms of duration of exercise, in individuals who are overweight or obese and aiming for weight loss or in individuals with metabolic syndrome, the evidence supports as much as 60 minutes of daily moderate-intensity physical activity [49].

Pharmacological Approaches

Thus far, this chapter has discussed the non-pharmacologic approaches to obesity and T2D with a focus on inflammation (Table 10.2). The remainder of this chapter will focus on pharmacologic interventions specific to obesity and T2D that have been shown to reduce inflammation.

Metformin

Metformin is a first-line medication for the treatment of T2D and is increasingly used off-label for obesity due to its efficacy and favorable safety profile [52]. Its primary therapeutic effect results from improving glycemic control by inhibiting hepatic gluconeogenesis and reducing endogenous glucose production [53]. On a cellular level, metformin has pleiotropic properties and several proposed mechanisms of action [52]. One of metformin's major mechanisms of action is the activation of hepatic AMPK, which is a chief regulator of cellular glucose and lipid metabolism and is thought to be an essential component of the signaling cascade leading to the inhibition of gluconeogenesis [54]. Moreover, chronic AMPK activation is hypothesized to indirectly inhibit gluconeogenesis by improving hepatic insulin sensitivity [52]. Another key mechanism of action of metformin independent of AMPK is the inhibition of mitochondrial respiratory chain complex I (MRCC-I) [55]. MRCC-I is thought to trigger changes in the cellular oxidation-redox state and energy charges that later result in the inhibition of gluconeogenesis [55].

Metformin also plays a vital role in obesity-related tissue inflammation or "meta-inflammation" [52]. Specifically, metformin ameliorates meta-inflammation and improves insulin sensitivity by inhibiting the differentiation of monocytes to macrophages and by promoting the activation of the anti-inflammatory T regs [56]. Mechanistically, this is hypothesized to occur via both AMPK-dependent and AMPK-independent pathways [56]. Furthermore, metformin was found to inhibit the release of pro-inflammatory cytokines TNFα and IL-6 in response to LPS in both human and animal models [52, 57]. From a clinical perspective, a couple of randomized controlled trials investigating the impact of metformin on pro-inflammatory cytokines in individuals with obesity and insulin resistance and individuals with T2D revealed that metformin was associated with a significant reduction in TNFα, IL-6, and CRP [58, 59]. In addition, one of the trials showed that the non-metformin group had lower adiponectin levels [58]. These anti-inflammatory effects were coupled with improved glycemic control and insulin sensitivity [59]. Moreover, another randomized controlled trial demonstrated that the anti-inflammatory action of metformin is also seen in healthy individuals without diabetes and is independent of the diabetes status [60], indicating that metformin has a significant inherent anti-inflammatory potential.

In addition to metformin's effects on hepatic gluconeogenesis, an increasing body of evidence points toward a gut-mediated mechanism of action [52]. One

Table 10.2 Anti-obesity medications and their effects on various inflammatory markers

Obesity medication	Inflammatory markers					
	TNFα	IL-1β	IL-6	CRP	Leptin	Adiponectin
Metformin	↓		↓	↓		
Exenatide	↓	↓	↓	↓		↑
Liraglutide	↓		↔			
Semaglutide	↓		↓	↓		
Tirzepatide			↓	↓	↓	
Empagliflozin	↓		↓			↑
Dapagliflozin	↓			↓		
Canagliflozin		↓	↓			↑
Phen/Top				↓		↑
Bup/Nal				↔		

example supporting the gut-mediated activity of metformin is that the single-daily-dosing of extended-release metformin was shown to be as effective as the regular, twice-daily-dosing immediate-release formulation in improving glycemic control in patients with T2D [61]. Given that the delayed-release metformin is released gradually in the ileum where low absorption occurs, the similar efficacy profile of the delayed-release and immediate-release strongly suggests that metformin has a gut-mediated, or more specifically, perhaps an ileum-mediated glucose-reducing effect [61].

This gut-mediated mechanism of action is hypothesized to rely on the secretion of incretins, namely glucagon-like peptide 1 (GLP-1) [52]. Recent data suggest that metformin stimulates the secretion of GLP-1 in T2D [62, 63]. Furthermore, stopping metformin in these trials resulted in a decrease in the total and active GLP-1 levels [63]. Metformin was also shown to upregulate the expression of the GLP-1 receptor in mice pancreatic islet cells [64]. As a result, metformin is considered an excellent therapeutic option for use in combination with other GLP-1 agonists due to its incretin-based effects [64] and may, therefore, additionally help to reduce inflammation akin to GLP-1 agonists as discussed below.

GLP-1 Agonists

GLP-1 is an incretin hormone secreted by the enteroendocrine L-cells in the small and large intestines in response to nutrients in the gut lumen [52, 65]. GLP-1 stimulates glucose-dependent insulin secretion, slows gastric emptying and gastrointestinal motility, and increases satiety [65]. As a result of these effects, GLP-1 agonists can reduce food intake and promote weight loss [65]. The role of these GLP-1 agonists in meta-inflammation has recently become a subject of interest. Three well-studied GLP-1 agonists, exenatide, liraglutide, and semaglutide, and their anti-inflammatory roles are discussed below.

Exenatide In a randomized controlled study exploring the anti-inflammatory effects of exenatide in patients with obesity and T2D, exenatide had a potent weight loss-independent anti-inflammatory response by suppressing mRNA expression of TNFα and IL-1β and lowering the plasma concentrations of IL-6 [66]. Moreover, given the reduction of HbA1c in the absence of weight loss, exenatide was thought to potentially enhance insulin sensitivity via the suppression of inflammatory cytokines that interfere with the physiological insulin signaling [66]. The lack of weight loss with exenatide was attributed to the short duration of the trial [66]. Another trial supported these findings and revealed that although exenatide led to a significant reduction in body weight and truncal fat mass, the exenatide-induced reduction in CRP and increase in adiponectin were independent of changes in body weight [67]. Furthermore, a few other studies in both humans and animal models illustrated that exenatide administration was associated with decreased levels of inflammatory cytokines such as TNFα and CRP, increased levels of adiponectin, and reduced markers of insulin resistance and T2D [68–70]. The elevated levels of adiponectin were hypothesized to contribute to the insulin-sensitizing effect of exenatide [70].

Liraglutide A prospective study investigating liraglutide in patients with T2D revealed that despite the reduction in body mass index (BMI) and improvement in glycemic control and insulin sensitivity that resulted from liraglutide administration, there was no statistically significant difference in the TNFα and IL-6 levels [65]. However, a couple of other studies, one in vitro in human umbilical vein endothelial cells [71] and one clinical study in patients with obesity and T2D [72], revealed that liraglutide had a profound anti-inflammatory effect by inhibiting TNFα and its downstream pro-inflammatory signaling pathways. Moreover, in mice models with hypoadiponectinemia and insulin resistance induced by a high-fat diet, liraglutide was shown to mitigate the hypoadiponectinemia-induced decline in insulin sensitivity through the prevention of the hypoadiponectinemia-induced suppression of PPARγ, the key regulator of insulin sensitivity in the body [73]. This suggests that liraglutide could potentially prevent the early stages of hypoadiponectinemia-induced and diet-induced insulin resistance, thereby preventing the development of T2D [73].

Semaglutide In a retrospective analysis of a weight management trial, semaglutide was associated with significantly reduced levels of CRP in patients with obesity and T2D [74]. Another exploratory analysis of multiple trials investigating the efficacy of semaglutide in patients with T2D illustrated that semaglutide decreased CRP levels, partially via a reduction in body weight and improvement in HbA1c but also potentially through a direct anti-inflammatory effect of the drug itself [75]. Furthermore, one study in mice models with atherosclerosis revealed that semaglutide reduced the recruitment of macrophages into aortic plaques and decreased gene expression of TNFα and IL-6 [76]. Those anti-inflammatory effects were thought to explain the reduced risk of atherosclerosis seen with semaglutide, indicating that semaglutide's anti-inflammatory benefits are not just implicated in ameliorating insulin resistance but also in cardiovascular disease risk modification [76].

GLP-1/GIP Dual Agonists

GLP-1 agonists have been previously described. The glucose-dependent insulinotropic polypeptide (GIP) is another incretin hormone secreted by the enteroendocrine K cells in the small intestine [77]. GIP enhances post-prandial insulin secretion in adults in a glucose-dependent manner, along with GLP-1. GIP additionally has a direct effect on lipid homeostasis and stimulates glucagon during periods of hypoglycemia [78]. It has been further suggested that GIP may lead to weight loss by acting centrally to potentiate the GLP-1-induced reduction of food intake while also signaling satiety to hypothalamic receptors. Early studies have shown that the dual agonism of GLP-1 and GIP leads to more weight loss and improved glycemic control in patients with T2D than existing GLP-1 receptor agonists can alone [79]. The first GLP-1/GIP dual agonist, tirzepatide, was approved by the Food and Drug Administration (FDA) in May 2022 for the treatment of T2D. The phase 3 trials of tirzepatide for chronic weight management are ongoing but have been fast-tracked by the FDA.

Tirzepatide In a phase 2b study in patients with T2D, tirzepatide was compared to dulaglutide (a GLP-1 receptor agonist approved for the treatment of T2D). Tirzepatide was found to be superior to dulaglutide for both glycemic control and weight loss [80]. A post-hoc analysis was conducted, which evaluated biomarkers of inflammation as a proxy to help ascertain the potential for tirzepatide to help reduce overall cardiac risk. At 26 weeks, there were dose-dependent reductions in hsCRP and leptin. IL-6 levels remained unchanged in all groups. While the decrease in hsCRP was rapid over 4 weeks, the reduction in leptin was more gradual. It had not plateaued by 26 weeks, which led the authors to argue that tirzepatide may suppress inflammation and improve endothelial function independent of weight loss [81]. The cardiovascular outcome trial for tirzepatide, SURPASS-CVOT, is ongoing and will further explore the relationship between tirzepatide, weight loss, glycemic control, and changes in inflammation.

SGLT-2 Inhibitors

Sodium-glucose cotransporter 2 (SGLT2) inhibitors are a class of glucose-reducing medications that primarily work by blocking the reabsorption of glucose in the proximal convoluted tubule in the kidney resulting in glucosuria and decreased blood glucose levels [82]. The glucosuria thereby leads to a caloric loss and an approximated 2–3% reduction in body weight [82]. Akin to the other glucose-lowering agents, the role of SGLT2 inhibitors in the chronic inflammation of obesity and T2D has lately become an area of interest. However, given the novelty of this drug class, there is a paucity of clinical studies relating SGLT2 inhibitors to inflammation; hence, the majority of studies available involve animal models [82]. Three of the established SGLT2 inhibitors (empagliflozin, dapagliflozin, and canagliflozin) and their inflammatory roles are discussed below.

Empagliflozin Multiple studies in mice models elucidated that empagliflozin treatment reduced pro-inflammatory macrophage differentiation and infiltration within adipose tissue, decreased the mRNA expression and circulating plasma levels of TNFα and IL-6, and increased adiponectin levels [83, 84]. Moreover, despite empagliflozin being an SGLT2 inhibitor whose mechanism of action is independent of insulin, there was a notable decline in insulin resistance associated with empagliflozin [83, 84]. One proposed mechanism for the reduced insulin resistance seen with empagliflozin is the reversal of the pancreatic β-cell glucotoxicity and hence, the restoration of normal β-cell function [85]. Empagliflozin was also shown to attenuate certain CVD pathologies, including atherosclerosis and cardiac interstitial fibrosis [84, 86]. These cardiovascular benefits were attributed to the potential anti-inflammatory and insulin-sensitizing effects of empagliflozin [84, 86]. Another study in mice models fed a high-fat, high-sugar diet illustrated that empagliflozin reduced body weight, improved glycemic control and insulin sensitivity, and ameliorated diet-induced renal tubular damage [87]. This was hypothesized to occur via empagliflozin-induced inhibition of the NLRP-3 inflammasome signaling pathway implying that empagliflozin's anti-inflammatory effects may be contributing to its therapeutic benefits [87].

Dapagliflozin In a study exploring the cardioprotective effects of dapagliflozin in mice models with T2D, dapagliflozin mitigated the development of cardiac fibrosis and diabetic cardiomyopathy by counteracting the deleterious effects of TNFα, CRP, and the NLRP-3 inflammasome on myocardial tissue [88]. The underlying mechanism of action was thought to be an AMPK-dependent inhibition of the NLRP-3 inflammasome [88]. Similarly, dapagliflozin treatment was shown to markedly suppress the gene expression of pro-inflammatory cytokines and the infiltration of macrophages into the renal mesangium and glomeruli of diabetic mouse models, thereby attenuating diabetic nephropathy [89]. This indicates that the dapagliflozin-induced anti-inflammatory response is likely a major contributor to the drug's cardioprotective and renoprotective benefits.

Canagliflozin A study investigating the metabolic and anti-inflammatory effects of canagliflozin showed that canagliflozin lowered the IL-1β levels via an AMPK-dependent pathway. In contrast, the metabolic effects of reduced adiposity and increased fatty acid oxidation were AMPK-independent illustrating the central role of AMPK in canagliflozin's anti-inflammatory effect [90]. In an exploratory post-hoc analysis assessing the effects of canagliflozin on inflammatory biomarkers, canagliflozin treatment was associated with an increase in adiponectin levels and a decrease in serum IL-6 levels [91]. Furthermore, these changes were independent of changes in body weight or HbA1c suggesting that canagliflozin has intrinsic anti-inflammatory benefits independent of its glucose-lowering effects [91].

Additional Anti-Obesity Medications and Anti-Diabetic Agents

Two additional anti-obesity medications, phentermine/topiramate extended-release (phen/top ER) and bupropion/naltrexone (bup/nal), are FDA-approved for the chronic treatment of obesity. They are not treatments for T2D, but their impact on glycemic control was assessed in the clinical trials for these drugs. In the clinical trials for both medications, there was an improvement in glycemic control, along with an improvement in other cardiovascular and metabolic markers [92, 93]. Specifically, in the clinical trials of phen/top ER, aside from clinically significant weight loss and enhancement in glycemic control, there were also significant improvements in both hsCRP and adiponectin compared to placebo [92]. Similarly, bup/nal was studied in subjects who were overweight or obese with T2D [93]. In this study, while subjects did illustrate a significant reduction in weight and HbA1c compared to the placebo, there were no significant differences in the hsCRP levels between the two groups [93]. Another common, though now less frequently used, class of anti-diabetic medications is the thiazolidinediones which often lead to weight gain and can prevent weight loss and hence have not been included in this review.

Conclusion

The role of inflammation in the development of several diseases, including obesity and T2D, is an area of increasing interest. Chronic low-grade inflammation is a feature of both obesity and T2D, and improvement in these diseases has been shown to be associated with an improvement in inflammation. There is mounting evidence that diet and exercise interventions can improve inflammation. Though it is at times unclear if it is the diet itself that improves inflammation or improvement in the disease that reduces inflammation, studies have shown that diet can influence inflammation independently of weight change. Furthermore, there is no one specific "anti-inflammatory" diet or exercise routine that is known to be most effective, though many interventions discussed in this chapter have shown to be highly effective. In addition, pharmacotherapy for the treatment of obesity and T2D may help to reduce inflammation. Ultimately, the treatment of obesity and T2D should be individualized based on the patient's needs and goals. Lifestyle interventions and pharmacotherapy can improve obesity and T2D and may potentially decrease overall inflammation, which may, in turn, reduce the risk of developing other comorbid conditions associated with increased inflammation.

References

1. Weisberg SP, McCann D, Desai M, Rosenbaum M, Leibel RL, Ferrante AW. Obesity is associated with macrophage accumulation in adipose tissue. J Clin Invest. 2003;112(12):1796–808.
2. Esser N, Legrand-Poels S, Piette J, Scheen AJ, Paquot N. Inflammation as a link between obesity, metabolic syndrome and type 2 diabetes. Diabetes Res Clin Pract. 2014;105(2):141–50.
3. Minihane AM, Vinoy S, Russell WR, Baka A, Roche HM, Tuohy KM, et al. Low-grade inflammation, diet composition and health: current research evidence and its translation. Br J Nutr. 2015;114(7):999–1012.
4. Ouchi N, Parker JL, Lugus JJ, Walsh K. Adipokines in inflammation and metabolic disease. Nat Rev Immunol. 2011;11(2):85–97.
5. Calder PC, Ahluwalia N, Brouns F, Buetler T, Clement K, Cunningham K, et al. Dietary factors and low-grade inflammation in relation to overweight and obesity. Br J Nutr. 2011;106(Suppl):S5–78.
6. Hotamisligil GS, Arner P, Caro JF, Atkinson RL, Spiegelman BM. Increased adipose tissue expression of tumor necrosis factor-alpha in human obesity and insulin resistance. J Clin Invest. 1995;95(5):2409–15.
7. Rohm TV, Meier DT, Olefsky JM, Donath MY. Inflammation in obesity, diabetes, and related disorders. Immunity. 2022;55(1):31–55.

8. Esser N, L'homme L, De Roover A, Kohnen L, Scheen AJ, Moutschen M, et al. Obesity phenotype is related to NLRP3 inflammasome activity and immunological profile of visceral adipose tissue. Diabetologia. 2013;56(11):2487–97.
9. Dominguez H, Storgaard H, Rask-Madsen C, Steffen Hermann T, Ihlemann N, Baunbjerg Nielsen D, et al. Metabolic and vascular effects of tumor necrosis factor-alpha blockade with etanercept in obese patients with type 2 diabetes. J Vasc Res. 2005;42(6):517–25.
10. Marra M, Campanati A, Testa R, Sirolla C, Bonfigli AR, Franceschi C, et al. Effect of etanercept on insulin sensitivity in nine patients with psoriasis. Int J Immunopathol Pharmacol. 2007;20(4):731–6.
11. Gonzalez-Gay MA, De Matias JM, Gonzalez-Juanatey C, Garcia-Porrua C, Sanchez-Andrade A, Martin J, et al. Anti-tumor necrosis factor-alpha blockade improves insulin resistance in patients with rheumatoid arthritis. Clin Exp Rheumatol. 2006;24(1):83–6.
12. Schroder K, Zhou R, Tschopp J. The NLRP3 inflammasome: a sensor for metabolic danger? Science. 2010;327(5963):296–300.
13. Larsen CM, Faulenbach M, Vaag A, Vølund A, Ehses JA, Seifert B, et al. Interleukin-1-receptor antagonist in type 2 diabetes mellitus. N Engl J Med. 2007;356(15):1517–26.
14. Wang X, Bao W, Liu J, Ouyang Y-Y, Wang D, Rong S, et al. Inflammatory markers and risk of type 2 diabetes: a systematic review and meta-analysis. Diabetes Care. 2013;36(1):166–75.
15. Rosenbaum M, Leibel RL. The role of leptin in human physiology. N Engl J Med. 1999;341(12):913–5.
16. Friedman JM, Halaas JL. Leptin and the regulation of body weight in mammals. Nature. 1998;395(6704):763–70.
17. Santos-Alvarez J, Goberna R, Sánchez-Margalet V. Human leptin stimulates proliferation and activation of human circulating monocytes. Cell Immunol. 1999;194(1):6–11.
18. Maeda N, Shimomura I, Kishida K, Nishizawa H, Matsuda M, Nagaretani H, et al. Diet-induced insulin resistance in mice lacking adiponectin/ACRP30. Nat Med. 2002;8(7):731–7.
19. Ouchi N, Kihara S, Funahashi T, Nakamura T, Nishida M, Kumada M, et al. Reciprocal association of C-reactive protein with adiponectin in blood stream and adipose tissue. Circulation. 2003;107(5):671–4.
20. Yamauchi T, Kamon J, Minokoshi Y, Ito Y, Waki H, Uchida S, et al. Adiponectin stimulates glucose utilization and fatty-acid oxidation by activating AMP-activated protein kinase. Nat Med. 2002;8(11):1288–95.
21. Takemura Y, Ouchi N, Shibata R, Aprahamian T, Kirber MT, Summer RS, et al. Adiponectin modulates inflammatory reactions via calreticulin receptor-dependent clearance of early apoptotic bodies. J Clin Invest. 2007;117(2):375–86.
22. Lopez-Garcia E, Schulze MB, Fung TT, Meigs JB, Rifai N, Manson JE, et al. Major dietary patterns are related to plasma concentrations of markers of inflammation and endothelial dysfunction. Am J Clin Nutr. 2004;80(4):1029–35.
23. Hariharan R, Odjidja EN, Scott D, Shivappa N, Hébert JR, Hodge A, et al. The dietary inflammatory index, obesity, type 2 diabetes, and cardiovascular risk factors and diseases. Obes Rev. 2022;23(1):e13349.
24. Esmaillzadeh A, Azadbakht L. Major dietary patterns in relation to general obesity and central adiposity among Iranian women. J Nutr. 2008;138(2):358–63.
25. Nanri A, Yoshida D, Yamaji T, Mizoue T, Takayanagi R, Kono S. Dietary patterns and C-reactive protein in Japanese men and women. Am J Clin Nutr. 2008;87(5):1488–96.
26. Sharman MJ, Volek JS. Weight loss leads to reductions in inflammatory biomarkers after a very-low-carbohydrate diet and a low-fat diet in overweight men. Clin Sci (Lond). 2004;107(4):365–9.
27. Mirabelli M, Chiefari E, Arcidiacono B, Corigliano DM, Brunetti FS, Maggisano V, et al. Mediterranean diet nutrients to turn the tide against insulin resistance and related diseases. Nutrients. 2020;12(4):1066.

28. Chrysohoou C, Panagiotakos DB, Pitsavos C, Das UN, Stefanadis C. Adherence to the Mediterranean diet attenuates inflammation and coagulation process in healthy adults: the ATTICA study. J Am Coll Cardiol. 2004;44(1):152–8.

29. Shai I, Schwarzfuchs D, Henkin Y, Shahar DR, Witkow S, Greenberg I, et al. Weight loss with a low-carbohydrate, Mediterranean, or low-fat diet. N Engl J Med. 2008;359(3):229–41.

30. Appel LJ, Moore TJ, Obarzanek E, Vollmer WM, Svetkey LP, Sacks FM, et al. A clinical trial of the effects of dietary patterns on blood pressure. DASH Collaborative Research Group. N Engl J Med. 1997;336(16):1117–24.

31. Juraschek SP, Kovell LC, Appel LJ, Miller ER, Sacks FM, Chang AR, et al. Effects of diet and sodium reduction on cardiac injury, strain, and inflammation: the DASH-sodium trial. J Am Coll Cardiol. 2021;77(21):2625–34.

32. O'Neill BJ. Effect of low-carbohydrate diets on cardiometabolic risk, insulin resistance, and metabolic syndrome. Curr Opin Endocrinol Diabetes Obes. 2020;27(5):301–7.

33. Hu Y, Block G, Norkus EP, Morrow JD, Dietrich M, Hudes M. Relations of glycemic index and glycemic load with plasma oxidative stress markers. Am J Clin Nutr. 2006;84(1):70–6.

34. Paniagua JA, Pérez-Martinez P, Gjelstad IMF, Tierney AC, Delgado-Lista J, Defoort C, et al. A low-fat high-carbohydrate diet supplemented with long-chain n-3 PUFA reduces the risk of the metabolic syndrome. Atherosclerosis. 2011;218(2):443–50.

35. Tierney AC, McMonagle J, Shaw DI, Gulseth HL, Helal O, Saris WHM, et al. Effects of dietary fat modification on insulin sensitivity and on other risk factors of the metabolic syndrome--LIPGENE: a European randomized dietary intervention study. Int J Obes. 2011;35(6):800–9.

36. Szeto YT, Kwok TCY, Benzie IFF. Effects of a long-term vegetarian diet on biomarkers of antioxidant status and cardiovascular disease risk. Nutrition. 2004;20(10):863–6.

37. Lederer A-K, Maul-Pavicic A, Hannibal L, Hettich M, Steinborn C, Gründemann C, et al. Vegan diet reduces neutrophils, monocytes and platelets related to branched-chain amino acids - a randomized, controlled trial. Clin Nutr. 2020;39(11):3241–50.

38. Sutliffe JT, Wilson LD, de Heer HD, Foster RL, Carnot MJ. C-reactive protein response to a vegan lifestyle intervention. Complement Ther Med. 2015;23(1):32–7.

39. Shah B, Newman JD, Woolf K, Ganguzza L, Guo Y, Allen N, et al. Anti-inflammatory effects of a vegan diet versus the American Heart Association-recommended diet in coronary artery disease trial. J Am Heart Assoc. 2018;7(23):e011367.

40. Mantzoros CS, Williams CJ, Manson JE, Meigs JB, Hu FB. Adherence to the Mediterranean dietary pattern is positively associated with plasma adiponectin concentrations in diabetic women. Am J Clin Nutr. 2006;84(2):328–35.

41. Lutsey PL, Jacobs DR, Kori S, Mayer-Davis E, Shea S, Steffen LM, et al. Whole grain intake and its cross-sectional association with obesity, insulin resistance, inflammation, diabetes and subclinical CVD: the MESA study. Br J Nutr. 2007;98(2):397–405.

42. Esposito K, Nappo F, Giugliano F, Di Palo C, Ciotola M, Barbieri M, et al. Meal modulation of circulating interleukin 18 and adiponectin concentrations in healthy subjects and in patients with type 2 diabetes mellitus. Am J Clin Nutr. 2003;78(6):1135–40.

43. Bhupathiraju SN, Tucker KL. Greater variety in fruit and vegetable intake is associated with lower inflammation in Puerto Rican adults. Am J Clin Nutr. 2011;93(1):37–46.

44. Moldogazieva NT, Mokhosoev IM, Mel'nikova TI, Porozov YB, Terentiev AA. Oxidative stress and advanced Lipoxidation and glycation end products (ALEs and AGEs) in aging and age-related diseases. Oxidative Med Cell Longev. 2019;2019:3085756.

45. Chow LS, Gerszten RE, Taylor JM, Pedersen BK, van Praag H, Trappe S, et al. Exerkines in health, resilience and disease. Nat Rev Endocrinol. 2022;18(5):273–89.

46. Safdar A, Saleem A, Tarnopolsky MA. The potential of endurance exercise-derived exosomes to treat metabolic diseases. Nat Rev Endocrinol. 2016;12(9):504–17.

47. Ostrowski K, Rohde T, Asp S, Schjerling P, Pedersen BK. Pro- and anti-inflammatory cytokine balance in strenuous exercise in humans. J Physiol. 1999;515(Pt 1):287–91.

48. Pedersen BK. Anti-inflammatory effects of exercise: role in diabetes and cardiovascular disease. Eur J Clin Investig. 2017;47(8):600–11.

49. Fischer CP, Berntsen A, Perstrup LB, Eskildsen P, Pedersen BK. Plasma levels of interleukin-6 and C-reactive protein are associated with physical inactivity independent of obesity. Scand J Med Sci Sports. 2007;17(5):580–7.
50. Pedersen BK, Saltin B. Exercise as medicine - evidence for prescribing exercise as therapy in 26 different chronic diseases. Scand J Med Sci Sports. 2015;25(Suppl 3):1–72.
51. Yang Z, Scott CA, Mao C, Tang J, Farmer AJ. Resistance exercise versus aerobic exercise for type 2 diabetes: a systematic review and meta-analysis. Sports Med. 2014;44(4):487–99.
52. Foretz M, Guigas B, Viollet B. Understanding the glucoregulatory mechanisms of metformin in type 2 diabetes mellitus. Nat Rev Endocrinol. 2019;15(10):569–89.
53. Hundal RS, Krssak M, Dufour S, Laurent D, Lebon V, Chandramouli V, et al. Mechanism by which metformin reduces glucose production in type 2 diabetes. Diabetes. 2000;49(12):2063–9.
54. Zhou G, Myers R, Li Y, Chen Y, Shen X, Fenyk-Melody J, et al. Role of AMP-activated protein kinase in mechanism of metformin action. J Clin Invest. 2001;108(8):1167–74.
55. Owen MR, Doran E, Halestrap AP. Evidence that metformin exerts its anti-diabetic effects through inhibition of complex 1 of the mitochondrial respiratory chain. Biochem J. 2000;348(Pt 3):607–14.
56. Vasamsetti SB, Karnewar S, Kanugula AK, Thatipalli AR, Kumar JM, Kotamraju S. Metformin inhibits monocyte-to-macrophage differentiation via AMPK-mediated inhibition of STAT3 activation: potential role in atherosclerosis. Diabetes. 2015;64(6):2028–41.
57. Kim J, Kwak HJ, Cha J-Y, Jeong Y-S, Rhee SD, Kim KR, et al. Metformin suppresses lipopolysaccharide (LPS)-induced inflammatory response in murine macrophages via activating transcription factor-3 (ATF-3) induction. J Biol Chem. 2014;289(33):23246–55.
58. Evia-Viscarra ML, Rodea-Montero ER, Apolinar-Jiménez E, Muñoz-Noriega N, García-Morales LM, Leaños-Pérez C, et al. The effects of metformin on inflammatory mediators in obese adolescents with insulin resistance: controlled randomized clinical trial. J Pediatr Endocrinol Metab. 2012;25(1–2):41–9.
59. Fidan E, Onder Ersoz H, Yilmaz M, Yilmaz H, Kocak M, Karahan C, et al. The effects of rosiglitazone and metformin on inflammation and endothelial dysfunction in patients with type 2 diabetes mellitus. Acta Diabetol. 2011;48(4):297–302.
60. Cameron AR, Morrison VL, Levin D, Mohan M, Forteath C, Beall C, et al. Anti-inflammatory effects of metformin irrespective of diabetes status. Circ Res. 2016;119(5):652–65.
61. DeFronzo RA, Buse JB, Kim T, Burns C, Skare S, Baron A, et al. Once-daily delayed-release metformin lowers plasma glucose and enhances fasting and postprandial GLP-1 and PYY: results from two randomised trials. Diabetologia. 2016;59(8):1645–54.
62. Mannucci E, Tesi F, Bardini G, Ognibene A, Petracca MG, Ciani S, et al. Effects of metformin on glucagon-like peptide-1 levels in obese patients with and without type 2 diabetes. Diabetes Nutr Metab. 2004;17(6):336–42.
63. Napolitano A, Miller S, Nicholls AW, Baker D, Van Horn S, Thomas E, et al. Novel gut-based pharmacology of metformin in patients with type 2 diabetes mellitus. PLoS One. 2014;9(7):e100778.
64. Maida A, Lamont BJ, Cao X, Drucker DJ. Metformin regulates the incretin receptor axis via a pathway dependent on peroxisome proliferator-activated receptor-α in mice. Diabetologia. 2011;54(2):339–49.
65. Díaz-Soto G, de Luis DA, Conde-Vicente R, Izaola-Jauregui O, Ramos C, Romero E. Beneficial effects of liraglutide on adipocytokines, insulin sensitivity parameters and cardiovascular risk biomarkers in patients with type 2 diabetes: a prospective study. Diabetes Res Clin Pract. 2014;104(1):92–6.
66. Chaudhuri A, Ghanim H, Vora M, Sia CL, Korzeniewski K, Dhindsa S, et al. Exenatide exerts a potent antiinflammatory effect. J Clin Endocrinol Metab. 2012;97(1):198–207.
67. Bunck MC, Diamant M, Eliasson B, Cornér A, Shaginian RM, Heine RJ, et al. Exenatide affects circulating cardiovascular risk biomarkers independently of changes in body composition. Diabetes Care. 2010;33(8):1734–7.

68. Viswanathan P, Chaudhuri A, Bhatia R, Al-Atrash F, Mohanty P, Dandona P. Exenatide therapy in obese patients with type 2 diabetes mellitus treated with insulin. Endocr Pract. 2007;13(5):444–50.

69. Derosa G, Putignano P, Bossi AC, Bonaventura A, Querci F, Franzetti IG, et al. Exenatide or glimepiride added to metformin on metabolic control and on insulin resistance in type 2 diabetic patients. Eur J Pharmacol. 2011;666(1–3):251–6.

70. Li L, Yang G, Li Q, Tan X, Liu H, Tang Y, et al. Exenatide prevents fat-induced insulin resistance and raises adiponectin expression and plasma levels. Diabetes Obes Metab. 2008;10(10):921–30.

71. Shiraki A, Oyama J, Komoda H, Asaka M, Komatsu A, Sakuma M, et al. The glucagon-like peptide 1 analog liraglutide reduces TNF-α-induced oxidative stress and inflammation in endothelial cells. Atherosclerosis. 2012;221(2):375–82.

72. Savchenko LG, Digtiar NI, Selikhova LG, Kaidasheva EI, Shlykova OA, Vesnina LE, et al. Liraglutide exerts an anti-inflammatory action in obese patients with type 2 diabetes. Rom J Intern Med. 2019;57(3):233–40.

73. Li L, Miao Z, Liu R, Yang M, Liu H, Yang G. Liraglutide prevents hypoadiponectinemia-induced insulin resistance and alterations of gene expression involved in glucose and lipid metabolism. Mol Med. 2011;17(11–12):1168–78.

74. Newsome P, Francque S, Harrison S, Ratziu V, Van Gaal L, Calanna S, et al. Effect of semaglutide on liver enzymes and markers of inflammation in subjects with type 2 diabetes and/or obesity. Aliment Pharmacol Ther. 2019;50(2):193–203.

75. Mosenzon O, Capehorn MS, De Remigis A, Rasmussen S, Weimers P, Rosenstock J. Impact of semaglutide on high-sensitivity C-reactive protein: exploratory patient-level analyses of SUSTAIN and PIONEER randomized clinical trials. Cardiovasc Diabetol. 2022;21(1):172.

76. Rakipovski G, Rolin B, Nøhr J, Klewe I, Frederiksen KS, Augustin R, et al. The GLP-1 analogs liraglutide and semaglutide reduce atherosclerosis in ApoE−/− and LDLr−/− mice by a mechanism that includes inflammatory pathways. JACC Basic Transl Sci. 2018;3(6):844–57.

77. Jepsen MM, Christensen MB. Emerging glucagon-like peptide 1 receptor agonists for the treatment of obesity. Expert Opin Emerg Drugs. 2021;26(3):231–43.

78. Rosenstock J, Wysham C, Frías JP, Kaneko S, Lee CJ, Fernández Landó L, et al. Efficacy and safety of a novel dual GIP and GLP-1 receptor agonist tirzepatide in patients with type 2 diabetes (SURPASS-1): a double-blind, randomised, phase 3 trial. Lancet (London, England). 2021;398(10295):143–55.

79. Frías JP, Davies MJ, Rosenstock J, Pérez Manghi FC, Fernández Landó L, Bergman BK, et al. Tirzepatide versus semaglutide once weekly in patients with type 2 diabetes. N Engl J Med. 2021;385(6):503–15.

80. Frias JP, Nauck MA, Van J, Kutner ME, Cui X, Benson C, et al. Efficacy and safety of LY3298176, a novel dual GIP and GLP-1 receptor agonist, in patients with type 2 diabetes: a randomised, placebo-controlled and active comparator-controlled phase 2 trial. Lancet (London, England). 2018;392(10160):2180–93.

81. Wilson JM, Lin Y, Luo MJ, Considine G, Cox AL, Bowsman LM, et al. The dual glucose-dependent insulinotropic polypeptide and glucagon-like peptide-1 receptor agonist tirzepatide improves cardiovascular risk biomarkers in patients with type 2 diabetes: a post hoc analysis. Diabetes Obes Metab. 2022;24(1):148–53.

82. Bonora BM, Avogaro A, Fadini GP. Extraglycemic effects of SGLT2 inhibitors: a review of the evidence. Diabetes Metab Syndr Obes. 2020;13:161–74.

83. Xu L, Nagata N, Nagashimada M, Zhuge F, Ni Y, Chen G, et al. SGLT2 inhibition by empagliflozin promotes fat utilization and browning and attenuates inflammation and insulin resistance by polarizing M2 macrophages in diet-induced obese mice. EBioMedicine. 2017;20:137–49.

84. Han JH, Oh TJ, Lee G, Maeng HJ, Lee DH, Kim KM, et al. The beneficial effects of empagliflozin, an SGLT2 inhibitor, on atherosclerosis in ApoE −/− mice fed a western diet. Diabetologia. 2017;60(2):364–76.

85. Papaetis GS. Empagliflozin therapy and insulin resistance-associated disorders: effects and promises beyond a diabetic state. Arch Med Sci Atheroscler Dis. 2021;6:e57–78.
86. Lin B, Koibuchi N, Hasegawa Y, Sueta D, Toyama K, Uekawa K, et al. Glycemic control with empagliflozin, a novel selective SGLT2 inhibitor, ameliorates cardiovascular injury and cognitive dysfunction in obese and type 2 diabetic mice. Cardiovasc Diabetol. 2014;13:148.
87. Benetti E, Mastrocola R, Vitarelli G, Cutrin JC, Nigro D, Chiazza F, et al. Empagliflozin protects against diet-induced NLRP-3 inflammasome activation and lipid accumulation. J Pharmacol Exp Ther. 2016;359(1):45–53.
88. Ye Y, Bajaj M, Yang H-C, Perez-Polo JR, Birnbaum Y. SGLT-2 inhibition with dapagliflozin reduces the activation of the Nlrp3/ASC inflammasome and attenuates the development of diabetic cardiomyopathy in mice with type 2 diabetes. Further augmentation of the effects with saxagliptin, a DPP4 inhibitor. Cardiovasc Drugs Ther. 2017;31(2):119–32.
89. Terami N, Ogawa D, Tachibana H, Hatanaka T, Wada J, Nakatsuka A, et al. Long-term treatment with the sodium glucose cotransporter 2 inhibitor, dapagliflozin, ameliorates glucose homeostasis and diabetic nephropathy in db/db mice. PLoS One. 2014;9(6):e100777.
90. Day EA, Ford RJ, Lu JH, Lu R, Lundenberg L, Desjardins EM, et al. The SGLT2 inhibitor canagliflozin suppresses lipid synthesis and interleukin-1 beta in ApoE deficient mice. Biochem J. 2020;477(12):2347–61.
91. Garvey WT, Van Gaal L, Leiter LA, Vijapurkar U, List J, Cuddihy R, et al. Effects of canagliflozin versus glimepiride on adipokines and inflammatory biomarkers in type 2 diabetes. Metabolism. 2018;85:32–7.
92. Gadde KM, Allison DB, Ryan DH, Peterson CA, Troupin B, Schwiers ML, et al. Effects of low-dose, controlled-release, phentermine plus topiramate combination on weight and associated comorbidities in overweight and obese adults (CONQUER): a randomised, placebo-controlled, phase 3 trial. Lancet (London, England). 2011;377(9774):1341–52.
93. Hollander P, Gupta AK, Plodkowski R, Greenway F, Bays H, Burns C, et al. Effects of naltrexone sustained-release/bupropion sustained-release combination therapy on body weight and glycemic parameters in overweight and obese patients with type 2 diabetes. Diabetes Care. 2013;36(12):4022–9.

Correction to: Genetic and Epigenetic Basis of Obesity-Induced Inflammation and Diabetes

Radoslav Stojchevski, Sara Velichkovikj, and Todor Arsov

Correction to: Chapter 6 in: D. Avtanski, L. Poretsky (eds.), *Obesity, Diabetes and Inflammation*, Contemporary Endocrinology, https://doi.org/10.1007/978-3-031-39721-9_6

Owing to an unfortunate oversight, the book was inadvertently published with errors in a few author affiliations.

The corrections are listed below.

Radoslav Stojchevski:

- Friedman Diabetes Institute, Lenox Hill Hospital, New York, NY, USA

- Donald and Barbara Zucker School of Medicine at Hofstra/Northwell, Hempstead, NY, USA

Sara Velichkovikj:

- Faculty of Natural Sciences and Mathematics, Institute of Biology, Ss. Cyril and Methodius University, Skopje, Macedonia

- Department of Medicine, Lenox Hill Hospital, New York, NY, USA

The updated version of the book can be found at https://doi.org/10.1007/978-3-031-39721-9_6

© The Author(s), under exclusive license to Springer Nature Switzerland AG 2023
D. Avtanski, L. Poretsky (eds.), *Obesity, Diabetes and Inflammation*, Contemporary Endocrinology, https://doi.org/10.1007/978-3-031-39721-9_11

Index

© The Editor(s) (if applicable) and The Author(s), under exclusive license to
Springer Nature Switzerland AG 2023
D. Avtanski, L. Poretsky (eds.), *Obesity, Diabetes and Inflammation*,
Contemporary Endocrinology, https://doi.org/10.1007/978-3-031-39721-9

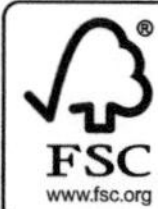

MIX
Papier aus verantwortungsvollen Quellen
Paper from responsible sources
FSC® C105338

If you have any concerns about our products,
you can contact us on
ProductSafety@springernature.com

In case Publisher is established outside the EU,
the EU authorized representative is:
Springer Nature Customer Service Center GmbH
Europaplatz 3, 69115 Heidelberg, Germany

Printed by Libri Plureos GmbH
in Hamburg, Germany